Studies in Computational Intelligence

Volume 936

Series Editor

Janusz Kacprzyk, Polish Academy of Sciences, Warsaw, Poland

The series "Studies in Computational Intelligence" (SCI) publishes new developments and advances in the various areas of computational intelligence—quickly and with a high quality. The intent is to cover the theory, applications, and design methods of computational intelligence, as embedded in the fields of engineering, computer science, physics and life sciences, as well as the methodologies behind them. The series contains monographs, lecture notes and edited volumes in computational intelligence spanning the areas of neural networks, connectionist systems, genetic algorithms, evolutionary computation, artificial intelligence, cellular automata, self-organizing systems, soft computing, fuzzy systems, and hybrid intelligent systems. Of particular value to both the contributors and the readership are the short publication timeframe and the world-wide distribution, which enable both wide and rapid dissemination of research output.

Indexed by SCOPUS, DBLP, WTI Frankfurt eG, zbMATH, SCImago.

All books published in the series are submitted for consideration in Web of Science.

More information about this series at http://www.springer.com/series/7092

Hrudaya Kumar Tripathy ·
Sushruta Mishra · Pradeep Kumar Mallick ·
Amiya Ranjan Panda
Editors

Technical Advancements of Machine Learning in Healthcare

Springer

Editors
Hrudaya Kumar Tripathy
School of Computer Engineering
KIIT University
Bhubaneswar, Odisha, India

Sushruta Mishra
School of Computer Engineering
KIIT University
Bhubaneswar, Odisha, India

Pradeep Kumar Mallick
School of Computer Engineering
KIIT University
Bhubaneswar, Odisha, India

Amiya Ranjan Panda
School of Computer Engineering
KIIT University
Bhubaneswar, Odisha, India

ISSN 1860-949X ISSN 1860-9503 (electronic)
Studies in Computational Intelligence
ISBN 978-981-33-4697-0 ISBN 978-981-33-4698-7 (eBook)
https://doi.org/10.1007/978-981-33-4698-7

This Springer imprint is published by the registered company Springer Nature Singapore Pte Ltd.
The registered company address is: 152 Beach Road, #21-01/04 Gateway East, Singapore 189721, Singapore

Preface

Artificial Intelligence and explicitly rising Machine Learning applications in Healthcare are giving big hopes to the human race in achieving more outstanding capabilities to diagnose and treat illness to establish a well-being society. Today, the healthcare industry is one of the leading sectors revolutionized by several machine learning approaches. Nowadays, healthcare data/image analysis is taking care of different machine learning approaches supported by various medical and Information Communication technologies. This edited book volume gives an insight into diverse machine learning-based techniques that broadly deal in delivery of quality, accurate, and affordable healthcare solutions. This book comprises different chapters addressing the potential for making faster advances in many scientific disciplines in many scientific fields and improving various enterprises' profitability and success. It also emphasizes advanced technologies like IoT and cloud computing, which can integrate with machine learning to assist in the healthcare sector. Initial chapters of this book focused on the general usability of Machine Learning in the healthcare system and services and the present big data applications in the healthcare domain. Subsequent chapters enlightened the usability of feature selection and extractions in computed Tomography Lung analysis and Hepatitis disease. Also, the authors discussed the classification procedure for predicting different conditions and using the cognitive neural network for Emphysema classification. Insight regarding the use of machine learning in drug discovery is highlighted in the succeeding chapter. Later, authors have assembled the effective techniques on Deep Learning models (Convolutional Neural Network) to design the frameworks in healthcare focused on the diagnosis of heart diseases, Medical Signal, and Image processing (such as mammogram analysis, detection of Glaucoma in Fundus Images). The authors focused on some optimization techniques for the analysis of Brain MRI along with different medical image representations and future challenges. The following chapter is also convergent towards the social sensing for crowd monitoring in any pandemic situations using IoT based Drone driven system. In another chapter, authors have centered their research into Medical Bots in Clinical Domain and movement controls of robotic arms in operation theaters. The final two chapters deal with disease and crisis forecasting frameworks using the machine learning approach. This book provides a futuristic approach and methodologies for healthcare solutions using machine learning approaches. The contents are organized very precisely and compact fully. This book will act as an educational and research guiding support for academicians, research scholars, students, and technical support to the software developers, data scientist aspirants, data analytics managers, business analysts, and information architects working in machine learning for healthcare domain.

The entire editorial board would like to express thanks and gratitude to all authors to consider and trust this book as the platform for publishing their valuable work and for their kind co-operation extended during the various stages of processing the manuscript. The reviewing of a chapter is essential to ensure the quality of the chapter published in any book. The board also expresses sincere thanks to all reviewers for their excellent contributions during the review process. We would also like to express our heartfelt thanks to the authorities of our university as this book would have been impossible without their support on all fronts and motivation to carry out the research.

Bhubaneswar, India

Dr. Hrudaya Kumar Tripathy
Dr. Sushruta Mishra
Dr. Pradeep Kumar Mallick
Dr. Amiya Ranjan Panda

Contents

Editors and Contributors

About the Editors

Dr. Hrudaya Kumar Tripathy is an Associate Professor of the School of Computer Engineering, KIIT University, Bhubaneswar, India. He has completed a Doctorate in Computer Science from Berhampur University, a Master in Computer Science Engineering from the Indian Institute of Technology, Guwahati, and received Post-Doctoral Fellowship from the Ministry of Higher Education Malaysia. He has 20 years of teaching experience with post doctorate research experience. He had been Visiting Faculty for a couple of years in Asia Pacific University, Kuala Lumpur, Malaysia, and the University of Utara Malaysia, Sintok, Malaysia. Dr. Tripathy awarded a Young IT professional award in 2013 on a regional level from the Computer Society of India (CSI). He has more than 100 research publications in different national/international journals and conferences to his credit.

Dr. Sushruta Mishra is an Indian by birth. He completed his B.Tech. from ITER, Bhubaneswar, in 2009. He pursued his M.Tech. degree from IIIT, Bhubaneswar, in 2012. He completed his Ph.D. from KIIT University, Bhubaneswar, in 2017. Currently, he is working as Assistant Professor in KIIT University, Bhubaneswar, in the School of Computer Engineering. He has a good 7 years of academic teaching experience. Her prime research area of interest includes machine learning, sentiment analysis, cognitive computing and robotics. Dr. Mishra has published more than 60 research and development articles in various reputed journals, conferences and book chapters.

Dr. Pradeep Kumar Mallick is currently working as Senior Associate Professor in the School of Computer Engineering , KIIT Deemed to be University, India. He has also served as Professor and Head Department of Computer Science and Engineering, Vignana Bharathi Institute of Technology, Hyderabad. He has completed his Post Doctoral Fellowship from Kongju National University South Korea,

PhD from Siksha Ó' Anusandhan University, India and Master degree from Bijupatnaik University, Odisha. Besides academics, he is also involved in various administrative activities, Member of Board of Studies, Member of Doctoral Research Evaluation Committee, Admission Committee etc. Now he is the editorial member of Korean Convergence Society for SMB. He has published 12 edited books, 1 text Book and more than 100 research papers in National and international journals and conference proceedings to his credit.

Dr. Amiya Ranjan Panda has seven years of research experience in DRDO Chandipur and more than three years of teaching experience. He received B.Tech. degree in Information Technology from Biju Patnaik University of Technology, Odisha, India, in 2009, M.Tech. degree in Computer Science and Engineering from the KIIT University, India in 2012. and Ph.D. degree from Siksha 'O' Anusandhan University, Odisha, in the year 2017. Currently, he is working as Assistant Professor in KIIT Deemed to be University, Bhubaneswar. His research interest is machine learning, IoT, data acquisition system and software-defined radio. He has published more than 25 articles in international journals. Currently he is working with a real-time project of DRDO.

Contributors

R. Arthi Department of ECE, SRM Institute of Science and Technology, Ramapuram Campus, Chennai, India

Rahul Kumar Barik Department of ECE, SRM Institute of Science and Technology, Ramapuram Campus, Chennai, India

Mandakini Priyadarshani Behera Department of Computer Science and Engineering, ITER, Siksha 'O' Anusandhan Deemed To Be University, Bhubaneswar, India

Aradhana Behura Computer Science and Engineering, Veer Surendra Sai University of Technology, Sambalpur, Odisha, India

Anuttam Dash Kalinga Institute of Industrial Technology, Bhubaneswar, Odisha, India

Satya Ranjan Dash School of Computer Applications, KIIT University, Bhubaneswar, India

Sujoy Datta School of Computer Engineering, KIIT Deemed University, Bhubaneswar, Odisha, India

Chinmaya Dehury University of Tartu, Tartu, Estonia

Somya Gupta Department of ECE, SRM Institute of Science and Technology, Ramapuram Campus, Chennai, India

Lambodar Jena Department of Computer Science and Engineering, ITER, Siksha 'O' Anusandhan (Deemed to be University), Bhubaneswar, India

Jin-Kyu Kang Department of Industrial and Management Engineering, Hanbat National University, Daejeon, Korea

Joon-Yong Kim Department of Liberal Arts (Computer Science), Seoul Theological University, Bucheon-si, South Korea

Santhosh Kumar UBDTCE, Davanagere, India

S. Lalithakumari School of EEE, Sathyabama Institute of Science and Technology, Chennai, Tamil Nadu, India;
Department of EIE, Sathyabama Institute of Science and Technology, Chennai, India

B. S. Mahanand Department of Information Science and Engineering, Sri Jayachamarajendra College of Engineering JSS Science and Technology University, Mysuru, Karnataka, India

Debolina Mahapatra Department of Computer Science and Engineering, Silicon Institute of Technology, Bhubaneswar, India

Pradeep Kumar Mallick School of Computer Science and Engineering, KIIT Deemed To Be University, Bhubaneswar, Odisha, India

Debahuti Mishra Department of Computer Science and Engineering, ITER, Siksha 'O' Anusandhan Deemed To Be University, Bhubaneswar, India

Shruti Mishra School of Computer Science and Engineering, VIT-AP University, Amaravati, India

Sushruta Mishra B. Tech in Computer Science and Systems Engineering-2021, KIIT University, Bhubaneswar, India;
School of Computer Engineering, Kalinga Institute of Industrial Technology, Bhubaneswar, Odisha, India

Mihir Narayan Mohanty Department of Electronics and Communication Engineering, ITER, Siksha 'O' Anusandhan (Deemed To Be University), Bhubaneswar, Odisha, India

Saumendra Kumar Mohapatra Department of Electronics and Communication Engineering, ITER, Siksha 'O' Anusandhan (Deemed To Be University), Bhubaneswar, Odisha, India

Deep Mukherjee B. Tech in Computer Science and Systems Engineering-2021, KIIT University, Bhubaneswar, India

Jai-Woo Oh Department of Health Management & Education, Kyungdong University, Wonju, Korea

Amiya Ranjan Panda School of Computer Engineering, KIIT Deemed to be University, Bhubaneswar, Odisha, India

Ganapati Panda Department of Electronics and Tele Communication, C V Raman Global University, Bhubaneswar, Odisha, India

Niranjan Panda Department of Computer Science and Engineering, Siksha 'O' Anusandhan, Bhubaneswar, India

Shivam Pandey Department of ECE, SRM Institute of Science and Technology, Ramapuram Campus, Chennai, India

R. Pandian Department of EIE, Sathyabama Institute of Science and Technology, Chennai, India;
School of EEE, Sathyabama Institute of Science and Technology, Chennai, Tamil Nadu, India

Parthasarathi Pattnayak School of Computer Applications, KIIT Deemed to be University, Bhubaneswar, India

A. Y. Prasad ACSCE, Bengaluru, India

A. Prashanthi VBIT, Hyderabad, India

Shyla Raj Department of Information Science and Engineering, Sri Jayachamarajendra College of Engineering JSS Science and Technology University, Mysuru, Karnataka, India

P. V. Rao VBIT, Hyderabad, India

Adyasha Rath Department of Computer Science and Engineering, Siksha 'O' Anusandhan (Deemed To Be) University, Bhubaneswar, Odisha, India

Ratula Ray School of Biotechnology, KIIT University, Bhubaneswar, India

Monideepa Roy School of Computer Engineering, KIIT Deemed University, Bhubaneswar, Odisha, India

Subhrojyoti Narayan Roy School of Computer Engineering, Kalinga Institute of Industrial Technology, Bhubaneswar, Odisha, India

Archana Sarangi Department of Computer Science and Engineering, ITER, Siksha 'O' Anusandhan Deemed To Be University, Bhubaneswar, India

Sandeep Kumar Satapathy School of Computer Science and Engineering, VIT University, Chennai, India

V. Sreepathi RRCE, Bengaluru, India

Hrudaya Kumar Tripathy B. Tech in Computer Science and Systems Engineering-2021, KIIT University, Bhubaneswar, India

D. S. Vinod Department of Information Science and Engineering, Sri Jayachamarajendra College of Engineering JSS Science and Technology University, Mysuru, Karnataka, India

Shafiz Mohd Yusof Faculty of Engineering and Information Sciences, University of Wollongong, Dubai, UAE

Innovation on Machine Learning in Healthcare Services—An Introduction

Parthasarathi Pattnayak and Amiya Ranjan Panda

Abstract The healthcare offerings in evolved and developing international locations are seriously important. The use of machine gaining knowledge of strategies in healthcare enterprise has a crucial significance and increases swiftly. In the past few years, there have been widespread traits in how system gaining knowledge can be utilized in diverse industries and research. The organizations in healthcare quarter need to take benefit of the system studying techniques to gain valuable statistics that could later be used to diagnose illnesses at a great deal in advance ranges. Present-day electronic wellness records (EHRs) offer realities to answer clinically noteworthy inquiries. The developing measurements in EHRs make human services ready for the use of gadget acquisition. In any case, acquisition in a logical putting offers exact requesting circumstances that confound the use of ordinary machine becoming acquainted with methodologies. This liquidation fills in as groundwork to enlighten these difficulties and features possibilities for contributors of the device learning network and also discusses the potential of utilizing gadget mastering technology in healthcare and descriptions numerous industry projects the usage of system studying initiatives to make contributions to healthcare area.

Keywords Healthcare · EHR · RCT · Machine learning · Big data · IoT

1 Introduction

Healthcare is one of the very important belongings inside society. However, due to speedy growth societies' wishes for healthcare exceeds the substances of low-cost and reachable care. As want for healthcare grows, imparting enough healthcare to the society is the primary priority of the rules in healthcare zone. The shape of the health

P. Pattnayak (✉)
School of Computer Applications, KIIT Deemed to be University, Bhubaneswar, India
e-mail: parthafca@kiit.ac.in

A. R. Panda
School of Computer Engineering, KIIT Deemed to be University, Bhubaneswar, Odisha, India
e-mail: amiya.pandafcs@kiit.ac.in

H. K. Tripathy et al. (eds.), *Technical Advancements of Machine Learning in Healthcare*,
Studies in Computational Intelligence 936,
https://doi.org/10.1007/978-981-33-4698-7_1

zone varies depending on the country's population, cultural development, natural sources, political and monetary device. Increase of significance given to healthcare and the high-quality degree of healthcare, increases opposition among health groups and offers a crucial contribution to the improvement of the world. Health issues sway human lives. During clinical consideration, well-being organizations secure clinical realities around every specific influenced individual, and influence information from the general populace, to decide how to deal with that patient. Data therefore performs an essential position in addressing health issues, and progressed statistics is essential to enhancing affected person care. Beyond any doubt, one of the most vital elements that affect healthcare region is era. Despite quick increase in societies and in societies' need for healthcare, today's advancing era can be one of the most vital elements that can respond to the want of healthcare offerings in societies. Luckily, these days we have a complicated generation in healthcare structures which could help in making decisions based on accumulated data. This capability of the generation in healthcare structures is already getting used to accumulate data approximately any symptom that an affected person has, to diagnose unique sicknesses before they occur at the affected person, and to prevent any of these illnesses with the aid of taking precautions. With the help of that technology, many sufferers have already been rescued from diverse deathly illnesses. Using facts, machine studying has driven advances in many domains inclusive of laptop imaginative and prescient, NLP, and automated speech popularity to supply puissant structures (For example, motors with driverless, non-public assistants activated voice, automated translation).

Considering quiet populaces to recognize causes, chance variables, powerful medications, and subtypes of illness has for quite some time been the domain of epidemiology. Epidemiological strategies, for example, case–control and irregular controlled preliminaries contemplates are the foundations of proof supported medication. Be that as it may, such strategies are tedious and costly, liberated from the predispositions they are intended to battle, and their outcomes may not be material to certifiable patient populaces [1]. Globally, the reception of electronic well-being records (EHRs) is expanding because of systems and organizations that boost their utilization strategies that influence EHRs to respond to questions handled by epidemiologists [2] and to build exactness in human services conveyance are currently commonplace [3].

Information examination approaches extensively fall into the accompanying classes: expressive, explorative, deductive, prescient, and causative [4]. An elucidating examination reports outlines of information without understanding and an explorative investigation distinguishes relationship between factors in an informational index. A deductive examination evaluates how much a watched relationship in a populace will hold outside the informational collection from which it was inferred, and a prescient report endeavors to measure the likelihood of an outcome at the degree of a person. At last, a causal examination decides how changes in a single variable influence another. It is vital to characterize the sort of inquiry being posed in an offered examination to decide the kind of information investigation that is fitting to use in addressing the inquiry. Prescient examinations used to anticipate results for people [4] by building a measurable model from watched information and utilizing this model to create an expectation for an individual dependent on their interesting highlights. Prescient displaying is a sort of algorithmic demonstrating, by which information are created to be obscure. Such displaying approaches measure execution by measurements, for example, accuracy, review, and adjustment, which evaluate various ideas of the recurrence.

AI is the way toward acquisition of a sufficient factual model utilizing watched information to foresee results or classify perceptions in future information. In particular, administered AI techniques string a model utilizing perceptions on tests where the classes or anticipated estimation of the result of intrigue are now known (the best quality level). The subsequent model—which is frequently a punished relapse of some structure—is normally applied to new examples to sort or foresee estimations of the result for beforehand inconspicuous perceptions, and its presentation assessed by contrasting anticipated qualities with real qualities for a lot of test tests. In this manner, AI "lives" in the realm of algorithmic demonstrating and ought to be assessed in that capacity. Relapse frameworks created utilizing AI techniques can't and ought not to be assessed utilizing measures from the universe of information demonstrating. To do so would create wrong evaluations of a model's presentation for its proposed task, conceivably deceptive clients into off base understanding of the model's yield.

EHRs give access to an enormous number and assortment of factors that empower top notch grouping and prediction, while AI offers the strategies to deal with the huge bulk of high-dimensional information that are common in a medicinal services setting. Subsequently, the utilization of AI to EHR information investigation is at the bleeding edge of current clinical informatics [5], filling propels in practice of medication and science. We portray the operational and methodological difficulties of utilizing AI in practice and research. Finally, our viewpoint on open doors for AI in medication and applications have the most noteworthy potential for affecting well-being and social insurance conveyance (Fig. 1).

This section spread the exceptional specialized difficulties that ought to be considered in AI frameworks for medicinal services undertakings, particularly as execution between prepared frameworks and human specialists narrows [6]. Inability to deliberately consider these difficulties can ruin the legitimacy and utility of AI for human services. We present a chain of command of clinical chances, sorted out into the accompanying general classifications: computerizing clinical undertakings, offering clinical help, and growing clinical limits. We close by delineating the open doors for looking into AI that have specific importance in medicinal services: pleasing movements in information sources and instruments, guaranteeing frameworks are interpretable, and distinguishing great portrayals.

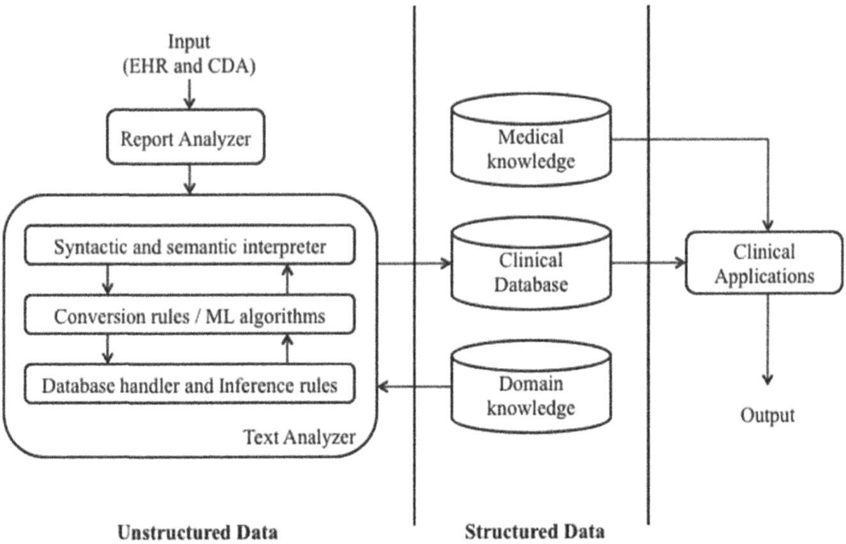

Fig. 1 EHR Frameworks information (both unstructured and structured)

2 The Requirement of Change in Healthcare

Much has been composed concerning the way where healthcare is changing, with a specific accentuation on how extremely huge amounts of information are presently being routinely gathered during the normal consideration of patients. The utilization of AI techniques to transform these ever-developing amounts of information into mediations that can improve persistent results appears as though it ought to be an undeniable way to take. Be that as it may, the field of AI in healthcare is still in its early stages. This book, compassionately upheld by the Institution of Engineering and Technology, means to give a "depiction" of the condition of ebb and flow explore at the interface between AI and medicinal services. Essentially, this is a fractional and one-sided testing of the condition of momentum examines, but then we have expected to give a wide-going prologue to the profundity and size of work that is being attempted around the world. In choosing material for this altered volume, we have set uncommon accentuation on AI extends that are (or are near) accomplishing improvement in persistent results. For some, reasons, revealed differently in a portion of the parts that follow, it is an axiom that "medicinal services is hard"; there are one of a kind limitations that exist, and contemplation that must be taken, when working with healthcare information. In any case, for every one of its troubles, working with medicinal services information is especially fulfilling, both as far as the computational difficulties that exist and as far as the yields of research having the option to influence the manner by which social insurance is conveyed. There are scarcely any application territories of AI that have such guarantee to profit society as does that of human services.

3 Verifiable Position and Tendency

The field of medicine has gone for immense strolls in its progress; the headway of vaccinations, hostile to microbial, and caused a course like effect on all patients and the possibility of purification have vexed the business pros drew in with social protection. Clearly, people have propelled a fantastic degree from past clinical thought. The human services industry is comprised of preventive, symptomatic, healing, and restorative parts. Each of these segments cooperates to give an extensive, widely inclusive experience for the propelled patients. Some huge examples are going on in the business today; the first incorporates the change to calm centered thought. Legitimate changes have caused advancement from being based on center consideration to being progressively subject to safety measure and outpatient driven thought. As medication arrives at the summit of its change to commercialization, there will be an innate need to furnish customers with the apparatuses to settle on insightful choices [7]. A crucial part of patient-orientated consideration is with respect to the quality of the connection between the doctors and their patients. Over the span of treatment (she had seen) a pulmonologist for her indications. James Rikert had performed pneumonic capacity tests, endorsed inhalers, and advised her to return if her side effects didn't improve. "She never returned, and the malignant growth was later found by her family specialist, by which time it was metastatic" [8]. The way that an advanced doctor cooperates with their patients decides their fulfillment with the consideration, their reaction to medicine, and their propensity to plan follow-up arrangements. In business as usual, specialists have an excessive number of patients to guarantee that every patient is healthy, much after the arrangement. As the need to build up associations with patient's increments couple with the improving figure of patients and requirement for care, specialists should use new innovation to achieve their objective of patient-focused consideration [9]. In the model above, innovation could have motioned to both the specialist and the inpatient that there was an evident need to plan a follow-up arrangement.

4 Exceptional Technical Challenges in Healthcare Tasks

Here the factors which are handling human services assignments that should be considered mindfully in the structure and appraisal of AI adventures: missingness, result definition, and causality. These considerations are noteworthy across both exhibiting frameworks (for example, administered versus unaided), and learning targets (e.g., order versus relapse).

A significant number of the most significant and energizing issues in social insurance require calculations that can answer causal, "imagine a scenario where?" inquiries regarding what will occur if a specialist directs a treatment [10]. These inquiries are past the range of old style AI calculations since they require a proper model of intercessions. To address this class of issues, we have to reason about and gain from information through the perspective of causal frameworks (e.g., see earlier work [11]. Gaining from information to respond to causal inquiries is most testing when the information are gathered observationally; that is, it might have been impacted by the activities of an operator whose strategy for picking activities isn't known. In social insurance, learning is done only utilizing observational information, which represents various difficulties to building frameworks that can respond to causal inquiries. For example, Simpson's Catch 22 portrays the perception that the connection between two factors can change headings if more data is remembered for the model. To all the more likely comprehend this issue, consider earlier work in which scientists found that asthmatic patients who were admitted to the medical clinic for pneumonia were all the more forcefully treated for the disease, bringing down the subpopulation mortality rate [12]. A model that predicts passing from asthma will discover that asthma is defensive. Assuming, in any case, an extra factor to represent the degree of care is incorporated, the model may rather find that having asthma expands the danger of death. This model shows that causal frameworks are valuable to assess medicines, however can likewise assist with building dependable prescient frameworks that don't make unsafe forecasts utilizing connections brought about by treatment arrangements in the preparation data. To represent these difficulties, solid suppositions must be made that can't be measurably checked or approved; i.e., assembling more information won't help [13]. The weaknesses of old style factual realizing while responding to causal inquiries are talked about in more noteworthy detail in earlier work [14].

5 Frameworks in Health Must Consider Missingness

Regardless of whether exceedingly significant factors are remembered for a social insurance data set, all things considered, numerous perceptions will be absent. Genuinely complete information is frequently illogical because of cost and volume. Gaining from deficient, or missing, information has gotten little consideration in the AI people group (despite the fact that special cases exist [15], however is an effectively examined subject in statistics [16]). Since human services is a powerful procedure where vitals are estimated and labs are requested after some time by specialists in light of past perceptions there are solid conditions between what factors are estimated and their qualities, which must be deliberately represented to maintain a strategic distance from one-sided results. There are three generally acknowledged arrangements of missing information components; i.e., the estimation instrument deciding if a worth is recorded or not [17]. The primary, missing totally aimlessly (MCAR), places a fixed likelihood of missingness. For this situation, dropping deficient perceptions—known as complete case examination—is generally utilized (though gullibly), and will prompt fair outcomes. Second, the information might be absent aimlessly (MAR), where the likelihood of missingness is irregular contingent on the watched factors. For this situation, regular strategies incorporate re-weighting information with techniques like converse likelihood of editing weighting or utilizing various ascription to in-fill [18]. At last, information might be absent not aimlessly (MNAR), where the likelihood of missingness relies upon the missing variable itself or other absent and imperceptibly factors.

5.1 Wellsprings of Missingness Must Be Painstakingly Comprehended

Wellsprings of missingness ought to be deliberately analyzed before sending a learning calculation. For instance, lab estimations are commonly requested as a major aspect of a symptomatic stir up, implying that the nearness of a data point passes on data about the patient's state. Consider an emergency clinic where clinical staff estimates persistent lactate level. In the event that a force blackout prompted a lot of lactate levels being lost, the information is MCAR. In the event that medical caretakers are more averse to gauge lactate levels in patients with horrible injury, and we record whether patients were conceded with injury, the information are MAR. Be that as it may, if medical caretakers are more averse to gauge lactate levels when accepted to be as of now, at that point the lactate estimates themselves are MNAR, and the estimation of the sign itself is significant. The key component of missing information is that there might be data passed on by the nonattendance of a perception, and disregarding this reliance may prompt frameworks that make off base, and even hurtful, expectations.

5.2 Incorporate Missingness in the Model

Counting missingness markers gives the most data to making predictions [19]. In any case, learning frameworks without a proper model of missingness prompts issues, for example, incorrect evaluation of highlight significance and frameworks that are weak to changes in estimation rehearses. For instance, troponin-T is normally estimated just when a myocardial dead tissue is viewed as likely. A model learned by treating troponin-T as MCAR would likely over predict the pace of myocardial localized necrosis on information where troponin-T was all the more consistently estimated. A model prepared with MAR troponin qualities would be increasingly powerful to this. Missingness can reflect human inclinations. We note that information may likewise be missing a result of contrasts in access, practice, or recording that reflects cultural biases [20]. frameworks prepared on such information may thus show unjustifiable execution for certain populaces if an AI expert is uninformed of this hidden variety; along these lines, checking frameworks across bunches is important [21].

5.3 Settle on Careful Choices in Defining Outcomes

Acquiring solid results for learning is a significant advance in characterizing undertakings. Results are frequently used to make the highest quality level marks required for administered forecast assignments, however are urgent in different settings also, e.g., to guarantee very much characterized accomplices in a grouping task. There are three key components to consider with result definitions: making solid results, understanding the significance of a result clinically, and the nuance of name spillage.

5.4 Comprehend the Result in Setting of a Social Insurance Framework

Clinical definitions are working frameworks utilizing ebb and flow logical comprehension of an infection. As understanding develops, so does the definition. The suggestion for AI is that acceptable prescient execution on names dependent on such definitions is just tantamount to the basic frameworks. For instance, intense kidney injury (AKI) is a significant basic sickness with two late definitions: RIFLE34 and KDIGO35. Thus, it is enticing to utilize the genuine conduct of clinicians as names, yet recall that they may not be right. For instance, work that objectives expectation of clinical activities should cautiously consider whether the medications are acceptable marks, and whether "erroneous forecasts" are in truth determining medicines that would have been given by different clinicians instead of medications that would ideally treat the patient [22].

5.5 Be Careful with Mark Spillage

The data gathered in a person's medical clinic experience is firmly coupled across time, and this can bring about data about the focused on task result spilling once again into highlights. While abusing such connections among highlights and targets is an objective of learning, data spillage can render an expectation aimless. Consider foreseeing mortality of emergency clinic patients utilizing every single accessible datum up until their season of death. Such an assignment could prompt a neurotic expectation rule—"on the off chance that the ventilator is killed in the previous hour, envision downfall." This conventionally takes place when families and their patients decide to pull back thought at a terminal period of sickness. High limit neural frameworks inspecting the whole EHR may likewise be liable to mark leakage; for instance, a last demonstrative name could use names that show up inside clinicians' underlying theories, affirming clinical consistency in speculations, as opposed to anticipating a determination dependent on pertinent information.

6 Statistical Frameworks from Scoring Systems

In medication, the utilization of scoring frameworks to classify patients into various hazard layers is very normal. For instance, the Charlson Comorbidity Index (CCI) [23] measures a person's weight of illness and comparing one year mortality chance. The utilized APACHE score [24] evaluates the seriousness of sickness patients admitted to escalated care units. The Apgar score sums up physiological measures as a pointer of newborn child dismalness [25]. An ongoing participant to chance scoring frameworks is the Rothman Index [26] that evaluates danger of death dependent on indispensable signs, nursing appraisals, and research center outcomes. Malady explicit scoring frameworks have additionally been grown, for example, the DLCN (Dutch Lipid Clinic Network) measures for diagnosing "impossible," "conceivable," "plausible," kin hypercholesterolemia [27]. The benefit of scoring frameworks being effectively explainable and are typically direct to oversee, yet not perform well at precisely mirroring the hazard for people. For instance, the DLCN measures for FH have explicitness running from 5.9 to 89.4% and affectability extending from 41.5 to 99.3% for foreseeing the aftereffects of a hereditary test for the disease [28]. In any case, because of the relationship among age and a few highlights of "unmistakable" FH, the scores are bound to misclassify more youthful people [29]. For instance, the amazing separation of the APACHE score makes it exceptionally valuable to conclude whether to move a patient out of an ICU or not. In any case, it is unseemly to utilize the score to evaluate that an individual patient should be revived with a 90% likelihood. Given such restrictions of customary scoring frameworks, moves toward that utilization AI to construct all around adjusted measurable frameworks that effectively order people and give exact appraisals of hazard are developing in notoriety. We have, for instance, as of late built up a measurable model—a punished calculated relapse model—to order patients as "improbable," "conceivable," "plausible," or "unmistakable" FH dependent on indistinguishable rules from the DLCN and EHR information. Our model enlarges the DLCN rules with factors that measure well-being framework usage and total insights levels of cholesterol and accomplishes 95% of an AUC with 86% review and 82% accuracy. Different methodologies have yielded equivalent outcomes for anticipating FH [30] and have huge potential cost reserve funds by decreasing superfluous hereditary testing and at the same time guaranteeing that genuine instances are not missed. Utilizing a comparable methodology, analysts in Canada refreshed and rethought the CCI with later managerial information and bigger progressively different patient populaces, and without depending on graph survey [31]. As opposed to supplanting the CCI out and out with a factual model, they utilized measurable frameworks to relegate new loads to comorbidities utilized in the CCI. Other hazard frameworks got the hang of utilizing EHR information incorporate PhysiScore [32], a framework that predicts preterm newborn child horribleness utilizing comparable physiological highlights as the Apgar score, and TrewScore [33], an early admonition framework for sepsis. Both accomplished improved execution contrasted with customary point-based scoring frameworks. Various different frameworks exist for frameworks that foresee sepsis

[34], postponed wound mending, danger of being discouraged [35], and cardiovascular antagonistic occasions [36]. These examinations exhibit that utilizing AI ways to deal with do the "hard work" of determining proper variable loads (and by and large, performing robotized variable determination) can create a model that beats the relating master inferred scoring framework and can refresh existing scoring frameworks as information change after some time. Appropriate utilization of AI strategies that can deal with enormous quantities of inadequately estimated factors and that can recognize which is the most critical impact on framework execution are pivotal to the achievement of frameworks worked from nonuniform and regularly untidy EHR information.

7 Difficulties EHR-Based Frameworks

The difficulties inalienable in reflectively breaking down EHR information gathered for clinical purposes and authoritative to inquire about have been very much described [37]. They incorporate inclinations because of utilizing information from people produced just at the point when they visit their medicinal services supplier (and are accordingly apt sick), inadequate records (and the affiliated issue of lost information disregarding the lost aimlessly suspicion), misfortune to development, the modification of evidences for charging potential, and purposes blunders acquainted with record of patients as they travel through a social insurance framework. Measurable techniques normally utilized to address these troubles remember attribution to fill for missing information and penchant score-based coordinating, weighting or delineation to choose tolerant examples [38]. These difficulties and predispositions that influence review concentrates additionally sway the utilization of AI to manufacture frameworks dependent on EHR information. An ongoing methodical audit of distributed research on creating prescient frameworks utilizing EHR information found that most prescient frameworks produced for social insurance applications didn't exploit the abundance of EHR information accessible. For instance, just about portion of the 60 investigations that anticipated a clinical result utilized data past determination codes to characterize the result, and just eight examinations utilized longitudinal estimations. The errand of precisely discovering whether a particular result happened is called electronic phenotyping [39] and the most significant advance in any measurable demonstrating workout finished with EHR information. A related report [40] recovered that in 4 out of 10 ailments inspected; the clinical records of fewer than 10% of examined patients known to have the condition contained the International Arrangement of Diseases analysis codes important to recognize the condition. For the rest that got from clinical notes or drug records (only two of numerous conceivable EHR-inferred sources) were required to decide the finding. Considering the significance of exact phenotype assurance—both for the result just as for the nearness of comorbidities—a few research endeavors are centered on utilizing AI techniques for the reason for phenotyping itself [41]. Another noteworthy issue looked at by analysts utilizing AI to get bits of knowledge from EHR information is that of outside legitimacy [42]—the exhibition of educated frameworks at locales differently which origin the information utilized for preparing. In this way, in the event that a model accomplishes adequate execution at a neighborhood site, at that point it has accomplished its motivation. So the conversation ought to be tied in with sharing the model structure work process to hold a model at another site, as opposed to about "outer legitimacy." Learning model utilizing site-explicit information and refreshing its parameters as an informational collection changes occasionally deliver the model which is most appropriate for forecast at that site and with that information [43]. The achievement of such a methodology over different locales is proof the model structure approach is valid. The achievement of building and conveying a measurable model at another site lays on the accessibility and reliable portrayal of information across sites. A universal coordinated effort of observational well-being analysts that has built up a CDM (Common Data Model) for EHR information as of now used to structure a huge number of patient records from in excess of 50 locales in 12 nations organized by the Observational Health Data Sciences and Informatics (OHDSI). A question to a CDM-agreeable database conveyed at some other OHDSI site can be built an associate at one site remain same. Such transportability has just presented the chance to create measurable frameworks that are versatile across locales and encouraged enormous scope examination into treatment pathways [44] (Fig. 2).

Scientist's allocation the work process used to build and train a model, to such an extent that it tends to be retrained utilizing information from another site and sent locally. Notwithstanding specialized difficulties around information frameworks, outer legitimacy, and the need to utilize different information types, arrangement of a measurable framework and development in a clinical setting additionally exist

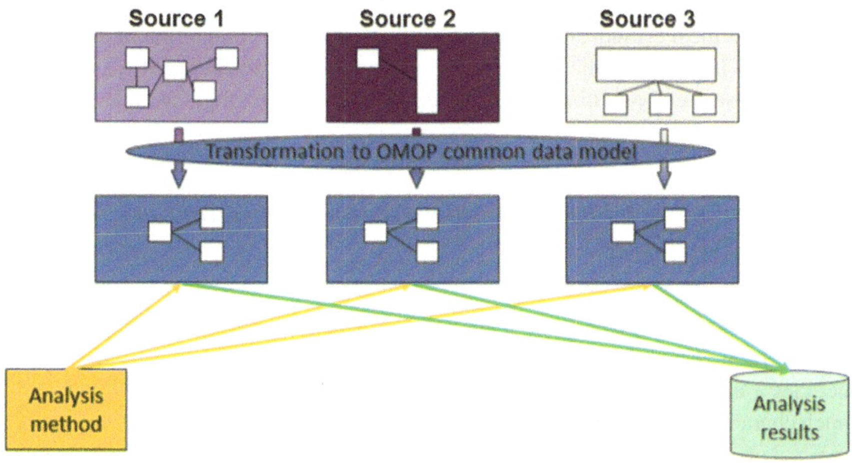

Fig. 2 CDM (Common Data Model) for EHR information. *Source* https://www.ohdsi.org/data-standardization/the-common-data-model

in operational difficulties. These challenges incorporate information get to, accessibility of staff with the important abilities to build up a model and decipher its yield, and, maybe generally basic, a framework for coordinating the model into the social insurance professional's work process it is intended to illuminate. Primary thought in surveying the utility of a prescient model manufactured utilizing EHR data by the accessibility of a compelling intercession. The achievement of frameworks sent for training the board in this way relies upon something beyond model execution—extra factors, for example, the framework are additionally important to consider the visibility and the expense of sending the framework of any activity is activated. For instance, variables examine and incorporate the size of the patient populace where mediation is conceivable, the predominance of the result being anticipated, the normal number of patients with the anticipated result, the cost investment funds per quiet presented to the intercession, the assessed cost of actualizing the intercession, the absolute objective reserve funds, moreover the quantity of patients exposed to the intercession required to meet that target. On the off chance that conveying a model is costly, or the influenced populace too little to even think about resulting in cost reserve funds for the training being referred to, the model won't be "valuable" regardless of whether its exhibition as estimated as far as accuracy, review, and adjustment is uncommon.

8 Inclined Opportunities in a Hierarchy of Healthcare

There are some high-sway open doors in human services. Prior to fitting frameworks, objectives ought to be plainly distinguished and approved as worth explaining. Here, we outline potential human services openings into three significant level classes: robotizing clinical errands, offering clinical help, and extending clinical limits. The subtleties of how a specialized arrangement is conveyed can change its expectation, and it is subsequently significant to connect with clinical partners at an early stage.

8.1 Automating Clinical Errands During Determination and Treatment

There are numerous errands right now performed by clinicians that current low-draping organic product for AI specialists. Clinical assignment mechanization includes a class of work that clinicians as of now do. These assignments are very much characterized (i.e., known information and yield spaces), and therefore require minimal measure of area adjustment and investment. The assessment of undertaking substitution is likewise clear—execution perhaps estimated against existing standards. We underline that calculations ought not to supplant clinical staff, but instead are utilized to advance the clinical work process. Clinical jobs will probably advance as these procedures improve, engaging staff to invest more energy with patients.

8.2 Computerizing Clinical Picture Assessment

Clinical imaging is a characteristic open door for AI since clinicians experience serious preparing to outline a fixed information space (for example the pictures) to a yield (for example the diagnosis). There have been a few late triumphs in applying profound figuring out how to clinical imaging undertakings. For instance, doctor level equality in the discovery of diabetic retinopathy, recognizing harmful and non-threatening skin injuries utilizing namely dermatoscopic images [45], identifying spleen hub metastases from bosom pathology slides2, and distinguishing hip cracks put x-beam images [46].

8.3 Robotizing Routine Procedures

Thus, robotizing irregular clinical procedures stands to diminish the weight set on clinical staff. For instance, organizing triage request in the crisis division is frequently left to staff [47], however should be possible algorithmically. In like manner, summing up the substance of patients' clinical records is a tedious, however significant, task. For instance, when emergency clinic personnel are uncertain about patient's ailment status, they may require an irresistible illness interview in which a pro carefully audits all the accessible patient information, and physically sums up unique place of origin into a progression of suggested tests and treatments. Specialists can use work from characteristic language age moving in the direction of producing outlines from organized her information, sparing truly necessary time [48].

8.4 Streamlining Clinical Choice and Practice Support

Another arrangement of chances center around supporting and increasing consideration. Instead of supplanting a very much characterized function, support requires understanding clinical torment focuses and working with clinical staff to comprehend proper information, yield targets, and assessment capacities. Open doors for help center around work that regularly endures because of certifiable requirements on schedule and assets, frequently prompting data misfortune and blunders (e.g., mixed up understanding recognizable proof, defective translations, or off base recall [49]. Within this setting, it is suitable to assess how frameworks improve down-stream results couple with clinical info as opposed to no holds barred correlations with clinical staff.

8.5 *Normalizing Clinical Procedures*

Varieties in clinical preparing furthermore experience lead to scopes of treatment decisions that may not be ideal for focusing on the hidden illnesses of a patient's state. For instance, clinical staff might be uncertain which medicine sets or portions are generally proper for a patient. To help such needs, past work has analyzed prescribing both normalized request sets to assist care with staffing rapidly evaluate what drugs they may have missed and default doses to maintain a strategic distance from perilous dosing [50]. Here notice that robotizing a static, existing, convention is fundamentally simpler than full choice help for complex clinical rules that may change after some time, and there is possibly much incentive in both medical clinic and wandering choice support [51], and at-home support.

8.6 *Incorporating Divided Records*

Limited assets can likewise prompt an absence of correspondence and coordination, influencing persistent consideration. For instance, it can take a very long time to recognize local maltreatment survivors in light of the fact that each and every unique medicinal visit in disconnection might be reliable with different causes (for example, an affirmation for wounding is reliable with an unconstrained fall). While conceivable without emotionally supportive networks on a fundamental level, AI can be an integral asset, e.g., distinguishing residential maltreatment as long as 30 months ahead of time of the human services system.

8.7 *Growing Medicinal Capacities: New Skylines in Screening, Analysis, and Treatment*

As social insurance records become progressively digitized, clinicians are confronted with an ever-expanding measure of novel information for patients and populaces. The outcome is a chance to give the social insurance framework another arrangement of abilities to convey medicinal services in better and more brilliant ways. Significantly, making new limits appropriate contribution with medical teammates and effect ought to be estimated both in development and medical worth.

8.8 *Growing the Inclusion of Proof*

While human services is an inalienably information driven field, most clinicians work with constrained proof directing their choices. Randomized preliminaries gauge normal treatment impacts for a preliminary populace, yet various everyday choices are not founded on top notch randomized control preliminaries (RCTs). For instance, most of regularly utilized ICU medications are not thoroughly exactly validated a few examiners have assessed that lone up to 20% of medicines are sponsored by an RCT. Indeed, even in settings where an RCT exists, the preliminary populace will in general be a restricted, centered subgroup characterized by the preliminary's incorporation criteria, yet that partner can not be illustrative of the different populace to which preliminary outcomes are then applied. At last, RCT results can't mirror the multifaceted nature of treatment variety in light of the fact that, practically speaking, tolerant consideration methods are profoundly individualized. Earlier work found that roughly 10% of diabetes and gloom patients and practically 25% of hypertension patients had a one of a kind medication pathway (i.e., zero closest neighbors) in an associate of 250 million patients. One path forward is influence this normally happening heterogeneity to structure regular experiments that estimated the aftereffects of an RCT utilizing less assets, consequently permitting a lot bigger arrangement of clinical inquiries to be explored.

8.9 Moving Toward Constant Social Checking

Phenotyping is a significant objective in healthcare, and wearable information gives a progressing approach to gadgets to gather consistent non-obtrusive information and give important arrangements or alarms once a patient needs consideration. Late work has concentrated on foreseeing such shifted results as cardiovascular failure frequently gathered data. There are further settings where non-intrusive observing might be the main handy approach to give location. For instance, programmed fall discovery aged patients, or authorizing hand washing consistence in a clinical setting. Critically, earlier difficulties recognized in name spillage, delicate names, bewildering including longing be considered cautiously. In phenotyping interminable conditions, patients are regularly previously being dealt with, thus early discovery may now and then add up to distinguishing a current care. Accuracy medication tries to individualize the treatment of every patient; this is especially significant for disorder—conditions characterized by an assortment of side effects whose causes are unknown. For example, intense kidney injury (AKI) is characterized by an assortment of manifestations portraying kidney disappointment, not a fundamental cause. Two people may have created AKI for various reasons on the grounds that reaper numerous reasons that kidneys can fall flat. More estimation of the two people could uncover the distinction in cause, which may thus recommend elective treatment strategies. By customizing after eventually, one can learn singular explicit care impacts that address the reason for the syndrome [52] in a specific person. This identifies with the thoughts from "N = 1" hybrid examinations in trial design [53]. Customized treatment is empowered by developing vaults of longitudinal information, where long haul movements of a person's well-being are available [54].

9 Technologies like Big Data in Medicinal Services

Huge information and examination have been causing disturbances in significant industry portions. As of late, huge information has become another omnipresent term. Enormous Data alludes to huge, complex datasets that are past the capacities of conventional information the board frameworks of putting away, overseeing, and handling in a convenient and practical way. Large information advances can deal with organized, semi-organized, and unstructured information in petabytes and the sky is the limit from there. Human services are one of the verticals that can essentially profit by the expanding measures of information and its accessibility. Elements including social insurance suppliers, pharmaceutical organizations, look into establishments, and government offices have started to accumulate gigantic measures of information from look into, clinical preliminaries, and general well-being and protection programs. The union of information from different sources has noteworthy potential [55]. Before, specialists have been treating patients dependent on side effects; nonetheless, doctors are starting to determine and get patients to have an idea known as proof-based medication. This includes surveying a lot of information totaled by medicinal preliminaries and other treatment pathways for the enormous scope and settling on choices dependent on the best data accessible [56]. For instance, as long as a patient comes in with a specific instance of seasonal influenza, a doctor in the past would depend on what the person thought about this season's flu virus as a rule or what different specialists in the zone knew. With enormous information advances, a doctor can take a gander at across the country drifts active treatment would work best for the patient to endorse the best drugs. The conglomeration of individual informational indexes that would somehow or another demonstrate good for nothing furnishes specialists with the data expected to improve, progressively comprehensive clinical choices (Fig. 3).

10 Common Machine Learning Applications in Healthcare

There are multiple and endless Machine learning applications in healthcare industry. Some of the most common applications are cited in this section. Machine learning helps streamlining the administrative processes in the hospitals. It also helps mapping and treating the infectious diseases for the personalized medical treatment. Machine learning will affect physician and hospitals by playing a very dominant role in the clinical decision support. For example, it will help earlier identification of the diseases and customize treatment plan that will ensure an optimal outcome. Machine learning can be used to educate patients on several potential disease and their outcomes with different treatment option. As a result it can improve the efficiency hospital and health systems by reducing the cost of the healthcare. Machine learning in healthcare can be used to enhance health information management and the exchange of the health

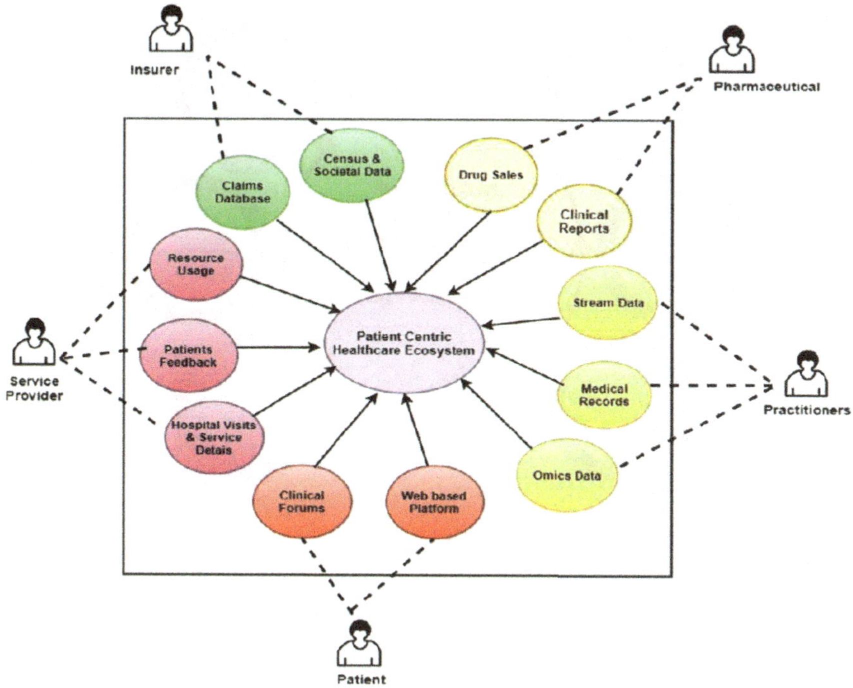

Fig. 3 Big data and medical services

information with the aim of improving and thus, modernizing the work-flows, facilitating access to clinical data and improving the accuracy of the health information. Above all it brings efficiency and transparency to information process (Fig. 4).

10.1 Machine Learning (ML) Application in Drug Discovery

Machine learning (ML) approaches, have played key role in the process of drug discovery in the recent times. It has helped minimize the high failure rate in drug development by leveraging the availability of huge high-quality data. There are multiple challenges in ML for drug development. One of the important challenges is to ensure drug safety. One of the challenging and complex tasks in the process of drug discovery is to analyze and interpret the available information of the known effects of the drugs and prediction of their side effects. Researchers from various reputed universities/institutions and of course, many pharmaceutical companies have been continuously using ML to obtain relevant information from clinical data used in clinical trials. Analyzing and interpreting these data using ML in the context of drug safety is an active area of research in recent times. Above all, the computational

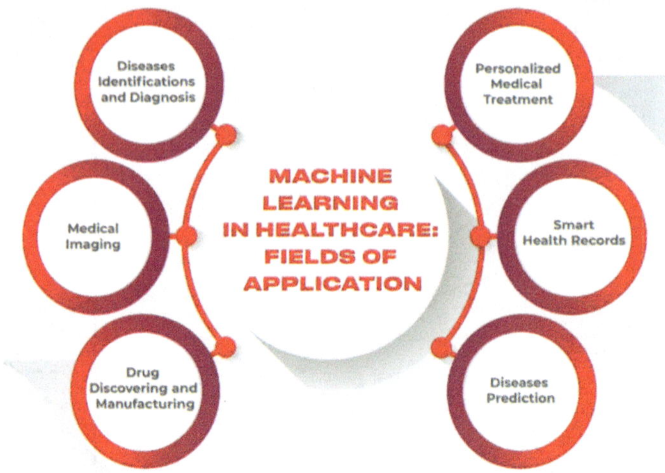

Fig. 4 Common machine learning applications in healthcare

solution in drug discovery has helped significantly reduce the cost of introducing drugs to the market.

10.2 Neuroscience and Image Computing

Neuroscience Image Computing (NIC) pays particular attention for the development of advanced imaging approaches, and its interpretation into clinical studies. NIC studies attempt to discover the etiology of brain disorders, including psychiatric disorders, neurodegenerative disorders, and traumatic brain injuries by using advanced technologies.

10.3 Cloud Computing Frameworks in Building Machine Learning-Based Healthcare

AI in general and ML in particular have seen tremendous growth in the recent times because of its ability to use huge volumes of data and produce accurate and deep understanding about the issues at hand. Cloud computing has made it possible that are more cost effective and its ability to handle increasing market demand. Models using ML are seen to be more robust that are using cloud computing resources. The cloud computing resources can track data from device wearable devices and health trackers. Then they can stream and aggregate it cost effectively in cloud-based storage. The large volume of data can be analyzed efficiently using cloud-based compute infrastructure. This allows the ML models to be more accurate and robust.

10.4 Applying Internet of Things and Machine Learning for Personalized Healthcare

Internet of Things (IoT) in healthcare has made it increasingly possible to connect a large number of people, things with smart sensors such as wearable and medical devices and environments. Patient vitals and various types of real-time data are captured by sensors and smart assets in IoT devices. Data analytics technologies, such as ML, can be used to deliver value-based care to the people. For instance, operational improvements enhance efficiencies that provide quality care at reduced costs. Similarly, clinical improvements ensure quicker and relatively accurate diagnoses. It also ensures more patient-centric, scientific determination of the best therapeutic approach to support better health outcomes. ML uses collected dataset to improve illness movement method and sickness forecast. Explanatory models by using ML are incorporated into various human services applications. These models typically break down the collected information from sensor gadgets and different sources to recognize personal conduct standards and clinical states of the patient.

10.5 Machine Learning in Outbreak Prediction

Multiple outbreak prediction models are widely used by researchers in the recent times to make most appropriate decisions and implement relevant measures to control the outbreak. For example, researchers are using some of the standard models such as epidemiological and statistical models for prediction of COVID-19. Prediction emerging from these models proved to be less robust and less accurate as it involves huge uncertainty and paucity of relevant data. Recently, many researchers are using ML models to make long-term prediction of this outbreak. Researchers have shown that machine learning-based models proved to be more robust compared to the alternative models for this outbreak.

10.6 Machine Learning in Patient Risk Stratification

In healthcare, risk stratification is understood as the process of classifying patients into types of risks. This status depends on data obtained from various sources such as medical history, health indicators, and the lifestyle of a population. The goal of stratifying risk include addressing population management challenges, individualizing treatment plans to lower risks, matching risk with levels of care, and aligning the practice with value-based care approaches. Traditional models for predicting risk mostly hinges on the expertise and experience of the practitioner. ML does not demand human inputs—to analyze clinical and financial data for patient risk stratification. By using the availability of volumes of data such as medical reports, patients' records, and insurance records, and apply ML to provide the best outcomes.

10.7 Machine Learning in Telemedicine

Tele-health in healthcare is an important industry. It makes the patient care process easier for both providers and patients. This industry is growing at a faster pace worldwide. The advancement of new technology such as ML in the healthcare has provided medical professionals with truly genuine tools and resources to manage the daily influx of patients. Machine Learning can help these professionals with a new way to analyze and interpret volumes of raw patient data and offer interesting insights and directions toward achieving better health outcomes.

10.8 Multimodal Machine Learning for Data Fusion in Medical Imaging

Multimodal medical image fusion technique is a useful and significant technique to investigate diseases by deriving the complementary information from different multimodality medical images. These strategies have been consistently and progressively applied in clinical practice. Multimodal picture investigation and troupe learning strategies are developing fast and carrying remarkable incentive to clinical applications. Driven by the ongoing achievement of applying these learning strategies to clinical picture handling, researchers have proposed algorithmic design to administer multimodal picture investigation with cross-methodology combination at the component learning level, classifier level, and at the dynamic level as well. At that point structure a picture division framework dependent on profound convolutional neural systems is executed to shape the injuries of delicate tissue sarcomas utilizing multimodal pictures, including those from attractive reverberation imaging, registered tomography, and positron discharge tomography. The system prepared with multimodal pictures shows better execution contrasted to systems prepared with single-modular pictures.

11 Machine Learning Opportunities in Healthcare

Tending to the pecking order of chances in medicinal services makes various open doors for advancement. Importantly, clinical staff and AI scientists frequently have integral aptitudes, and some high-sway issues must be handled by community-oriented endeavors. We note a few promising bearings of research, explicitly featuring such issues of information non-stationary, model interpretability, and finding proper portrayals.

Regardless of the methodological difficulties of working with EHR information and analysts have however to exploit the universe of EHR-determined factors accessible for prescient displaying, there are many energizing open doors for AI to improve well-being and human services conveyance frameworks that separate patients into various hazard classifications to advise practice the executives have tremendous potential effect on human services esteem and strategies that can anticipate results for singular patients bring clinical practice one bit nearer to exactness medication [57]. Distinguishing significant expense and high-hazard patients [58] so as to endeavor focused on intercession will turn out to be progressively essential as medicinal services suppliers assume the budgetary danger of handling their patients. AI address has just been utilized to portray and foresee an assortment of well-being dangers. Late work in our gathering utilizing punished strategic relapse to distinguish patients with undiscovered fringe corridor malady and foresee their mortality chance found that such a methodology beats an easier stepwise calculated relapse as far as precision, alignment, and net renaming. Such prescient frameworks have been executed in clinical work on, bringing about progressively proficient and better quality consideration. AI has additionally been applied to medical clinic and practice the board, to smooth out tasks and improve quiet results. For instance, frameworks have been created to anticipate interest for crisis division beds [55] and elective medical procedure case volume [20], to advise emergency clinic staffing choices. The Veterans Health Administration's Clinical Data Warehouse, which houses clinical information for in excess of 20 million patients, was utilized to create frameworks for danger of hospitalization and passing of individual patients with AUC esteems extending from 0.81 to 0.87 [58]. The hazard scores determined by these frameworks are introduced to Patient-Aligned Care Teams and are gotten to be in excess of 1200 social insurance suppliers for every month as a major aspect of their normal practice. In another effective model, a one-month readmission chance score for heart disappointment patients at the Parkland Health and Hospital System, called e-Score, was executed in an imminent report to survey the adequacy of a focused on mediation sick person with a high anticipated danger of readmission [20]. The examination found that the mediation, activated by the anticipated hazard score, brought about altogether diminished one-month readmission contrasted with a benchmark group. These frameworks exhibit that prescient frameworks can be sent in human services settings and utilized successfully to improve asset assignment and patient consideration.

At long last, AI isn't a panacea, and not everything that can be anticipated will be significant. For instance, we might have the option to precisely anticipate movement from stage 3 to arrange 4 constant renal disappointments. Without viable treatment alternatives—other than kidney transplant and dialysis—the expectation doesn't do a lot to improve the administration of the sick person. As another outrageous model, envision a model that predicts that treatment of a specific malignancy (state lung disease) will be ineffectual dependent on the genotypic profile of the tumor. Would we retain treatment dependent on such an expectation? Such extraordinary circumstances aside, there is abundant center ground where the utilization of prescient demonstrating in human services will empower proactive treatment, more effective utilization of assets, and convey better consideration at lower cost. Different ventures, for example, fund, retail, flight, web business, and political race battling—have made the change to fuse AI, and the subsequent prescient frameworks, into their separate work processes. It is the ideal opportunity for medicinal services to make that progress.

One territory, specifically, in which AI has conceivable boundless cultural effects are in the human services domain. In a developing industry of shrewd watches, fit bits, and gadgets that continually assemble a plentifulness of well-being information, the predominance of utilizing AI to dissect this information is picking up force [59, 64]. Organized well-being information is the data that is anything but difficult to classify put a database; they can incorporate a progression of measurements with classifications including however not restricted to quiet loads, temperatures, and even conventional indications like cerebral pain, stomach torment, etc. Most of clinical information is unstructured information as different various notes, reports, release rundowns, pictures, and sound and picture recording. It is exceptionally difficult to measure and arrange a discussion between the suppliers with the sick person; the discussion is customized and can take a wide range of bearings. Having the option to tackle and understanding this kind of information for an enormous scope will end up being very helpful in applying AI innovations in the medicinal services domain. Right now, an enormous number of fake information innovation exists for organized information; be that as it may, a lot littler level of current pioneers are concentrating on organized information, concentrating on the accounts present in the social insurance domain. AI, when applied adequately, can assist doctors with making close to consummate findings, pick the best drugs, and decide sick person expectation for poor results to prescription, together with better patients' general well-being while at the same time decreasing expense. As expenses for medicinal services deteriorate at truly significant expenses and the requirement for clinical oversight expands, AI for enormous scope unstructured information may end up being the answer for this ever-developing issue. Several organizations and people have set up itself in the market today with their AI innovation applied to present-day medication with both unstructured information and organized information. In social insurance, 0.5 of the all-out costs originate from 0.05 of absolute patients; furthermore, the quantity of incessant conditions requiring predictable, consistent consideration has continuously expanded the nation over. AI can demonstrate to distinguish patients who might be progressively inclined to repeating diseases and help analyze patients. Moreover, near

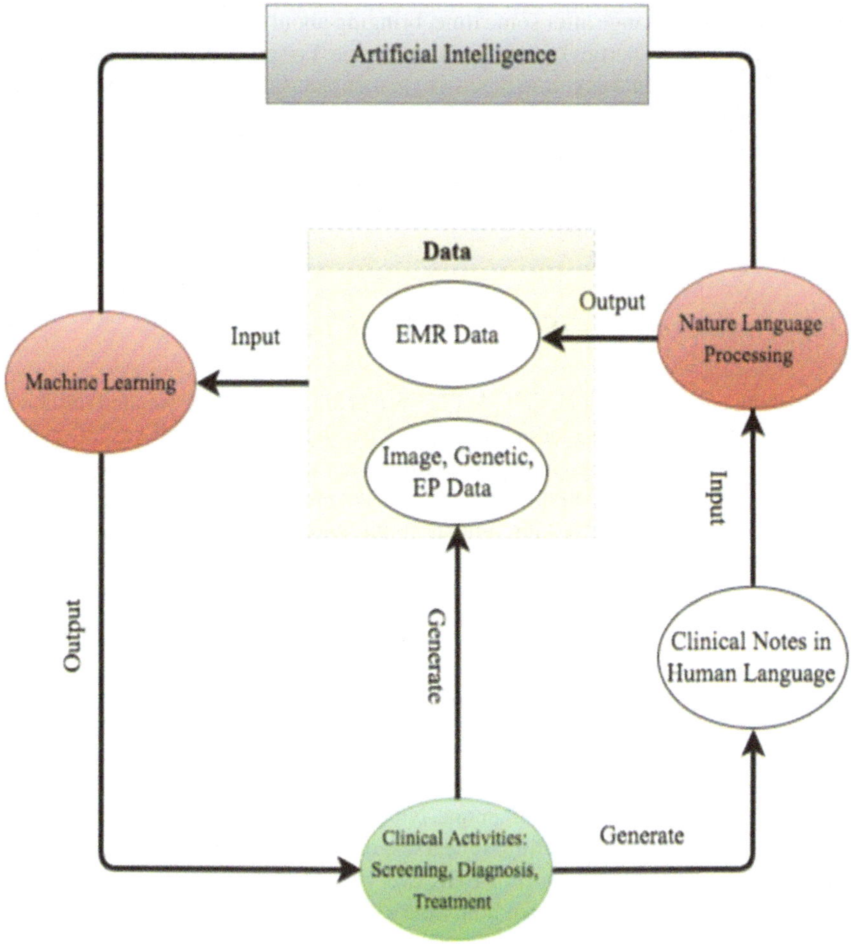

Fig. 5 Machine learning in clinical decision making [61]

0.9 visits crisis room are preventable. Utilization of AI help to analyze and straight patients to legitimate care all while minimizing expenses by retention patients out of costly, time concentrated crisis care focuses (Fig. 5).

11.1 Pleasing Data and Practice Non-stationarity in Learning and Deployment

In most existing work, frameworks are prepared on the biggest dataset conceivable and thought to be fit for arrangement, i.e., frameworks don't continue learning. This is tricky in clinical settings, since tolerant populaces and suggested treatment methodology will change after some time, bringing about corrupted prescient execution as the factual properties of the objective change. For instance, clinicians recently accepted that estrogen was cardio defensive in menopausal women [20] and hormone treatment was routinely endorsed as a protection measure until enormous preliminaries revealed either no advantage or an expansion in unfavorable heart events. In growing new frameworks for human services, frameworks must be made vigorous to these changes, or recognize their misalignment for the new population [60].

11.2 Inside Validity—Shift After Some Time

In a striking case of idea float, Google Flu Trends diligently overestimated influenza because of movements in search behaviors. The underlying model was an incredible achievement, utilizing Google search information to foresee influenza occurrence; notwithstanding, without update the model started to overestimate influenza frequency in resulting a very long time as client search practices had moved. While the float was inadvertent, the model rouses the requirement for frameworks that ceaselessly update.

11.3 Outside Validity—Shift Over Sources

There is additionally no motivation to accept from the earlier that a model gained from one clinic will sum up to another one. Numerous variables sway generalizability, including nearby emergency clinic rehearses, diverse patient populaces, accessible gear, and even the particular sort of EHR every utilization—advances starting with one EHR then onto the next make non-clear element mapping problems. This issue will stay until foundation to effectively test over numerous destinations gets common. The nonappearance of such normalization makes openings regarding information standardization and the improvement of frameworks that are powerful to contrasts in information assortment at various sites.

11.4 Making Frameworks Powerful to Criticism Circles

Frameworks that gain from existing clinical practice are vulnerable to intensifying the predispositions endemic to present-day human services. While not yet saw in human services, such input circles have been noted in the organization of prescient policing. Such inclinations reflected in sent expectations can spread into future preparing information, viably making an input circle that brings about additional bias. Work in algorithmic decency ought to be considered as it spurs the requirement for frameworks that are adequately mindful that they can make us aware of such undesirable conduct. Furthermore, frameworks prepared on EHR will gain from existing systems; instead speak to officially best-rehearse conventions, which might be tricky given low manual consistence in much clinical practice.

11.5 Making Interpretable Frameworks and Suggestions

In a clinical setting, discovery techniques present new difficulties. Generally, quantitative preparing has not been stressed in a doctor's broad clinical training and most doctors don't have a powerful comprehension of rubrics, for example, positive prescient value. Frameworks can't be sent "in the wild" with ease, and clinical staff must legitimize deviations in treatment to fulfill both clinical and legitimate prerequisites. An attribute optimization technique was developed in [62] for efficient diabetes prediction. Mishra et al. [63] presented a sampling-based method to deal with uneven datasets in healthcare domain.

11.6 Characterizing What Interpretability Implies

There are numerous potential approaches to interpretability, e.g., through component space minimization, model regularization, or an inclination for specific classes of frameworks that have notable post hoc investigation methods. For instance, giving a back dissemination over conceivable choice lists. Such records can give a characteristic method to clinicians to consider the overall dangers of their patient's condition.

11.7 Moving to Legitimization from Translation

In different areas, numerous types of interpretability depend on human aptitude, e.g., a model may feature a solitary sentence from a client survey ("The espresso is superb.") as the method of reasoning for an audit forecast. Clinicians are probably not going to have a comparable logical system, and it is probably not going to be evident what a specific example of lab estimations that maximally enacts model methods, organically or clinically. We contend that frameworks ought to rather give ''legitimacy"; past clarifying a particular expectation, frameworks ought to endeavor toward supporting the prescient way itself. For instance, late work has suggested that locally interpretable outcomes can be introduced for every individual prediction. Outside of consoling end clients, supporting an AI calculation's choice is likewise significant for security worries, as medication might be interestingly defenseless against "antagonistic attacks."

11.8 Adding Collaboration to AI and Assessment

AI work in medicinal services has a chance to make frameworks that interface and team up Clinical staff with human specialists. Give less than their skill; they likewise go about as parental figures, and sympathy is perceived as a significant component of clinical practice. Building shared frameworks can use the correlative qualities of doctors and learning frameworks. There are numerous strings of research in the AI writing that can fill in as an establishment for such frameworks. In dynamic learning, for instance, the objective is to use a prophet so as to master utilizing fewer samples]. The investigation of collective frameworks, where machine cooperate and the human is still in its beginning times.

11.9 Recognizing Multiple Source

Network Portrayal learning has provoked incredible advances in AI; for instance, the lower dimensional, subjectively important portrayals of imaging datasets learned by convolutional neural systems. Human services information needs such clearly characteristic structures, and examinations concerning suitable portrayals ought to incorporate multisource coordination, and learning area fitting portrayals.

12 Incorporating Expectations and Learning Significant Portrayals for the Space

Singular patient information has expanded to incorporate numerous sources and modalities, making mix additionally testing in frameworks as of now battling with overload. New memory frameworks are required for succession forecast undertakings, in light of the fact that so much records are not equally dispersed, can cover extremely long lengths, and early occasions can influence understanding state numerous years.

Learning significant state portrayals that give great prescient execution on various errands, and record for contingent connections of premium, is a significant territory. Managing portrayals unequivocally might be beneficial in light of the fact that they can helpfully communicate pandemic anterior that are not explicit to a solitary prescient job. There are a few potency chances to speech for portrayals for a medical institution scope. Initial, a solitary persevering information (for example, physiologic information) can compare to numerous conceivable right yields (for example, demonstrative codification), and this must be conceivable in the portrayals we investigate. There has likewise been some underlying investigation into education portrayals of other information types that all the while catch chain of importance and similarity.

13 Conclusion

Human services are one of the quickest developing divisions in the present economy; more individuals require care, and it is turning out to be increasingly costly. Government spending on social insurance has arrived at a record-breaking high while the intrinsic requirement for upgraded tolerant doctor association turns out to be promptly apparent. Technologies like enormous information and AI can possibly support the two licenses and suppliers as far as better consideration and lower costs.AI procedures applied to EHR information can create noteworthy bits of knowledge, from enhancing understanding danger score frameworks, to anticipating the beginning of malady, to smoothing out medical clinic activities. Measurable frameworks that influence the assortment and extravagance of EHR-determined information (rather than utilizing a little arrangement of master chose and additionally generally utilized highlights) are still moderately uncommon and offer an energizing road for additional exploration. New sorts of information, for example, from wearable's, bring their own chances and difficulties. Difficulties in successfully utilizing AI techniques incorporate the accessibility of staff with the aptitudes to construct, assess, and apply learned frameworks, just as the surveying this present reality money saving advantage exchange off of inserting a model in a social insurance work process.

References

1. Mason, E., Jain, S., Kendall, M., Mostashari, F., Blumenthal, D.: The regional extensioncenter program: helping physicians meaningfully use health information technology. Ann. Intern. Med. **153**, 666–670 (2010)
2. Mossialos, E., Wenzl, M., Osborn, R., Sarnak, D.: 2015 International Profiles of HealthCare Systems. The Commonwealth Fund (2016)
3. Parikh, R.B., Kakad, M., Bates, D.W.: Integrating predictive analytics into high-valuecare: the dawn of precision delivery. JAMA **315**, 651–652 (2016)
4. Kayyali, B., Knott, D., Kuiken, S.: The big DataRevolution in US health care: accelerating value and innovation. McKinsey & Company
5. Goldstein, B.A., Navar, A.M., Pencina, M.J., Ioannidis, J.P.: Opportunities and challengesin developing risk prediction models with electronic health records data: a systematicreview. J. Am. Med. Inform. Assoc. **27**(1), 198–208 (2016)
6. Jung, K., Covington, S., Sen, C.K., Januszyk, M., Kirsner, R.S., Gurtner, G.C., et al.: Rapid identification of slow healing wounds. Wound Repair Regen. **24**, 181–188 (2016)
7. Pencina, M.J., Peterson, E.D.: Moving from clinical trials to precision medicine: the role for predictive modeling. JAMA **315**, 1713–1714 (2016)
8. Bates, D.W., Saria, S., Ohno-Machado, L., Shah, A., Escobar, G.: Big data in health care: using analytics to identify and manage high-risk and high-cost patients. Health Aff. **33**, 1123–1131 (2014)
9. Escobar, G.J., Puopolo, K.M., Wi, S., Turk, B.J., Kuzniewicz, M.W., Walsh, E.M., et al.: Stratification of risk of early-onset sepsis in newborns $ 34 weeks' gestation. Pediatrics **133**, 30–36 (2014)
10. Greenland, S., Robins, J.M., Pearl, J.: Confounding and collapsibility in causal inference. Stat. Sci. 29–46 (1999)

11. Pearl, J.: Theoretical impediments to machine learning with seven sparks from the causal revolution. arXiv preprint arXiv:180104016 (2018)
12. Leek, J.T., Peng, R.D.: Statistics. What is the question? Sci. **347**, 1314–1315 (2015)
13. Marlin, B.M., Zemel, R.S., Roweis, S.T., Slaney, M.: Recommender systems, missing data and statistical model estimation. In: International Joint Conference on Artificial Intelligence (IJCAI), vol. 22, p. 2686 (2011)
14. Ding, P., Li, F.: Casual inference: a missing data perspective. Stat. Sci. **33**(2), 214–237 (2018)
15. Robins, J.M.: Robust estimation in sequentially ignorable missing data and causal inference models. Proc. Am. Stat. Assoc. **1999**, 6–10 (2000)
16. Miscouridou, X., Perotte, A., Elhadad, N., Ranganath, R.: Deep survival analysis: nonparametrics and missingness. In: Machine Learning for Healthcare Conference; pp. 244–256 (2018)
17. Rajkomar, A., Hardt, M., Howell, M.D., Corrado, G., Chin, M.H.: Ensuring fairness in machine learning to advance healthequity. Ann. Intern. Med. **169**(12), 866–872 (2018)
18. Chen, I.Y., Szolovits, P., Ghassemi, M.: Can AI help reduce disparities in general medical and mental health care? AMA J. Ethics **21**(2), 67–179 (2019)
19. Ghassemi, M., Wu, M., Feng, M., Celi, L.A., Szolovits, P., Doshi-Velez, F.: Understanding vasopressor intervention and weaning: risk prediction in a public heterogeneous clinical time series database. J. Am. Med. Inf. Assoc. 138 (2016)
20. Rajkomar, A., Oren, E., Chen, K., Dai, A.M., Hajaj, N., Liu, P.J., et al.: Scalable and accurate deep learning for electronichealth records. arXiv preprint arXiv:180107860 (2018)
21. Casey, B.M., McIntire, D.D., Leveno, K.J.: The continuing value of the Apgar score for the assessment of newborn infants. N. Engl. J. Med. **344**, 467–471 (2001)
22. Finlay, G.D., Duncan Finlay, G., Rothman, M.J., Smith, R.A.: Measuring the modified early warning score and the Rothman Index: advantages of utilizing the electronic medical record in an early warning system. J. Hosp. Med. **9**(2), 116-119 (2014)
23. Wei, W.-Q., Teixeira, P.L., Mo, H., Cronin, R.M., Warner, J.L., Denny, J.C.: Combining billing codes, clinical notes, and medications from electronic health records provides superior phenotyping performance. J. Am. Med. Inform., Assoc. **23**, e20–e27 (2016)
24. European Association for Cardiovascular Prevention and Rehabilitation, Reiner, Z., Catapano, A. L., De Backer, G., Graham, I., Taskinen, M.-R., et al.: ESC/EAS (2011)
25. Damgaard, D., Larsen, M.L., Nissen, P.H., Jensen, J.M., Jensen, H.K., Soerensen, V.R., et al.: The relationship of molecular genetic to clinical diagnosis of familial hypercholesterolemia in a Danish population. Atherosclerosis **180**, 155–160 (2005)
26. Besseling, J., Reitsma, J.B., Gaudet, D., Brisson, D., Kastelein, J.J.P., Hovingh, G.K., et al.: Selection of individuals for genetic testing for familial hypercholesterolaemia: development and external validation of a prediction model for the presence of a mutation causing familial hypercholesterolaemia. Eur. Heart J. **38**(8), 565–573 (2016)
27. Weng, S.F., Kai, J., Andrew Neil, H., Humphries, S.E., Qureshi, N.: Improving identification of familial hypercholesterolaemia in primary care: derivation and validation of the familial hypercholesterolaemia case ascertainment tool (FAMCAT). Atherosclerosis **238** (2015)
28. Quan, H., Li, B., Couris, C.M., Fushimi, K., Graham, P., Hider, P., et al.: Updating andvalidating the Charlson comorbidity index and score for risk adjustment in hospital discharge abstracts using data from 6 countries. Am. J. Epidemiol. **173**, 676–682 (2011)
29. Saria, S., Rajani, A.K., Gould, J., Koller, D., Penn, A.A.: Integration of early physiological responses predicts later illness severity in preterm infants. Sci. Transl. Med. **2** 48ra65 (2010)
30. Henry, K.E., Hager, D.N., Pronovost, P.J., Saria, S.: A targeted real-time early warningscore (TREWScore) for septic shock. Sci. Transl. Med. **7**, 299ra122 (2015)
31. Gultepe, E., Green, J.P., Nguyen, H., Adams, J., Albertson, T., Tagkopoulos, I.: From vitalsigns to clinical outcomes for patients with sepsis: a machine learning basis for a clinicaldecision support system. J. Am. Med. Inform. Assoc. **21**, 315–325 (2014)
32. Huang, S.H., Paea, L., Iyer, S.V., Ming, T.-S., David, C., Shah, N.H.: Toward personalizing treatment for depression: predicting diagnosis and severity. J. Am. Med. Inform. Assoc. **21**, 1069–1075 (2014)

33. Ross, E.G., Shah, N.H., Dalman, R.L., Nead, K., Cooke, J., Leeper, N.J.: The use of machine learning for the identification of peripheral artery disease and future mortality risk. J. Vasc. Surg. **64**, 1515–1522 (2016)
34. Patorno, E., Grotta, A., Bellocco, R., Schneeweiss, S.: Propensity score methodology forconfounding control in health care utilization databases. Epidemiol. Biostat., Public Health 10,(2013).
35. Hersh, W.R., Weiner, M.G., Embi, P.J., Logan, J.R., Payne, P.R.O., Bernstam, E.V., et al.: Caveats for the use of operational electronic health record data in comparative effectiveness research. Med. Care **51**, S30–S37 (2013)
36. Richesson, R.L., Jimeng, S., Jyotishman, P., Abel, K., Denny, J.C.: A survey of clinicalphenotyping in selected national networks: demonstrating the need for high-throughput, portable, and computational methods. Artif. Intell. Med. **71**, 57–61 (2016)
37. Agarwal, V., Vibhu, A., Tanya, P., Banda, J.M., Veena, G., Leung, T.I., et al.: Learningstatistical models of phenotypes using noisy labeled training data. J. Am. Med. Inform. Assoc. **23**, 1166–1173 (2016)
38. Iezzoni, L.I.: Statistically derived predictive models. Caveat Emptor. J. Gen. Intern. Med. **14**, 388–389 (1999)
39. Lee, J., Maslove, D.M.: Customization of a severity of illness score using local electronic medical record data. J. Intensive Care Med. **32**(1), 38–47 (2015)
40. Applod, K.: Five big industry changes to watch in 2016
41. Kayyali, B., Knott, D., Kuiken, S.: The Big data revolution in US health care: accelerating value and innovation. McKinsey & Company
42. Brown, B.: Top 7 healthcare trends and challenges from our financial expert
43. Esteva, A., Kuprel, B., Novoa, R.A., Ko, J., Swetter, S.M., Blau, H.M., et al.: Dermatologist-level classification of skin cancer with deep neural networks. Nature **542**(7639), 115 (2017)
44. Gale, W., Oakden-Rayner, L., Carneiro, G., Bradley, A.P., Palmer, L.J.: Detecting hip fractures with radiologist-level performance using deep neural networks, arXiv preprint arXiv:171 106504. (2017)
45. McCoy, T.H., Yu, S., Hart, K.L., Castro, V.M., Brown, H.E., Rosenquist, J.N., et al.: High throughput phenotyping for dimensional psychopathology in electronic health records. Biol. Psychiatry (2018)
46. Shneiderman, B., Plaisant, C., Hesse, B.W.: Improving healthcare with interactive visualization. Computer **46**(5), 58–66 (2013)
47. Pivovarov, R., Coppleson, Y.J., Gorman, S.L., Vawdrey, D.K., Elhadad, N.: Can patient record summarization support quality metric abstraction? In: AMIA Annual Symposium Proceedings.American Medical Informatics Association, vol. 2016, p. 1020 (2016)
48. Fishbane, S., Niederman, M.S., Daly, C., Magin, A., Kawabata, M., de Corla-Souza, A., et al.: The impact of standardized order sets and intensive clinical case management on outcomes in community-acquired pneumonia. Arch. Intern. Med. **167**(15), 1664–1669 (2007)
49. Bates, D.W., Gawande, A.A.: Improving safety with information technology. N. Engl. J. Med. **348**(25), 2526–2534 (2003)
50. Beam, A.L., Kohane, I.S.: Big data and machine learning in health care. JAMA (2018). https://doi.org/10.1001/jama.2017.18391
51. Poplin, R., Varadarajan, A.V., Blumer, K., Liu, Y., McConnell, M.V., Corrado, G.S., et al.: Prediction of cardiovascular risk factors from retinal fundus photographs via deep learning. Nat. Biomed. Eng. **1** (2018)
52. Che, Z., Purushotham, S., Cho, K., Sontag, D., Liu, Y.: Recurrent neural networks for multivariate time series with missing values. Sci. Rep. **8**(1), 6085 (2018)
53. Pearl, J.: Causality: models, reasoning, and inference. Cambridge University Press (2009)
54. Schulam, P., Saria, S.: Reliable decision support using counterfactual models. In: Neural Information Processing Systems (NIPS) (2017)
55. Lin, C., Jain, S., Kim, H., Bar-Joseph, Z.: Using neural networks for reducing the dimensions of single-cell RNA-Seq data. Nucleic Acids Res. **45**(17), e156–e156 (2017)

56. Choi, E., Bahadori, M.T., Song, L., Stewart, W.F., Sun, J.: GRAM: graph-based attention model for healthcare representation learning. In: International Conference on Knowledge Discovery and Data Mining (KDD). ACM, pp. 787–795 (2017)
57. Nickel, M., Kiela, D.: Poincare embeddings for learning hierarchical representations. arXiv preprint arXiv:170508039 (2017)
58. Chen, R., Michael, S.: Promise of personalized omics to precision medicine. Wiley Interdisc. Rev.: Syst. Biol. Med. **5**(1), 73–82 (2013)
59. Bengio, Y., Courville, A., Vincent, P.: Representation learning: a review and new perspectives. IEEE Trans. Pattern Anal. Mach. Intell. **35**(8), 1798–1828 (2013)
60. Abbeel, P., Ng, A.Y.: Apprenticeship learning via inverse reinforcement learning. In: Proceedings of the twenty-first international conference on Machine learning. ACM, p. 1 (2004)
61. Jiang, F., Jiang, Y., Zhi, H., et al.: Artificial intelligence in healthcare: past, present and future. Stroke Vasc. Neurol. **2**(4), 230–243 (2017)
62. Mishra, S., Tripathy, H.K., Mallick, P.K., Bhoi, A.K., Barsocchi, P.: EAGA-MLP—an enhanced and adaptive hybrid classification model for diabetes diagnosis. Sensors **20**, 4036 (2020)
63. Mishra, S., Mallick, P.K., Jena, L., Chae, G.S.: Optimization of skewed data using sampling-based preprocessing approach. Front. Public Health **8**, 274 (2020). https://doi.org/10.3389/fpubh.2020.00274
64. Mallick, P.K., Mishra, D., Patnaik, S., Shaw, K.:A hybrid approach for simultaneous gene clustering and gene selection for pattern classification. Indian J. Sci. Technol. **9**(21), 1–10 (2016)

Big Data Application in Health Care: A Study

Saumendra Kumar Mohapatra, Pradeep Kumar Mallick, and Mihir Narayan Mohanty

Abstract Day by day the size of the digital data is increasing due to the rapid advancement of information technology. This is happening in every digitalized sector. Analysis and processing of this big quantity of data are very challenging. Big data is one of advanced data analysis technology that has been introduced by the researchers for handling the data having large volume, velocity, variety, value, and veracity. Due to the digitalization in the healthcare sector, the generation of different health-related data is growing day by day. Use of big data in the healthcare sector helps physicians to process as well as extract useful information from these large amounts of data. The authors in this chapter have discussed several applications of big data in the healthcare sector. Also, a case study on big data technology for classifying the cardiac data in the multi-agent framework is proposed. This system is classifying different cardiac abnormalities by using a support vector machine (SVM). From the result, it is observed that the multi-agent system providing better performance and can be considered for any real-time application for cardiac disease detection.

Keywords Big data · Healthcare sector · Cardiac data · SVM · Multi-agent system

1 Introduction

Different figures and facts accessed and stored by computer are generally referred as data. From a report it has been analyzed that an amount of five exabytes data was generated by humankind from starting of civilization until 2003. But nowadays,

---

S. K. Mohapatra · M. N. Mohanty (✉)
Department of Electronics and Communication Engineering, ITER, Siksha 'O' Anusandhan (Deemed To Be University), Bhubaneswar, Odisha, India
e-mail: mihir.n.mohanty@gmail.com

S. K. Mohapatra
e-mail: saumendra95@yahoo.com

P. K. Mallick
School of Computer Engineering, KIIT Deemed To Be University, Bhubaneswar, Odisha, India
e-mail: pradeepmallick84@gmail.com

H. K. Tripathy et al. (eds.), *Technical Advancements of Machine Learning in Healthcare*, Studies in Computational Intelligence 936,
https://doi.org/10.1007/978-981-33-4698-7_2

five exabytes data is producing in every two days and the amount is also accelerating day by day. These data are of different types like human activity data, image and video data, multiple sensor generated data, conversion data, and data generated through different IoT enabled devices [1]. Processing and storing of these data is a challenging task in current scenario and for this research based on large-scale data processing is growing day by day [2]. Big data has been considered to be a breakthrough technological development over few years. Regardless, we have up till now constrained comprehension of how associations make an interpretation of its potential into real social and financial worth. Big data has increased critical impulse as a leap forward innovative advancement in scholarly and business networks. Big Data in this way alludes to our capacity to utilize the ever-expanding volumes of information [3, 4].

Definition of big data can be derived from the dimension of data. A data set can is considered as "big data," if it satisfies the following three high degree discrete dimensions: volume, velocity, and variety. Also there two other V dimensions value and veracity which are recently added to the big data definition [5]. The definition of big data can be defined through these five V as follows;

- **Velocity**: data generation speed
- **Volume**: generated data size
- **Variety**: assorted variety or various sorts of the data
- **Value**: data worth
- **Veracity**: quality, precision, or reliability of the data.

Generally these large datasets are available in two kinds of format such as structured data and unstructured data. The data generated from machine or human having a specific size, shape, and model is referred to as structured data. These data defined with well-structured data types. Integer, float, string type data are the examples of structured data stored in database columns. The data don't having any specific structure, shape, or model are referred to as the unstructured data category. Different text files, social media posts, mobile phone data, media, data, and log files are the basic examples of unstructured data. In current days every organization is producing huge amount of data which is increasing in every minute and it is essential to adopt different advanced technology to manage these high volume data. In the field of data analysis, big data technology is a new revolution. For getting important information and secret patterns from large quantity of data, big data technology plays a significant role. This can be helpful for understanding different information more accurately. Different organizations strap up their data and new opportunities can be identified. It can help different organizations for more proficient operations, adopting smart business moves, more profit, and customer satisfaction [6, 7].

In smart business system, big data plays an important role for identifying new opportunities. Different organizations are adopting this technology for improving their business process. It can help for boosting the business process with minimum complexity in operation. It has the capability to increase the business efficiency, that can help for profit increment as well as customer satisfaction. The following factors are the main cause behind the popularity of big data.

Reduced cost: This advanced data processing technique is more cost effective for handling large quantity of data and can be useful for effective business processing.

Quick decision making: Big data technology is the combination of high power memory and capable of analyzing different types of data. These features help in making any decision faster than before. Also the organizations can take any smart decision with the help of analytical learning strategy.

New products and features—Big data technology has the ability to identify the customer's need and satisfaction level. Some of the organizations also using this technology for creating new products for satisfying their customers.

A basic structure of factors for adopting big data technology is presented in Fig. 1. Due to the aforementioned factors of big data concept, numerous organizations are increasing their sale, operation, efficiency, customer service, and risk management.

Data isn't just about discovering answers, it's the place where the thoughts start. Each huge organizations faces multiple challenges of getting to tremendous measures of data and effectively placing them into utilization for business profitability. Data is put away in various frameworks and storehouses that make it hard for the associations to get to that information and upgrade their day by day activities and significant choices. Examination of this large data by utilizing the intensity of the cloud can transform it into noteworthy bits of knowledge. Dynamic comprehends this test by investigating, mining, picturing, and examining your large information (both inside and outside). Utilizing progressed diagnostic procedures against broad, differing

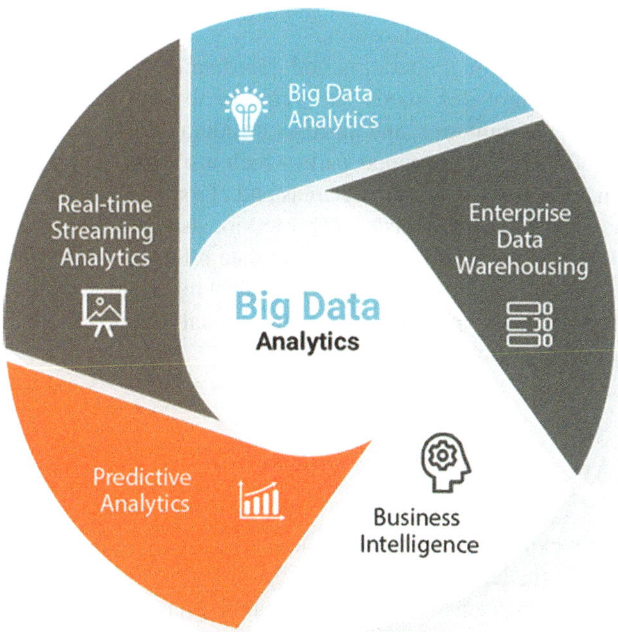

Fig. 1 Factors behind adopting big data technology

informational collections, we transform the information into new experiences and assist you with improving your business forms alongside dynamic. Our large information examination capacities assist you with enabling everybody in your association with better and more profound experiences to settle on information driven choices. According to industry expertise, academicians, and other entrepreneurs, big data is acting as a great game changer in most of the sectors in last few years. Though big data keeps on oversupplying our daily exists, there has been enormous progress of center from the publicity surrounding it to finding out genuine incentive in its operation. Big data is most likely at the forefront of everybody's thoughts for a long while now. Also, the truth of the matter is Big Data has fanned out quickly and is very nearly vanquishing each domain of the world. It isn't just a decision that the IT world yet has assumed control over different enterprises also. Huge Data on account of the advantages it outfits the different enterprises with, is presently turning into a fundamental piece of them. Large Data, on the other side, is step by step vanquishing the more established out of date advances and is a major matter of worry for those experts who are as yet dealing with it. The necessary intentions of Big Data applications is to assist organizations with settling on increasingly educational business choices by examining enormous volumes of information.

Associations from the various areas are putting resources into Big Data applications, for analyzing huge informational collections to reveal every single concealed example, ambiguous relationships, advertise patterns, client tendencies, and other cooperative business information. The basic application areas of big data technology are retail organizations, healthcare sector, finance, telecom, automobile, media and entertainment, e-commerce, and education.

Healthcare sector is a conglomeration and coordination of segments inside the financial support that provides goods and ventures to treat patients with therapeutic, preventative, rehabilitative, and gesture consideration. The advanced healthcare sector includes three fundamental parts which are supervisions, objects, and financials and may be isolated into many areas and classifications and relies on the different sectors of arranged specialists and professionals to tackle medical issues of persons and populaces. The term healthcare big data refers to assembly, dissecting and exploiting customer, patient, physical, and clinical information that is extremely huge or compound to be comprehended by conventional techniques for biomedical data processing and analysis.

2 State of Art

Size of the data has expanded in different fields in the course of the most recent two decades; henceforth, the term "big data" has been introduced. It has been generally foreseen that the size of data will keep on expanding enormously in the coming a long time right now, where tremendous measures of information are continually being produced from a few sources. The entirety of this information makes new chances to separate more esteem. In this way, "enormous information" could be characterized as a quickly developing measure of information from different sources that inexorably represents a test to mechanical associations and furthermore presents them with an unpredictable scope of significant use, stockpiling, and examination issues. Research dependent on enormous information is turning out to be progressively famous nowadays. In this way, the effect, execution, and difficulties of huge information have been examined generally over all the different segments.

The rise of shrewd urban communities targets relieving the difficulties raised because of the constant urbanization advancement and expanding populace thickness in urban areas. To confront these difficulties, governments and chiefs embrace shrewd smart city projects focusing on maintainable financial development and better personal satisfaction for the two occupants and guests. Data and Communication Technology is a key empowering innovation for city tiding. Removing experiences and concealed relationships from huge amount of data is a developing pattern in data frameworks to offer better types of assistance to residents and bolster the dynamic procedures. Notwithstanding, to separate significant experiences for creating city level shrewd data benefits, the produced datasets from different city areas should be incorporated and broke down. This procedure for the most part alluded to as large information examination or huge information esteem chain. A novel big data analytics-based smart city framework was introduced in [8]. Their proposed approach is to answer the different questions related to big data enabled smart city framework. In order to answer such type of questions, authors have conducted an organized review of literature on big data enabled smart cities. Their planned system acquaints new objectives with huge data examination structures spoke to in data model administration and conglomeration. The estimation of the proposed structure was talked about in contrast with customary information disclosure draws near. A review on application of big data in smart cities was discussed in [9]. Their review examines and looks at changed meanings of the savvy city and enormous information and investigates the chances, difficulties and advantages of fusing large information applications for brilliant urban areas. Furthermore it endeavors to recognize the prerequisites that help the usage of large information applications for shrewd city administrations. Because of the colossal volume of information produced by urban reconnaissance frameworks, big data technology has arranged low intricacy programmed foundation subtraction strategies are in extraordinary interest. A big data enabled novel background image analysis technique for urban surveillance system was introduced in [10]. In their proposed automatic system, computer was enabled for renewing an image with a new background at the time when there was no object in an image. There proposed method was designed in simple and robust properties with respect to changes in light condition. Customer investigation is at the focal point of a big data insurgency. Innovation helps catch rich and copious information on customer marvels progressively. To all the more likely comprehend the result of big data on multiple supporting movements, allowing resolved to all the more likely endeavor its benefits, a designed organization that gets bigger on asset-based hypothesis was discussed in [11]. Three benefits such as objective, human, and hierarchical assets—moderate the supplementary: (1) the path for assembling and putting away proof of buyer movement as Big Data, (2) the way toward extricating shopper knowledge from Big Data, and (3) the way toward using purchaser understanding to improve dynamic/versatile capacities. Moreover, one of a kind asset necessities for firms to profit by Big Data are examined. Traffic clog is a state of a portion in the street organize where the traffic request is more noteworthy than the accessible street limit. The recognition of uncommon traffic designs including blockages is a critical research issue in the information mining and information disclosure network. Notwithstanding, as far as we could possibly know, the disclosure of proliferations, or causal collaborations among identified traffic clogs has not been suitably researched previously. In [12], authors have presented calculations which build causality trees from clogs and gauge their engendering probabilities dependent on fleeting and spatial data of the blockages. Visit substructures of these causality trees uncover repeating associations among spatio-transient blockages, yet potential bottlenecks or defects in the plans of existing traffic systems. Their proposed calculations have been approved by investigates a movement time informational index recorded from an urban street organize. IoT is a basic strategy aim to decide data and support purpose for radiant dwellings. Connected machines and tools within the keen home create plenty of information about customers and how they move toward their day by day exercises. IoT processing can help in customizing applications that advantage the two mortgage holders and the regularly developing ventures that need to take advantage of shoppers profiles. Application of big data on IoT-based data collected form smart homes was presented in [13]. Fog node and cloud system was considered for data-driven and addressing different challenges on online and offline data processing and analysis. Smart Farming is a development that accentuates the exploitation of data and communication modernization in the digital substantial farmhouse the board cycle. Advanced innovations, for example, the IoT and Cloud Computing are required to exploit this enhancement and nearby more robots and man-made brainpower in humanizing. This is incorporated by the wonder of Big Data, monstrous amount of information with a wide assortment that can be caught, examined, and utilized for dynamic. A few authors have also proposed that Big Data will basis significant moves in jobs and force relations among various players in current nourishment production network systems. The scene of partners displays an intriguing game between groundbreaking tech organizations, investors, and regularly little new companies and new contestants [14]. For extending the business strategy, analysis of data is an important asset. It can be useful for analyzing and further processing of the data generated from different operations. An overview of big data technology in manufacturing sector was derived in [15] by using IoT. Also authors have discussed about some challenges and necessities of big data technology for manufacturing data. Large information examination has as of late developed as a significant research territory because of the prevalence of the Internet and the approach of the Web 2.0 advances. Besides, the multiplication and reception of web-based social networking applications have given broad chances and difficulties to scientists and specialists. The gigantic measure of information produced by clients utilizing online networking stages is the consequence of the mix of their experience subtleties and everyday exercises. This colossal volume of produced information known as "large information" has been seriously looked into as of late. A review on role of big data for social media data was discussed in [16]. The literature was classified based on different useful aspects. Enormous information is progressively turning into a significant hierarchical endeavor power to deal with right now for all sizes of ventures. It is a slanting new endeavor framework or stage which apparently offers more highlights for getting, putting away, and investigating voluminous created information from different sources to acquire esteem increases. In any case, momentum look into uncovers that there is constrained understanding with respect to the presentation of "big data" Therefore, this paper endeavors to completely explore "big data" its application and investigation in tasks or store network the board, just as the patterns and viewpoints right now [17]. The fast predominance and potential effect of big data analysis have started an enthusiasm among various experts and the scholarly world. Assembling associations are especially appropriate to profit by information examination stages in their whole item lifecycle the board for keen data preparing, performing producing exercises, and making esteem chains. This needs a deliberate re-architecting approach joining cautious and careful assessment of objectives for coordinating assembling inheritance data frameworks with information investigation stages. Besides, improving the vulnerability of the effect the new enormous information engineering on framework quality objectives is expected to keep away from cost victory in the usage and testing stages [18]. The significance of large information examination, computerized reasoning, and AI has been at the front line of research for tasks and store network the executives. Writing has revealed the impact of large information investigation for improved operational execution, yet there has been a lack of research in regard to the job of enterprising direction on the selection of enormous information examination. To address this hole, creators have drawn on the dynamic abilities perspective on firms and on possibility hypothesis to create and test a model that depicts the job of EO on the appropriation of huge information examination controlled by man-made consciousness and operational execution [18]. They have tried their examination theories utilizing an overview of 256 reactions assembled utilizing a pre-tried poll from assembling firms in India with the assistance of the outcomes from their examination demonstrate that EO empowers an association to abuse and further investigate the BDA-AI abilities to accomplish predominant OP. Further, their outcomes give observational proof dependent on information investigation that EO is firmly connected with higher request capacities, (for example, BDA-AI) and OP under differential impacts of natural dynamism. These discoveries broaden the dynamic ability view and possibility hypothesis to make better comprehension of dynamic capacities of the association while likewise giving hypothetically grounded direction to the administrators to adjust their EO to their innovative capacities inside their organizations. China Unicom, the biggest WCDMA 3G administrator in China, meets the prerequisites of the verifiable Mobile Internet Explosion, or the flooding of Mobile Internet Traffic from versatile terminals. As indicated by the interior insights of China Unicom, portable client traffic has expanded quickly with a Compound Annual Growth Rate (CAGR) of 135%. Right now China Unicom month to month stores in excess of 2 trillion records, information volume is more than 525 TB, and the most elevated information volume has arrived at a pinnacle of 5 PB. Since October 2009, China Unicom has been building up a home-blended large information stockpiling and investigation stage dependent on the open-source Hadoop Distributed File System (HDFS) as it has a long haul technique to utilize this Big Data. All Mobile Internet Traffic is all around served utilizing this large information stage. At present, the setting up speed has arrived at 1 390 000 accounts for each second, and the record recovery time in the table that contains trillions of records is under 100 ms. To make the most of this chance to be a Big Data Operator, China Unicom has grown new capacities and has various developments to unravel reality requirement challenges introduced in information preparing [19]. The challenges for designing a novel architectural solution to managing the social media data quality in each stage of the big data structure was addressed in [20]. Their approach can give a real-time solution in different decision-making problems for the users. Enormous information progressively advantage both research and modern territory, for example, medicinal services, money administration, and business suggestion. Topical bundle space including delegate labels, the dispersions of cost, visiting time, and visiting period of every theme, is mined to connect the jargon hole between client travel inclination and travel courses. To prescribe customized POI grouping, first, celebrated courses were positioned by the similitude between client bundle and course bundle. At that point top positioned courses were additionally advanced by social comparable clients' movement records. Delegate pictures with perspective and occasional assorted variety of POIs were appeared to offer an increasingly extensive impression [21].

With the quickly expanding notoriety of monetary exercises, a lot of financial information is being gathered. Albeit such information offers super open doors for monetary examination, its low quality, high dimensionality, and tremendous volume present incredible difficulties on effective investigation of financial enormous information. The current techniques have fundamentally broke down financial information from the point of view of econometrics, which includes constrained markers and requests earlier information on market analysts. When grasping enormous assortments of monetary variables, these strategies will in general yield unacceptable execution. Big data based a new feature selection method for analyzing the huge amount of economic data was presented in [22]. In particular, the structure joins the strategies for monetary element choice and econometric model development to uncover the shrouded designs for financial advancement. The usefulness lays on three columns: (i) novel information pre-handling systems to get ready top notch financial information, (ii) an inventive appropriated highlight recognizable proof answer for find significant and delegate monetary markers from multidimensional informational collections, and (iii) new econometric models to catch the shrouded designs for financial advancement. The exploratory outcomes on the monetary information gathered in Dalian, China, exhibit that their proposed structure and strategies have unrivaled execution in breaking down gigantic financial information. Propelled communication and information handling advancements carry incredible advantages to the brilliant lattice. In any case, digital security dangers likewise stretch out from the data framework to the savvy matrix. The current security works for keen lattice center around conventional insurance and recognition strategies. Be that as it may, a great deal of dangers happen in an extremely brief timeframe and disregarded by leaving security segments. These dangers typically impact sly affect shrewd brace and upset its ordinary activity. Additionally, it is past the point where it is possible to make a move to safeguard against the dangers once they are distinguished, and harms could be hard to fix. An awareness structure for security issues in big data application in smart grid technology was introduced by the authors in [23]. With the quick development of advanced distributing, reaping, overseeing, and investigating academic data have gotten progressively testing. The term Big Scholarly Data is begat for the quickly developing academic information, which contains data including a huge number of creators, papers, references, figures, tables, just as insightful systems and advanced libraries. These days, different insightful information can be handily gotten to and amazing information investigation innovations are being created, which empower us to investigate science itself with another point of view. A background study about the role of big scholarly data was discussed in [24]. Application of the big scholarly data in different related technology as well as the analysis method was discussed by them. They have also addressed various research issues and findings in respective areas. Power value estimating is a critical piece of keen lattice since it makes shrewd framework cost proficient. By and by, existing techniques for value gauging might be hard to deal with colossal value information in the network, since the excess from include choice can't be turned away and an incorporated framework is likewise needed for organizing the systems in power value determining. To tackle such an issue, a novel power value gauging model was created [25]. In particular, three modules were incorporated in the proposed model. To start with, by converging of Random Forest (RF) and Relief-F calculation, they have proposed a half and half element selector dependent on Gray Correlation Analysis (GCA) to dispense with the element excess. Second, a combination of Kernel capacity and Principle Component Analysis (KPCA) was utilized in highlight extraction procedure to understand the dimensionality decrease. At long last, to figure value characterization, they have advanced a differential evolution (DE) based Support Vector Machine (SVM) classifier. Their proposed power value gauging model was acknowledged through these three sections. Numerical outcomes show that our proposition has unrivaled execution than different strategies. Complex Big Data frameworks in present-day associations are logically turning out to be assault focuses by existing and rising danger operators. Detailed and concentrated assaults will progressively be created to misuse vulnerabilities and shortcomings. With the ever-expanding pattern of cybercrime and episodes because of these vulnerabilities, successful defenselessness the executives is basic for present-day associations paying little mind to their size. In any case, associations battle to deal with the sheer volume of vulnerabilities found on their systems. Additionally, powerlessness the board will in general be progressively responsive practically speaking. Thorough measurable models, mimicking foreseen volume and reliance of defenselessness exposures, will without a doubt give significant bits of knowledge to associations and assist them with getting progressively proactive in the administration of digital dangers [26].

Resting state functional magnetic resonance imaging (rfMRI) can be utilized to gauge useful availability and afterward distinguish mind organizes and related cerebrum issues and maladies. To investigate these unpredictable systems, be that as it may, immense measures of information are important. Late advances in neuro-imaging advances, and the one of a kind methodological methodology of rfMRI, have empowered us to a time of Biomedical Big Data. The ongoing advancement of enormous information imparting undertakings to their difficulties are examined. This expanding measure of neuro-imaging information has extraordinarily expanded the significance of creating preprocessing pipelines and progressed expository procedures, which are better at dealing with huge scope datasets. Before applying any examination strategy on rfMRI information, a few preprocessing steps should be applied to lessen every undesirable impact. Three elective approaches to gain admittance to huge preprocessed rfMRI information are introduced including the insignificant preprocessing pipelines. There are a few generally utilized strategies to look at useful availability. In any case, they become restricted in the investigation of enormous information, and another device to investigate such information is vital. Different novel rfMRI data analysis methods were introduced by the authors in [27]. The expanded utilization of digital empowered frameworks and Internet of Things (IoT) prompted a monstrous measure of information with various structures. Most huge information arrangements are based on the Hadoop eco-framework or utilize its disseminated document framework (HDFS). Be that as it may, contemplates have indicated wastefulness in such frameworks when managing the present information. Some examination conquered these issues for explicit kinds of chart information, yet the present information are more than one sort of information. Such productivity issues may prompt huge scope issues, remembering bigger space necessities for server farms, and waste in assets (like force utilization), that thusly lead to natural issues, (for example, more carbon discharge), according to researchers. For this Hadoop ecosystem a data analysis model was proposed in [28]. Also they have introduced a distributed encoding system for genetic algorithm-based data analysis. Their proposed system permits the Hadoop to handle the delivery of the data based on their clusters. Their system was also capable of handling large amount of data. The medicinal providing industry has formed a lot of information, determined by keeping record, managerial requirements, and patient contemplation. As mot information is forwarded in printing format, the current prototype is running toward rapid digitization [29].

3 Application of Big Data in Health Care

In the present period of smartphones and wearable gadgets, huge measures of patient wellbeing information records framing Big Data are being set into enormous databases where they can be gotten to by various clients including specialists, parental figures, and patients. In Fig. 2, the application of big data in healthcare domain is displayed. The evaluated spending on medicinal services in 2015 in the U.S. is around $3.2 trillion, which triggers the topic of progress of patient consideration while containing the expenses. The target of the current examination is to survey a couple of uses of investigation of Big Data in the human services field and

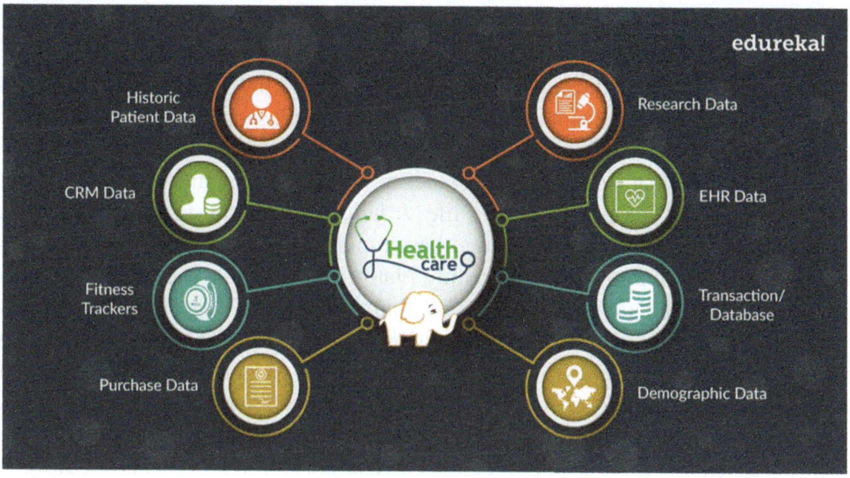

Fig. 2 Big data application in healthcare sector

the related results. Large Data is for the most part described by the volume, speed, assortment, and veracity of complex information. Numerous emergency clinics have applied examination to huge information from different sources including persistent wellbeing records to accomplish by and large improvement in human services. Operationally, the greater part of the appropriate information of patients are caused accessible on request so specialists to can perceive how different medications have functioned all around and apply important outcomes to encourage better dynamic and mediations. Utilizing large information investigation in medicinal services can prompt improvement in care conveyance combined with noteworthy cost reserve funds. Simultaneous difficulties to be tended to incorporate availability, protection, security, ease of use, usage costs, transportability, interoperability, and normalization. All in all, utilizing effective and streamlined investigation to large information will add to snappy and precise conclusion, suitable treatment, diminished expenses, and improved generally speaking medicinal services quality [30].

The quickly developing volume of multimodal electrophysiological signal information is assuming a basic job in understanding consideration and clinical research over different illness areas, for example, epilepsy and rest medication. To encourage optional utilization of these information, there is a dire need to create novel calculations and informatics approaches utilizing new distributed computing innovations just as ontologies for community-oriented multicenter examines. A cloud-based strategy for designing an algorithm to analyze the cardiac measurement as well as to process large amount of ECG was presented by the authors in [31]. Their system also helps to visualize the features of the original data set. Due to the development of big data in biomedical and medicinal services networks, precise examination of clinical information benefits early sickness recognition, persistent consideration, and network administrations. Notwithstanding, the examination precision is diminished when the nature of clinical information is deficient. In addition, various locales show interesting attributes of certain local maladies, which may debilitate the forecast of sickness episodes. A modified disease prediction model for analysis of real-life biomedical data collected from a hospital was developed in [32]. As deep learning is capable of handling huge amount of data, authors have used a convolutional neural network model for predicting the risk factors from both structured and unstructured data. In the current situation mobile devices are becoming the most important asset in the daily life of the people's daily life. It helps to perform different operations in minimum time and expenses. Cloud-based mobile communication system joins together the mobile and cloud computing platform to increase the performance as well as conquers the use of CPU, memory, and battery. A mobile cloud computing-based big data analysis system for processing the huge amount of biomedical data was proposed in [33]. These days, wearable clinical gadgets assume an essential job in numerous conditions, for example, persistent wellbeing checking of people, street traffic the executives, climate determining, and brilliant home. These sensor gadgets ceaselessly produce a tremendous measure of information and put away in distributed computing. An IoT-based big data enabled system was designed by the authors in [34] for clinical application. Their proposed system was also enabled of MetaFog-Redirection (MF-R) and Grouping & Choosing (GC) technique. For overcoming this problem, MapReduce-based logistic regression technique was designed to handle huge amount of data. Research on bioinformatics is described by voluminous and gradual datasets and complex information examination techniques. Several issues and problems arising due to the application of big data in bioinformatics was discussed in [35]. They have also presented different challenges as well as future research scopes in this domain. Huge Data is an aggregation of informational indexes which are copious and mind boggling in character. They include both organized and unstructured information that develop bounteous, so expedient they are not advantageous by traditional social database frameworks or current scientific devices. Enormous Data Analytics isn't directly ready to extend. It is a predefined composition. Presently enormous information is exceptionally useful for reinforcement of information not for everything else. There is constantly an information presenting. It likewise assists with taking care of India's large issues. It additionally assists with filling the information hole. Social insurance is the preservation or headway of wellbeing along the evasion, translation, and clinical consideration of turmoil, terrible wellbeing, misuse, and other generous and otherworldly weakening in mortal. Social insurance is communicated by wellbeing specialists in joined wellbeing specialists, pros, doctor partners, mid-spouse, nursing, anti-microbial, drug store, brain research, and other wellbeing.

In [36], a diagram of ongoing developments in big data with observation to bioinformatics and patient information was given. Additionally, a portion of the current exercises and future open doors identified with huge information for wellbeing, delineating a portion of the key fundamental issues that should be handled was examined. As of now, the exponential development of biomedical information alongside the complexities of overseeing high dimensionality, imbalanced appropriation, inadequate properties induces a troublesome test of successfully applying utilitarian systems as another enormous scope prescient demonstrating in social insurance and biomedicine. In [37], utilitarian systems dependent on inclination score and Newton Raphson-greatest probability improvements as another enormous scope AI classifier to upgrade its exhibition in tending to these difficulties inside huge biomedical information was proposed. Diverse use-cases situations dependent on incorporated phenotypic and genomics enormous biomedical information were proposed: Real-life biomedical information, (i) ideal plan of malignant growth chemotherapy; (ii) recognize inpatient-affirmation of people with essential conclusion of disease; (iii) distinguish extreme asthma worsening youngsters utilizing coordinated phenotypic and SNP vault information; and (iv) blend models recreation contemplates. Near examinations were conveyed to think about the presentation of the new worldview versus the basic state-of-the-craft of AI, information mining, and insights plans. The consequences of execution of the new classifier with the most widely recognized classifiers on the four benchmark databases have been recorded in tables and charts. They got aftereffects of the new classifier beat a large portion of existing cutting edge factual AI plans with solid and productive execution. The new prescient demonstrating classifier is sparing the computational time and having dependable exhibitions alongside future road for expansion to manage cutting edge sequencing information on superior figuring stages. Entering clinical experience information by hand is tedious. What's more, information are frequently not gone into the database in an auspicious enough manner to empower their utilization for consequent crucial. The Patient Informatics Processing Software semi-robotizes the information assortment process locally available boats. At that point information inside these pictures are caught and used to populate a database, after which different boat databases are utilized for detailing and investigation. In [38], the Patient Informatics Processing Software Hybrid Hadoop Hive to organize database handling by means of different boats, by marshaling the circulated servers, running the different undertakings in equal, dealing with the entirety of the correspondences and information moves between the different pieces of the framework, and accommodating excess and adaptation to internal failure was utilized. At that point they have utilized the Apache Hive as an information stockroom foundation based on Hadoop for information outline, inquiry, and examination to recognize awful mind injury (TBI) just as other injury cases. At long last, a proposed Misdiagnosis Minimization Approach strategy was utilized for information examination. They have gathered information on three boat factors (Byrd, Boxer, Kearsage) and wounds to four body districts (head, middle).

In this day and age, the colossal data in social insurance is to be prepared so as to distinguish, analyze, recognize, and forestall the different infections. Enormous information investigation is the difficult one on the grounds that huge information contain huge measure of records. It was proposed to build up a unified patient observing framework utilizing enormous information. In [39], enormous arrangement of clinical records were taken as information. From this clinical dataset, it was intended to extricate the required data from the record of heart patients utilizing map decrease system. Coronary illness is a significant medical issue and it is the main sources of death all through the world. Early recognition of coronary illness has become a significant issue in the clinical research fields. For coronary illness location, a few highlights are examined, for example, RR interim, QRS interim, and QT interim. The arrangement procedure states whether the patient is ordinary or strange and in the location step utilizing map diminish strategy to recognize the sickness and decrease the dataset. Subsequently, the proposed framework assists with grouping an enormous and complex clinical dataset and distinguish the coronary illness. Diabetes is one of the top needs in clinical science and medicinal services the board, and a plenitude of information and data is accessible on these patients. Regardless of whether information come from factual models or complex example acknowledgment models, they might be melded into prescient models that join persistent data and prognostic result results. Such information could be utilized in clinical choice help, ailment reconnaissance, and general wellbeing the executives to improve quiet consideration. The point was to survey the writing and give a prologue to prescient models in screening for and the administration of common short- and long-haul confusions in diabetes [40]. Prescient models have been produced for the executives of diabetes and its confusions, and the quantity of productions on such models has been becoming over the previous decade. Frequently numerous calculated or a comparable direct relapse was utilized for forecast model turn of events, perhaps attributable to its straightforward usefulness. Eventually, for expectation models to demonstrate valuable, they should show sway, to be specific, their utilization must create better patient results. Albeit broad exertion has been placed into building these prescient models, there is a noteworthy shortage of effect considers. The adjustment in the DNA is a type of hereditary variety in the human genome. Likewise, the DNA duplicate number change is additionally connected with the movement of many developing sicknesses. Cluster-based Comparative Genomic Hybridization (CGH) is considered as a significant undertaking when estimating the DNA duplicate number change over the genome. Additionally, DNA duplicate number change is a fundamental measure to analyze the malignancy sickness. Cutting edge sequencing is a significant technique for contemplating the spread of irresistible infection subjectively and quantitatively. CGH was broadly utilized in persistent observing of duplicate number of thousands of qualities all through the genome. As of late, the size of the DNA arrangement information is huge. Consequently, there is a need to utilize a versatile AI way to deal with conquer the different issues in DNA duplicate number change identification. In [41], a Bayesian concealed Markov model (HMM) with Gaussian Mixture (GM) Clustering way to deal with model the DNA duplicate number change over the genome was proposed. The proposed Bayesian HMM with GM Clustering approach was contrasted and different existing methodologies, for example, Pruned Exact Linear Time strategy, double segmentation technique, and fragment neighborhood technique. Exploratory outcomes exhibit the adequacy of our proposed change discovery calculation. Populace wellbeing the executives and explicitly constant illness the executives rely upon the capacity of suppliers to forestall improvement of significant expense and high-chance conditions, for example, diabetes, cardiovascular breakdown, and incessant respiratory infections and to control them. The coming of large information investigation can possibly engage social insurance suppliers to make opportune and really proof-based educated choices to give increasingly viable and customized treatment while diminishing the expenses of this consideration to patients. The objective of the work [42] was to distinguish true social insurance uses of large information examination to decide its viability in both patient results and the help of money related weights. The strategy for this examination was a writing audit using 49 articles. Proof of huge information investigation being generally valuable in the zones of hazard expectation, demonstrative exactness, and patient result improvement, clinic readmission decrease, treatment direction, and cost decrease was noted. Introductory uses of enormous information examination have demonstrated valuable in different periods of ceaseless sickness the board and could help lessen the interminable malady trouble. The productive programmed identification of cardiovascular arrhythmia utilizing a half breed strategy from ECG enormous information was proposed in [43] with novel component extraction procedure utilizing large amount of ECG signals were taken from MIT-BIH arrhythmia database for discovery two kinds of arrhythmias LBBB and RBBB Their proposed method can precisely identify and order LBBB and RBBB alongside typical heartbeat. An epic and crossbreed strategy for discovery of cardiovascular arrhythmia have four principle stages: denoising of crude ECG, pattern meander evacuation, proposed include extraction, and identification of anomalous pulses utilizing MPNN neural classifier. 8600 ECG beats were chosen, including 4200 ordinary and 4400 anomalous beats (2200 LBBB and 2200 RBBB) were used for testing the proposed strategy. The discovery result utilizing MPNN was contrasted and other two neural classifiers: Feed Forward neural system (FFNN) and Back Propagation Neural Network (BPNN) classifiers. Ongoing advances in data innovation have prompted a touchy development of information, making another time of huge information. Sadly, conventional AI calculations can't adapt to the new attributes of huge information. In [44], the issue of bosom disease expectation in the large information setting. We thought about two assortments of information, specifically, quality articulation (GE) and DNA methylation (DM) was proposed. The goal was proportional to the AI calculations that were utilized for grouping by applying each dataset independently and mutually. For this reason, Apache Spark as a stage was picked. Three distinctive arrangement calculations, specifically, bolster vector machine (SVM), choice tree, and irregular timberland, to make nine models that help in anticipating bosom malignant growth was thought of. A far-reaching similar examination utilizing three situations with the GE, DM, and GE and DM consolidated, so as to show which of the three sorts of information would deliver the best outcome as far as precision and mistake rate was finished. Also, a trial correlation between two stages (Spark and Weka) so as to show their conduct when managing enormous arrangements of information was performed. The trial results demonstrated that the scaled SVM classifier in the Spark condition beats different classifiers, as it accomplished the most elevated exactness and the least mistake rate with the GE dataset. With the headway of innovation in information science and system innovation, the world has ventured into the Era of Big Data, and the clinical field is wealthy in information reasonable for investigation. In this manner, as of late, there has been a lot of research in clinical huge information, basically focusing on information assortment, information investigation, and perception. Notwithstanding, not many works give a full review of the clinical large information on incessant infections and wellbeing checking. The review in [45] explores late research endeavors and leads a complete diagram of the work on clinical huge information, particularly as identified with constant sicknesses and wellbeing observing. It centers around the full patterns of the large information handling, which incorporates clinical huge information preprocessing, enormous information instruments and calculations, huge information perception, and security issues in huge information. It additionally endeavors to join regular enormous information advances with unique clinical needs by examining in detail existing works of clinical large information. Apparently, this is the primary study that objectives interminable infections and wellbeing observing enormous information advancements.

4 Big Data Technology Advantages

Big data in wellbeing informatics can be accessible to foresee outcome of diseases and scourges, increment activity and personal satisfaction, and shield from less than ideal deaths and sickness development. The primary element of large information is to offer information identified with ailment and it additionally gives forewarning insights to the treatment that should have been controlled. By utilizing enormous information mankind is secured as well as the expense of disease treatment is decreased to exceptionally huge wiped out. As the fundamental capacity of the huge information is to offer enormous amount of data so it is getting advantageous for both clinical medicine and epidemiological research. It has claims on medicinal services on patients, laborers, researchers, and constitution masters. This information has been utilized by different associations, organizations to make define systems, plans, intervention, or restorative treatment, for example, meds development. Hence wherever large information is having generally excellent advantages particularly in wellbeing office. In the present time patients giving information identified with medicinal services choices are exceptionally demandable and need commitment in their wellness evaluation creation. The primary capacity of the large information is to keep patients consistently refreshed with the goal that they can generally settle on best decision in medicinal services. Likewise it additionally encourages them to satisfy with the wellbeing related management. Big data has capacity to diminish the recency predisposition or recency impact inclination. Recency inclination implies when the present measures are considered more profoundly than past measures so as to recoup the condition, however it may bring about inappropriate decisions. The ongoing information can likewise be joined into this procedure called enormous information. It has different advantages, for example, a few errors or issues in an affiliation could be perceived straightforwardly. Likewise the usable hazardous issues can be overpowered. It will bring about sparing time, cost and upgrade the yield. The offices likewise can be also redesigned in light of the fact that the modern information on specific subject substance is advertised. For instance, it is simpler to give the entire information on the patients and furthermore it will be conceivable to regulate restorative contribution without any suspension. It is likewise castoff in prognostic examination which is to perceive and talk the restorative issues before it turning into a wild issue. Medicinal services pros are fit to diminish the risk and overpowered the issue with the material imitative from the enormous information. Huge information is too fit to even consider aiding perceive misdirections in social insurance especially on repayment rights. Phony, error, and misleading privileges can be featured. This will ease repayment companies to keep away from harms. It can likewise help human services by means of information association, electrical therapeutic narratives, and archives request. It will profit to find and perceive the right masses or target group. It contains differed assortment of masses and unmistakable assortment can be perceived for chance valuation and communicates. Its essence would likewise allow development as well as change of any product bundle or inclusion to point the wellness issue. It would likewise let the clinical indictments to be started momentarily. Large information would offer a more grounded picture on the sort of masses and restorative problem. The plan of the scattering or disease information would have the option to offer quick development of mediation programming and furthermore coordinating the influenced assortment right away. Data advancements of pharmacological creations were assessed from patients, parental figures, stores, and Research and improvement. It could facilitate the pharmacological partnerships to perceive new planned and ostensible drugs and carry it to the clients at the earliest opportunity.

5 Applications of Big Data in Health Care

Significant instances of big data in healthcare services are talked about in Table 1. There are a few activities using the capability of Big Data in healthcare services. A portion of the models are:

Each Electronic Health Records (EHRs): It's the best broad programming project of enormous information in medicine region. All patients that are assuming medications from that position have their information spared in this purpose which contains socioeconomics, therapeutic records, hostilities, exam results, and so on.

Real-time caution: It gives a fundamental element which is called as constant alarming. In medicals, a purpose known as clinical decision support analyzes restorative data one after another, offering wellness specialists with direction since they can make unbending ends.

Advance patient appointment system: Various clients have a consideration in high innovation procedures that determine and monitor each stage they mirror. This overwhelming information might be gotten together with included recordable reports that can check conceivable wellness perils in future. Clients are normally observed for their wellbeing, and temptations from wellness protections can inspire them to have a fit and solid life.

Application of biomedical data for improved strategic planning: The use of Big data grants for planned readiness thanks to enhanced dreams into open's enthusiasms. Care officials can look at registration results among people in different segment assortments and group what issues dampen people from assuming control over fix.

Table 1 Some instances of Big data for biomedical applications

Example	Description
Asthma polis	For cure of asthma, different organizations have made a tracker called global positioning system (GPS) which screens utilization of inhaler by patients. Little top like gadget is to be put at the highest point of the inhaler that at as a sensor and help in giving valuable data. The patient that is utilizing such sort of inhaler when whenever experiences asthma assault and uses shrouded inhaler that time that gadget will record the time and put and pass on the data to site. This information is then made accessible to Center for Disease Control. The CDC'S take the review for why and from which hypersensitive source the assault of asthma was caused to quiet. In this way all the important information about the assault is accumulated through the assistance of gadget. The advantage of this gadget to client is that he can create the report of his assault and will know the source he is confronting assault of asthma. Also, presently patient will know to confront them and will be prepared with all the precautionary measures of asthma. In this way specialists can be very much aware of the continuous reports of their patient and give them better judgments
Battling the flu	Community for Disease Control have become solid column in huge information for flu. Longer than seven days 6, 80,000 influenza reports are gotten by CDC. Every one of these reports which are assembled by CDC incorporate the explanation behind ailment of the patient, what medicines are given to them, and whether that treatment is successful or not. The CDC encourages overall population to make this data accessible to them. Specialists additionally get the advantages of this by getting the more clear image of how and why the ailment is spreading over the world. It helps the guardians to get the data about antibodies and other antiviral medications that can be given to patients for their quicker recuperation. This use of huge information isn't just confined to specialists utilize just yet the patient can himself helps for better recuperation. The main impediment of this application is in the event that a few clients are putting some bogus information or erroneous information, at that point wrong analysis will make negative impact on different clients too
Diabetes and big data	In big data insurgency diabetes patients have likewise got up with part of advantages. Normal Sensing organization have given GoCap application, that not just assistance in recording the day by day dose of insulin yet in addition at what time measurements is given to the patient is recorded. This data is then fed over cell phones where persistent and different individuals can get this data. Along these lines information become simpler for other social insurance experts to get to and permits them for distinguishing where the issue is and what can be the correct finding for it. Another innovation that has developed with the blend of diabetes and Big Data is served by Allazo Health. Prescient examination is being utilized for improving drug program in this framework

(continued)

Table 1 (continued)

Example	Description
GNS Health Care and Aetna	Big data processing organizations have helped part in GNS human services; it has raised medical coverage organization Aetna to help the individuals that are having metabolic disorders. An innovation called as Reverse Engineering and Forward Simulation has been created by GNS. This innovation help in giving information identified with Aetna who have bought in for protection. Right off the bat the application will check for 5 signs in the patients which are: hypertension, low High thickness Lipoprotein, enormous midriff size, high glucose, and high triglycerides. Any patient who has the mix of these three signs leads to the outcome that the patient is experiencing Aetna. An alternate mix of these signs prompts various ends. Like if any patient whose report incorporate low High thickness Lipoprotein and high triglycerides may experience the ill effects of high-hazard hypertension inside the following not many months

Predictive analytics: Analysis of big data are presently exceptionally well known and supportive for each field. Prescient investigation are principle business intellectual competence right now. Prescient examination will have the option to improve patient's consideration and treatment. Optum Labs, U.S. explore co-agents have made electronic wellbeing records out of more than 40 billion individuals who are experiencing any sort of infection or disease. It has been done to make a databank for prescient examination instruments that would recoup the arrangement of treatment. The point of medicinal services business knowledge is to coordinate specialists settle on information driven decisions in milliseconds and recuperate individuals' fix.

Decrease fraud and improve information security: Misrepresentation and harm are huge issue in each field. So as to shield social orders from these glitches, various have thought to utilize investigation to help stop security threats by characterizing varieties in arrange course, or another movement that drives a digital assault.

Practice telemedicine: Telemedicine is the accessible available spot from 40 years however it was not all that mainstream and its advantages were not featured. Presently advancements, for example, film courses, telephones, remote approaches, and wearable and so on have shown up and they have made telemedicine increasingly famous. All the offices of centers are presently offered by these systems. It is castoff for fundamental conversations and early investigation, remote patient nursing, and therapeutic coaching for wellbeing experts.

Stop needless ER appointments: Securing period, cash, and essentialness by huge information examination in the field of medicinal services is fundamental. It is the condition in California, where a woman who was having mental malady and material abuse went to an assorted variety of local hospices on ordinary premise.

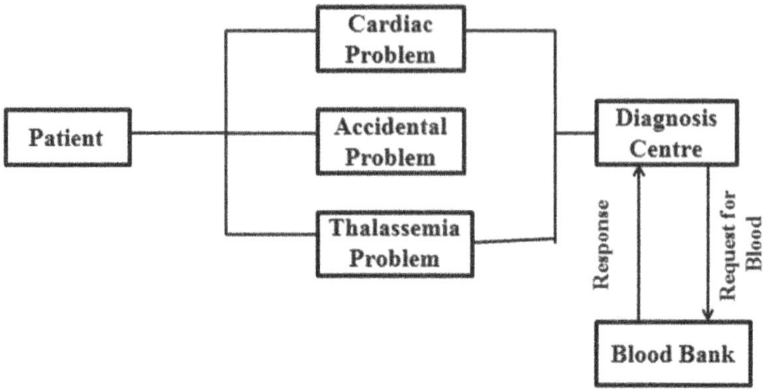

Fig. 3 Proposed Multi-Agent Intelligent system

6 Multi-agent System for Biomedical Data Processing

A multi-agent system for processing the cardiac data is proposed that can classify different cardiac abnormalities. This approach is designed for the application of big data in cardiac data analysis system. Different blocks in the proposed multi-agent system are presented in Fig. 3. The multi-agent system consists of the intelligent module for automatic disease detection along with the communication module with the blood bank. Once the abnormalities are detected it will communicate to the physician as well as to the patient. If the patient requires blood then diagnosis center will send a request to blood bank [46, 47].

Patient Agent—A Patient, who suffers from any disease, consults in the hospital. Different pathological tests will be performing by physicians' advice. Test result data will communicate with the server.

Physician Agent—This agent will communicate with the doctors. After diagnosis, the decision will be sent to patients by mail or SMS.

Diagnostic Center Agent—Data generated from the pathological tests will communicate to the diagnosis center for analysis and future diagnosis.

Blood Bank Agent—Control the blood bank and responses to the diagnosis center.

7 Multi-agent System for the Detection of Cardiac Abnormalities

The proposed multi-agent framework is considered for the detection of heart abnormalities from the norm. Human services research recommends that cardiovascular variation from the norm starts with harm to the inward layers of heart arteries. Because of the following factors the harm may happen.

(i) High blood pressure
(ii) High cholesterol
(iii) High blood sugar
(iv) Inflammation in the blood vessel.

These days, coronary illness is the most widely recognized type of cardiovascular malady. Diverse related tests might be attempted so as to make a precise analysis. Normally doctors endorse the accompanying insignificant tests for any heart patients. A blood test is required to know the levels of various factors such as electrolytes, blood cells, hormones in the blood, and clotting factors. Also, the sugar level in blood can be verified. Electrocardiogram (ECG) may show changes that indicate the heart muscle is not receiving enough oxygen.

Collection of biomedical data can be conducted directly from the patients or from any open-source databases. UCI cleveland cardiac data is considered in the proposed case study.

UCI machine learning repository is one of the open-source data repository where different types of databases are freely available. Here in our work, we have used the Cleveland heart disease data collected from the Cleveland clinical foundation. The dataset contains the cardiac sample of a total of 303 patients with 13 features. The detail description of the data set is presented in Table 2. The last attribute in the database corresponds to the cardiac class. Besides these clinical information electro-cardiogram (ECG) is also another pathological information that can help physicians to detect cardiac problems. In Figs. 4 and 5 the difference between normal and abnormal ECG plots are visualized.

Table 2 Detail description about the dataset

Features	Explanation
Age	Age of the patient
Sex	1 for male patient and 0 for female patient
Cp	Different chest pain symptoms (For typical angina, atypical angina, non-angial pain asymptomatic)
Trestbps	Patient hospitalization time blood pressure
Chol	Cholesterol of the patient in mg/dl
Fbs	Fasting blood sugar
Restecg	ECG report (normal = 0, ST-T abnormality = 1 left ventricular = 2
Thalch	Pulse rate of the patient
Exang	Exercise optimistic angina (Yes or No)
Oldpeak	ST depression induced by exercise ST segment
Slope	peak exercise slope (up sloping = 1, flat = 2, down sloping = 3
Ca	amount of main vessels (0–3) colored by fluoroscopy
Thal	3 shows the normal, fixed defect is denoted as 6 and reversible defect is denoted as 7

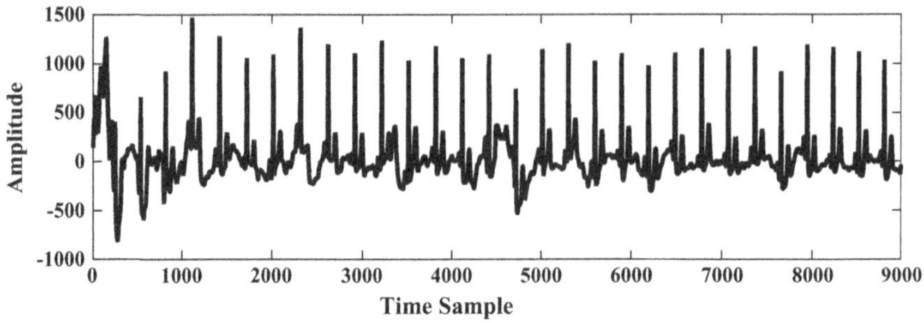

Fig. 4 Normal ECG

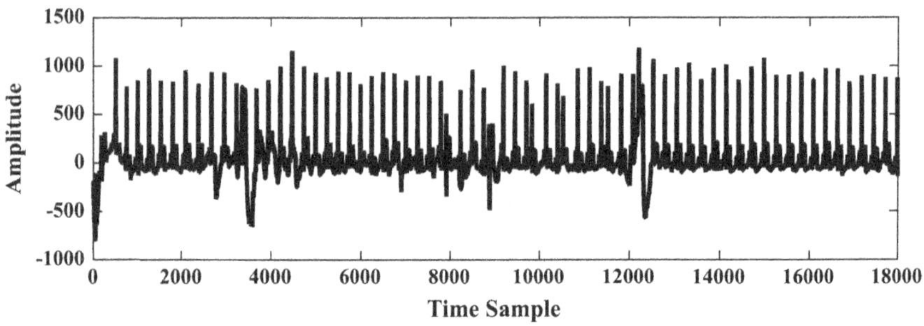

Fig. 5 Abnormal ECG

8 Classification Algorithm

SVM is one of the most popular linear machine learning classifier with some nice properties. This technique is mostly based on the structural risk minimization method where a hyperplane/decision boundary is created in such a manner that the positive and negative class separation margin can be maximized. Let us consider $\left\{\left(\mathbf{x}_j, o_j\right)\right\}_{j=1}^{N}$ is the training data set for the SVM classifier where $\mathbf{x}_j$ is the input feature for jth example and o_j is the corresponding output (target). Before beginning the classification process let us assume that, the output classes are linearly separable and are represented by $+1$(Positive class) and -1(Negative class). The output pattern separation process in the hyperplane or decision boundary can be represented by,

$$\mathbf{w}^{*}\mathbf{x} + d = 0 \tag{1}$$

The output of the SVM classifier can be defined by,

$$\begin{aligned} \mathbf{w}^{*} + d \geq 0 \qquad for\ \ o_j = +1 \\ \mathbf{w}^{*} + d \leq 0 \qquad for\ \ o_j = -1 \end{aligned} \tag{2}$$

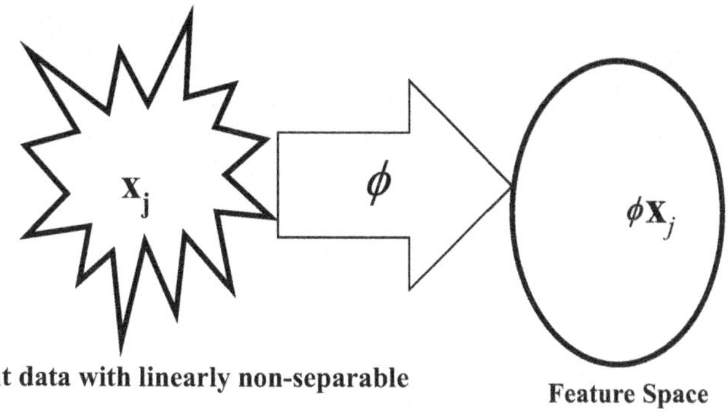

Fig. 6 Transformation of linearly non-separable data to feature space

where **x** is the input feature vector, $\mathbf{w}^*$ is the corresponding adjustable weight vector, and d is the bias or threshold. In linear SVM the separation between two classes in **x** is done by maximizing the separation margin in the optimal hyperplane. In the case of nonlinear SVM, the two classes are first mapped with the kernel function in feature space with a high dimension. The representation is presented in Fig. 6 [48, 49]. The mathematical representation for nonlinear SVM is,

$$\sum_{j=1}^{N} \mathbf{w}_j^* \phi_j(\mathbf{x}) + d \tag{3}$$

where $\phi(.)$ is the mapping function. The main goal is to develop an efficient classifier by using a set of training data $\left\{(\mathbf{x}_j, o_j)\right\}_{j=1}^{N}$. The optimized value of the weight vector $\mathbf{w}^*$ and bias d can be stated as,

$$o_j\left(\mathbf{w}^* \mathbf{x}_j + d\right) \geq 1 - \xi_j \qquad for\ j = 1, 2, 3, \ldots\ldots, N \tag{4}$$

where ξ is the slack variable for all j [50]. The weight vector $\mathbf{w}^*$ and the slack variable minimizes the cost function which can be represented by,

$$\varphi\left(\mathbf{w}^*, \xi\right) = \frac{1}{2}\left\|\mathbf{w}^*\right\|^2 + R\sum_{j=1}^{N} \xi_j \tag{5}$$

where R is a regularized parameter, i.e., used to control the discriminant function size. The final output of the SVM classifier is represented as,

$$o(x) = \sum_{j=1}^{N} K\left(\mathbf{x}_j, \mathbf{x}\right) \tag{6}$$

The kernel function $K(\mathbf{x}_j, \mathbf{x})$ is a special case of Mercer's theorem which arises at the time of functional analysis. In the proposed work the performance of the SVM is measured for four types of kernels like polynomial, linear, sigmoid, and linear. The polynomial kernel is one type of non-stationary kernel and it performs well for normalized training data. It can be represented as,

$$K(\mathbf{x}_j, \mathbf{x}) = (\mathbf{x}_j.\mathbf{x} + 1)^b \tag{7}$$

where b is the degree of the polynomial and is specified a priori by the user. Linear kernel another type of kernel in which the training of the SVM classifier is much faster as compared to other kernels. The mathematical equation of the linear kernel is,

$$K(\mathbf{x}_j, \mathbf{x}) = \mathbf{x}_j \cdot \mathbf{x} \tag{8}$$

Sigmoid is another type of kernel function of SVM which is also used as the proxy for neural network classifiers. It is represented as,

$$K(\mathbf{x}_j, \mathbf{x}) = \tanh(\beta \mathbf{x}_j \mathbf{x} + A) \tag{9}$$

where β is the slope and A is the intercept constant respectively. An RBF kernel is one of the most general kernels used in many neural network problems. The performance of this kernel is better when there is no earlier knowledge about the data. It is represented as,

$$K(\mathbf{x}_j, \mathbf{x}) = \exp\left(-\delta \left\|\mathbf{x}_j - \mathbf{x}\right\|^2\right) \tag{10}$$

where δ is a parameter inversely proportional to the width of the Gaussian kernel.

9 Result and Discussion

After collecting the data, the classification is done by using SVM classifier. These 13 features are considered as the input to the proposed SVM classifier whereas attribute number 14 is considered as the target class of the classifier. The original data set is divided into training and testing sets. 90% data (272 samples) are considered as the training set and the rest 10% (31 samples) data are kept for testing purposes. For measuring the performance of the classifier different measuring parameters are considered like precision, recall, accuracy, and F-1 score. The formula for calculating these parameters are,

$$\Pr ecision = \frac{TP}{TP + FP} \quad (11)$$

$$\text{Recall} = \frac{TP}{TP + FN} \quad (12)$$

$$F - 1Score = 2 * \frac{\Pr ecision * \text{Recall}}{\Pr ecision + \text{Recal}} \quad (13)$$

$$Accuracy = \frac{TP + TN}{N} \quad (14)$$

The corresponding confusion matrixes generated from SVM classifier with different kernels are shown in Fig. 7. In Table 3 the performance measuring parameters calculated from the confusion matrix are presented.

It can be observed that the classification performance of SVM with the polynomial kernel is better as compared to the other three types of kernels. Classification accuracy is around 87.5% for SVM with polynomial kernel function.

Confusion matrix SVM with Polynomial Kernel

	Normal	Cardiac
Normal	18	2
Cardiac	1	10

Confusion matrix SVM with Linear Kernel

	Normal	Cardiac
Normal	16	2
Cardiac	3	10

Confusion matrix SVM with Sigmoid Kernel

	Normal	Cardiac
Normal	12	5
Cardiac	5	9

Confusion matrix withRBF Kernel

	Normal	Cardiac
Normal	11	7
Cardiac	5	8

Fig. 7 Confusion matrix obtained from the SVM classifier

Table 3 SVM classification result

Kernel types	Precession (%)	Recall (%)	F1 score (%)	Accuracy (%)
SVM with Polynomial kernel	83.33	96.90	86.26	87.5
SVM with Linear kernel	83.33	76.92	79.99	83.87
SVM with Sigmoid kernel	64.28	64.25	62.27	67.74
SVM with RBF kernel	53.33	61.53	57.13	61.26

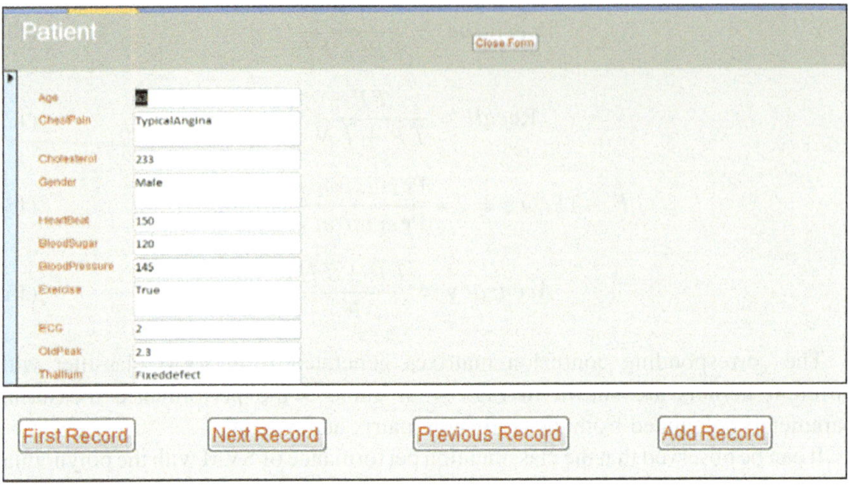

Fig. 8 Screenshot of the proposed multivalent system for cardiac abnormalities detection

The proposed classifier is then applied in a multi-agent system that can classify the cardiac abnormalities. In Fig. 8, the screenshot of the output screen of the multi-agent system for cardiac abnormalities detection was displayed. After providing the required information this system displays the cardiac risk factors and classes to the patients as well as to the doctors. The proposed multi-agent system is also connected with the blood bank system for urgent requirement of the blood for the patients admitted due to cardiac illness.

10 Conclusion

Big data has a major role in healthcare domain. Hospital sectors are getting more benefit by adopting this technology. It will help for the disease diagnosis, different electronics health record (EHR) handling in patient service sector. A case study on big data application in cardiac data analysis is provided in the proposed chapter. Classification of different cardiac abnormalities with the application of a multi-agent system is provided by the authors. Proposed system is providing a better classification result with SVM classifier. In future, other machine learning classifiers can be used for processing of different biomedical data to improve the performance of the classifier.

References

1. Russom, P.: Big data analytics. TDWI best practices report, fourth quarter. **19**(4), 1–34 (2011)
2. Ji, C. et al.: Big data processing: Big challenges and opportunities. J. Interconnect. Netw. **13**(03n04), 1250009 (2012)
3. Gupta, H.K., Parveen, R.: Comparative Study of Big Data Frameworks. In: 2019 International Conference on Issues and Challenges in Intelligent Computing Techniques (ICICT). IEEE (2019)
4. Deshai, N. et al.: A study on big data processing frameworks: spark and storm, in smart intelligent computing and applications, pp. 415–424. Springer (2020)
5. De Mauro, A., Greco, M., Grimaldi, M.: A formal definition of Big Data based on its essential features. Lib. Rev. (2016)
6. Kaisler, S. et al.: Big data: Issues and challenges moving forward. In 2013 46th Hawaii International Conference on System Sciences. IEEE (2013)
7. Hajirahimova, M.S., Aliyeva, A.S.: About big data measurement methodologies and indicators. Int. J. Modern Educ. Comput. Sci. **9**(10), 1 (2017)
8. Osman, A.M.S.: A novel big data analytics framework for smart cities. Future Gener. Comput. Syst. **91**, 620–633 (2019)
9. Al Nuaimi, E., et al.: Applications of big data to smart cities. J. Internet Serv. Appl. **6**(1), 25 (2015)
10. Hu, L., Ni, Q., Yuan, F.: Big data oriented novel background subtraction algorithm for urban surveillance systems. Big Data Mining Analyt. **1**(2), 137–145 (2018)
11. Erevelles, S., Fukawa, N., Swayne, L.: Big data consumer analytics and the transformation of marketing. J. Bus. Res. **69**(2), 897–904 (2016)
12. Nguyen, H., Liu, W., Chen, F.: Discovering congestion propagation patterns in spatio-temporal traffic data. IEEE Trans. Big Data **3**(2), 169–180 (2016)
13. Yassine, A., et al.: IoT big data analytics for smart homes with fog and cloud computing. Future Gener. Comput. Syst. **91**, 563–573 (2019)
14. Wolfert, S., et al.: Big data in smart farming–a review. Agric. Syst. **153**, 69–80 (2017)
15. Dai, H.-N. et al.: Big data analytics for manufacturing internet of things: opportunities, challenges and enabling technologies. Enterprise Inf. Syst. 2019, 1–25
16. Ghani, N.A., et al.: Social media big data analytics: a survey. Comput. Hum. Behav. **101**, 417–428 (2019)
17. Addo-Tenkorang, R., Helo, P.T.: Big data applications in operations/supply-chain management: a literature review. Comput. Ind. Eng. **101**, 528–543 (2016)
18. Fahmideh, M., Beydoun, G.: Big data analytics architecture design—an application in manufacturing systems. Comput. Ind. Eng. **128**, 948–963 (2019)
19. Huang, W., et al.: Mobile Internet big data platform in China Unicom. Tsinghua Sci. Technol. **19**(1), 95–101 (2014)
20. Immonen, A., Pääkkönen, P., Ovaska, E.: Evaluating the quality of social media data in big data architecture. IEEE Access **3**, 2028–2043 (2015)
21. Jiang, S., et al.: Personalized travel sequence recommendation on multi-source big social media. IEEE Trans. Big Data **2**(1), 43–56 (2016)
22. Zhao, L., et al.: Distributed feature selection for efficient economic big data analysis. IEEE Trans. Big Data **4**(2), 164–176 (2016)
23. Wu, J., et al.: Big data analysis-based security situational awareness for smart grid. IEEE Trans. Big Data **4**(3), 408–417 (2016)
24. Xia, F., et al.: Big scholarly data: a survey. IEEE Trans. Big Data **3**(1), 18–35 (2017)
25. Wang, K., et al.: Robust big data analytics for electricity price forecasting in the smart grid. IEEE Trans. Big Data **5**(1), 34–45 (2017)
26. Tang, M., Alazab, M., Luo, Y.: Big data for cybersecurity: vulnerability disclosure trends and dependencies. IEEE Trans. Big Data (2017)

27. Phinyomark, A., Ibanez-Marcelo, E., Petri, G.: Resting-state fmri functional connectivity: Big data preprocessing pipelines and topological data analysis. IEEE Trans. Big Data **3**(4), 415–428 (2017)
28. Hajeer, M., Dasgupta, D.: Handling big data using a data-aware HDFS and evolutionary clustering technique. IEEE Trans. Big Data **5**(2), 134–147 (2017)
29. Priyanka, K., Kulennavar, N.: A survey on big data analytics in health care. Int. J. Comput. Sci. Inf. Technol. **5**(4), 5865–5868 (2014)
30. Krishnan, S.M.: Application of analytics to big data in healthcare. In: 2016 32nd Southern Biomedical Engineering Conference (SBEC). IEEE (2016)
31. Sahoo, S.S., et al.: Heart beats in the cloud: distributed analysis of electrophysiological 'Big Data' using cloud computing for epilepsy clinical research. J. Am. Med. Inform. Assoc. **21**(2), 263–271 (2014)
32. Chen, M., et al.: Disease prediction by machine learning over big data from healthcare communities. IEEE Access **5**, 8869–8879 (2017)
33. Lo'ai, A.T. et al.: Mobile cloud computing model and big data analysis for healthcare applications. IEEE Access **4**, 6171–6180 (2016)
34. Manogaran, G. et al.: Big data analytics in healthcare Internet of Things, in Innovative healthcare systems for the 21st century, pp. 263–284. Springer (2017)
35. Kashyap, H. et al.: Big data analytics in bioinformatics: A machine learning perspective. (2015). arXiv:1506.05101
36. Andreu-Perez, J., et al.: Big data for health. IEEE J. Biomed. Health Inf. **19**(4), 1193–1208 (2015)
37. Elsebakhi, E., et al.: Large-scale machine learning based on functional networks for biomedical big data with high performance computing platforms. J. Comput. Sci. **11**, 69–81 (2015)
38. Rodger, J.A.: Discovery of medical Big Data analytics: improving the prediction of traumatic brain injury survival rates by data mining Patient Informatics Processing Software Hybrid Hadoop Hive. Inf. Med. Unlock. **1**, 17–26 (2015)
39. Vaishali, G., Kalaivani, V.: Big data analysis for heart disease detection system using map reduce technique. In: 2016 International Conference on Computing Technologies and Intelligent Data Engineering (ICCTIDE'16). IEEE (2016)
40. Cichosz, S.L., Johansen, M.D., Hejlesen, O.: Toward big data analytics: review of predictive models in management of diabetes and its complications. J. Diabetes Sci. Technol. **10**(1), 27–34 (2016)
41. Manogaran, G., et al.: Machine learning based big data processing framework for cancer diagnosis using hidden Markov model and GM clustering. Wireless Pers. Commun. **102**(3), 2099–2116 (2018)
42. Bhardwaj, N., et al.: The impact of big data on chronic disease management. Health Care Manager **37**(1), 90–98 (2018)
43. Rai, H.M., Chatterjee, K.: A novel adaptive feature extraction for detection of cardiac arrhythmias using hybrid technique MRDWT & MPNN classifier from ECG big data. Big Data Res. **12**, 13–22 (2018)
44. Alghunaim, S., Al-Baity, H.H.: On the scalability of machine-learning algorithms for breast cancer prediction in big data context. IEEE Access **7**, 91535–91546 (2019)
45. Lin, R., et al.: Chronic diseases and health monitoring big data: a survey. IEEE Rev. Biomed. Eng. **11**, 275–288 (2018)
46. Sarangi, L., Mohanty, M.N., Patnaik, S.: Design of ANFIS based e-health care system for cardio vascular disease detection. In: International Conference on Intelligent and Interactive Systems and Applications. Springer (2016)
47. Sarangi, L., Mohanty, M.N., Pattnaik, S.: Design of diagnosis and monitoring system of heart related diseases using fuzzy inference system. Ann. Comput. Sci. Inf. Syst. **10**, 321–327 (2017)
48. Vapnik, V., Guyon, I., Hastie, T.: Support vector machines. Mach. Learn **20**(3), 273–297 (1995)
49. Haykin, S.: Neural networks: a comprehensive foundation. Prentice Hall PTR (1994)
50. Mohanty, M.N., et al.: Power quality disturbances classification using support vector machines with optimised time-frequency kernels. Int. J. Power Electron. **4**(2), 181–196 (2012)

Development of Algorithm for Distinguishing of Malignancy in Computed Tomography Lung Using Feature Extraction and Artificial Neural Network

R. Pandian and S. Lalithakumari

Abstract Prior conclusion of malignancy cell development prompts spare bunches of valuable human lives. It is important to build up some mechanized instrument, so as to distinguish dangerous state toward the starting stage itself. Numerous calculations had been proposed before by numerous analysts previously, at the same time, the exactness of forecast is consistently a difficult undertaking. In this work, a counterfeit neural system based philosophy is proposed to locate the irregular development of lung tissues. Higher likelihood of discovery is taken as a target to get a robotized apparatus, with extraordinary exactness. Manual translation consistently prompts misdiagnosis. An undeniable Computer Tomography picture set of lung of 10 unique people, with typical and threatening wellbeing states have been considered in this work. The three unique perspectives on the CT examining framework, for example, pivotal, coronal, and sagittal have likewise been considered in the information base creation. Unmistakable textural highlights of the pictures give an intra class variety in its temperament, make a neural system, plausible for order of the typical pictures, recognizing ceaselessly from the threatening ones. Ideal capabilities got from Haralick Gray level co-event Matrix and utilized as the measurement decrease path for taking care of neural system. In this work, a paired Support Vector Machine Neural system has been proposed to recognize the typical pictures out of the considerable number of pictures. The capacity of the proposed neural system has been quantitatively processed utilizing disarray grid and found as far as arrangement exactness.

Keywords GLCM · Haralick · Classification accuracy · SVM classifier

---

R. Pandian (✉) · S. Lalithakumari
School of EEE, Sathyabama Institute of Science and Technology, Chennai, Tamil Nadu, India
e-mail: rpandianme@rediffmail.com

S. Lalithakumari
e-mail: lalithavengat@gmail.com

H. K. Tripathy et al. (eds.), *Technical Advancements of Machine Learning in Healthcare*, Studies in Computational Intelligence 936,
https://doi.org/10.1007/978-981-33-4698-7_3

1 Introduction

One of the most basic medical issues is malignant growth and the demise rate because of lung disease is the higher among the continuing kinds of malignancy. Lung disease prompts the smallest endurance rate after the determination, with a slow raise in the quantity of passings each. Prior recognition builds the odds of fruitful treatment are higher. Out of all the imaging modalities, Computer tomography picture gives better clearness, low clamor and twisting. CT imaging of lungs, give a low commotion, contrasted with ultrasonic image and CT image p [1]. Thus, it is chosen to utilize the CT images of lungs, in this proposed work. Huge improvement in ID prompts shield individuals from deadly circumstances. This could be accomplished by creating propelled picture preparing and neural system based calculations. Subsequently, this proposed work lead to accomplish the objective of mechanized determination. Ongoing literary works uncover that a little work just has been done in the zone. Many picture preparing methods were received to naturally decipher the data. As per the referred to writings, scarcely any works have been done in the region of automata particle of CT pictures. Pandian and Lalitha Kumar [2] actualized an arrangement calculation, in light of the lung locales extraction draws near. Highlight based drew closer have been utilized in CT lung picture [3]. Highlights like consistency, availability, and position highlights were separated to distinguish. In the highlights, for example, size, circularity, and mean brilliance of district of interests (ROIs) were extracted [4]. Zone, thickness, circularity, power, difference, confinement, and good ways from the lung divider are the removed highlights in [5]. Lung malignant growth is analyzed at a beginning period, it isn't excessively enormous and has not broaden, is more. Computer aided treatment is an attractive subject of studies into cancer disease. A fairly broad training database is used to base several implementations. Limited hospitals, however, are typically unable to obtain enough materials for rigorous identification training. Although the exchange of information in scientific research is growing, it is unclear if a system based on one database is very well adapted for other resources. Compared to a system based on the initial limited dataset, the accuracy improved by around 20 percent. The results showed that the proposed solution is an innovative and efficient method of CAD in clinics only with limited data set for learning. Continuous work is under way to accurately diagnose cancer disease focused on conventional machine learning methods, and deep learning-related strategies have become a common alternative for cancer diagnostics. However, it is time-consuming and difficult to gather evidence from various modalities, and certain modalities may have side effects on radioactivity. The object of our research is systemic magnetic resonance imaging. Their aims are as follows: to improve the degree of precision equivalent to the state-of-the-art techniques, to address the question of overcoming and, to examine established brain indications that have perceptible cancer diagnostic functionality. The specificity of an cancer assessment relies largely upon the disease's biological markers. A screening test acts as a safety and infection predictor; it is assessed and analyzed as an predictor of natural biological activities, pathogenic procedures, or pharmaceutical reactions to a medicinal intervention. Research showed a connection between behavioral differences in lung cancer and memory impairment. During the early stages of cancer, a very common and successful method is systemic CT Imaging. The effectiveness of software-aided models of diagnostic using systemic CT data largely depends on the two moment-consuming steps: (1) nonlinear identification through topics, and (2) clustering of brain tissue. To address this constraint, we suggest a method of extraction of landmarks dependent features that does not involve nonlinear identification and clustering of tissues. An innovative neighborhood filter that retains edge is suggested for image filtering. The filter's key objective is to suggest an adaptive filtering feature to compensate for the quality of the image although attempting to retain edge of the image. The proposed method uses image boundaries to filter the area in an edge-conserving way. Response of a variable, in a pixel area, in filtering, relies on the area between the object and the sensor. In addition, the measurement edge between it and the pixel does not lead to the calculation of the gray point. Image average decreases vibration which has other damaging consequences as blurring. In low noise level, the impact of image loss is greater than the impact of noise cancellation and grouping of the initial image yields better results than grouping the normal image. A threshold dependent on noise variation is being used to balance off between initial image and average image to resolve this deficiency. Developing image filtering methods is a very difficult problem as noise has to be eliminated without losing image attributes which are critical for clinical diagnosis. Verification of de-noising protocols may be done by means of a matrix calculation of image quality that takes into account noise cancellation and information conservation by reverting to a bubbling clustering of image information. Computer representations' findings demonstrate that the approach overcomes the drawbacks of modern approaches based on calculations of the vector image efficiency. It is also narrative basic and fast to deploy. While collection, these CT images are integrated with interference which reduces the image quality and restricts the diagnostic accuracy. Eliminating noise in clinical images is an essential activity in per-processing and various approaches occur to remove noise in clinical images. Various de-noising methods such as non-local measures, major component analysis, bilateral, and temporally adaptive non-local means (TANLM) filters are analyzed in this work to remove noise in CT. A structural association histogram is a grayscale-based study of the pixel brightness distribution degree by creating a correlation histogram which can increase the adaptive contrast improvement for different artifacts. The approach achieves important effects during pre-processing of contrast improvement and encourages corresponding procedures, thus reducing the time for detection and increasing accuracy. Popular approaches for improving contrast images include histogram equalization and selective eclipse of the adaptive histogram. It builds up the pixel values histogram in the image according to the initial exported image, and then shows all pixel functions in the image. It also adjusts the initial pixel quantities to increase the contrast between the images. The bright region is probably to be excessively exaggerated in a histogram equalization—processed shot; as a consequence, the shot highlight areas are hypersensitivity, the gap in image contrast is very big, and the pixel arrangement is irregular. CLAHE utilizes limited histogram distortion extension to prevent extreme variations in contrast after improvement or unnecessary image noise improvement. Pixels are improved systematically with CLAHE, and the histogram spectrum may be modified if needed to minimize superficiality after improvement of the image. HCHA, in images, will spontaneously improve three forms of large PD-affected atrophic brain cells. This algorithm uses the degree of pixel strength of every object's grayscale spread to create a connection histogram vector from the initial ROI. It then produces a portion of the histogram vector of association in which various frames convey each object's level of correlation propagation, as the same entities cannot be reflected in the histogram of general connection. The dynamic model focuses on individual artifacts to reflect the pixel similarity functions for optimization and governs the intensity of each single entity in an evolutionary way.

The filter design is a refinement of the bilateral filtering scheme which takes into account the resemblance of color pixels and their temporal range. Rather than direct measurement of the dissimilarity factor, therefore, the cost of a link is measured across a digital route that connects the fundamental pixel of the processing window and its surroundings. As in the traditional bilateral filter, the filter performance is measured as a weighted average of the pixels that are in the local relationship with the filtering window middle, and the weights are components of the marginal contact costs. The most commonly used filtering models are focused on the Vector Median Filter method, whose performance is determined using the vector organizing principle for a collection of pixels from the processing window. Sorting the accumulated ranges from a specified pixel to all other pixels through the filtering window determines the sorting of the vectors. The scalar number of ranges is then sorted and the related vectors may be arranged consequently. The VMF is very efficient in removing impulsive noise, but its performance is diminished when the image is skewed by Gaussian noise, and hence the VMF is typically paired with other filtering solutions in such a situation. This approach is focused on a semi-local average of the image pixels in such a way that the preserved image's new pixel value is measured as a weighted average of the pixels whose specific region is close to the pixel's local region being analyzed. There are various component-based transforms for momentum and magnetic data sets that can be used to illustrate related functionality. Nearly all of them, though, face the uncertainty issue in differential estimation. Hence, noise removal is sometimes implemented before implementing component-based transforms to increase the accuracy of the results. Nonetheless, traditional filter applications usually blur horizontal gradients in the results, which may negatively affect subsequent transformations, for example, that distort the precise borders of the correlative structures. The limitation of the above traditional de-noising approaches often occurs in weather data processing. To solve this issue, several seismologists have followed the kind of edge-preserving procedure, used in digital image analysis. Various experiments have shown that this type of system can efficiently remove the noise while retaining strong gradients. We intend to de-noise the original information without significantly disrupting the horizontal curve. In this way, the efficiency of derivative-based transformations can be enhanced by using variables derived from the de-noisy results. Using Bilateral Filter, the impulse noise and Rician noise in the clinical CT images are eliminated. Improved grasshopper simulation methodology is used to refine the BF variables.

The occurred impulse and Rician noises are used to mimic the clinical CT images. In checking areas of window height, space and strength scope, the EGOA is added to the noisy image in order to get the filter specifications efficiently. For optimization, the PSNR is used as the health benefit. After maximum certainty of variables, we analyzed the proposed effects of the methodology with other CT images. The findings of the suggested de-noising approach are compared with other previously used BFs, genetic algorithm (GA), generalized search algorithm (GSA) utilizing consistency parameters such as signal-to-noise ratio (SNR), the image quality metric is structural similarity index metric (SSIM), error parameter is mean squared error (MSE), and Peak Signal to Noise Ratio (PSNR) in order to explain the choice value of BF parameters. The test reveals that perhaps the EOGA approach with BF provides strong performance in both boundary protection and noise removal from clinical MR images as opposed to the previous approaches. The suggested technique updates an algorithmic bilateral filter to designate MR images using EGOA to significance. The popular nonlinear filter used in statistical domain for bottom-preserved filtering is bilateral filter. Here, the clinical images are taken as an input image and incorporate noises to create a noisy image, including Rician noise and impulse interference, with different noise variances. The noisy image is opposed using bilateral filter with optimization of parameters. The output level is measured by the parameters of PSNR, MSE and precision and the effects are then contrasted. The graphical attraction of the opposing pixel is known, and their gray level similarity. BF calculates the weighted number of pixels in a particular neighborhood. The surroundings weighted average of the pixel is used to remove the pixel. For this equation, the weights can be obtained by the physical and magnitude range of a pixel from its area. In a pixel neighborhood the spectral range is defined with the parameters of the field (spatial) filter while the weights of the filter set (intensity) are proportional to the isotopic range of the pixel. In cancer imaging research, the most popular technique has been design, where different lung areas/voxels are studied independently. Such methods are successful in other situations. However, they did not shed light on the interaction of the inner brain area correlated with brain activity or fascinating illness. Lung is, in essence, anatomically a rather complicated organ and the functional connections among its areas are much more so. Consequently, comprehension of this interdependence or connectivity between brain areas is required. The machine learning methodology named "Sparse Inverse Covariance Analysis" for learning functionality in the brain field, with limited computing expense and densely the correct degree. Within Gaussian hypothesis, any dimension of the vector of reverse covariance expresses conditional dependency between the pair of variables in the constituent, provided all parameters. Through implementing sparsity restriction, excessive/noisy structural constraints are abolished through placing the component factor at zero, participating in the factor pairs becoming conditionally autonomous. Many of the prevalent signs of cancer patients are cognitive problems and their activities, a lack of self-consciousness. Throughout the brain of entities with cancer disease, plaques and clumps can be seen which destroy the nerves and contribute to destruction of the total brain network. All radioactive CT and FDG-PET may be used to support doctors in the diagnostic process, i.e., assessing the brain areas and classifying the victim as Normal Controls

(NC's), MCI (Mild Cognitive Impairment), lung cancer. Visual representation of the image data is a moment-consuming operation and often vulnerable to mistake. The visual assessment has been suggested with mathematical methods in location (or in comparison to). Regional or voxel-wise approach has become the most widely employed numerical tool. Since regions of the brain are dynamically based on one another. Comprehending the brain network for correct interpretation of the lung cancer associated symptoms has been quite important. Traditional methods aim to grasp brain activity restricted to a few areas. Overall brain comprehension, taking into account all areas, is of utmost significance for treatment with lung cancer. Deep learning (DL) approaches have currently been used in the detection and diagnosis of radiography and have greatly enhanced method efficiency. Since Lung Cancers are among the most financially costly disorders, several scholars have focused on developing a high precision software system for the diagnosis of cancer and Normal Control instances. A modern computational approach focused on deep learning is used for diagnosing cancer disease. Here between DL networks, the Siamese Convolution Neural Network is introduced with triple ResNet-34 divisions to differentiate through the Structural CT among the lung cancer and the NC. A SCNN comprises rather than two CNN groups which are mostly similar to each other. The division contains convolution sequence, ReLU, accumulating, and totally linked surfaces. These dual-branches of CNNs are concurrently training on multiple image objects and are generating segments of the same direction function. The similitude of input objects is obtained by measuring the resemblance and range of the variables of the source function. This system includes three CNN brakes which are for one form of image of each section. In addition, the suggested system requires an indicator image for loading into one system CNN division which is randomly picked from the cancer learning dataset. Afterwards, the optimistic and bad images are sent to the show's two main CNN divisions. The positive image is the image chosen at random from the same indicator image mark. The negative image is likewise the randomly chosen item from the same anchor image mark. It has been common to assess cancer from moderate cognitive disorder (MCI) and executive norm (CN). Recent neuro-imaging developments in acceptance of machine learning technologies are particularly useful for pattern analysis in radiography to assist the doctor in early detection of lung cancer. Early pathological lung atrophy and stable brain atrophy are found to be similar. In our endeavor, we suggested a model that can more reliably distinguish MCI and CN to improve early detection of cancer. CT's are initially split into slides to conduct the clustering of T2 weighted CT images. Such images are preprocessed with Gaussian filter to remove chromatic aberrations and rising noise. Through skull stripped software, the non-brain substances are separated from the frames. Increases in brain shape and appearance are used to distinguish stable and deformed, and improved ICA is used to classify brain imaging into WM, GM, and Cerebrospinal Fluid (CSF). Atrophy of the brain tissue is required for the identification of stage cancer. Cancer is a chronic condition, improvements in the brain function perception of GM, structure and thickness of the WM, as well as blood vessel extension. We define the cancer in our job, based on GM degeneration. GM includes nerve cell bodies or glial cells, and semi-neuron neurons. GM undergoes production and development during infancy and adolescence; it is used to bring sugar to the brain; perception, voice, and cognitive function improves in this impact. In our research we concentrated primarily on the gray matter, in order to identify the cancer. We included CNN as a discriminator from the past few years that is used in various computer perception strategies. The definition of a combination model is implemented in our suggested Hybrid Improved ICA and it is defined in groups which are mutually dependent. Utilizing Markov Random Field Cognitive Knowledge is applied to GMM in the updated GMM method and takes into consideration temporal concentration. In Expectation Maximization (EM), Predicted phase is determined using mean log probability and deviation is measured using updated K-mean and endogenous factor is measured using Gibbs volume. The quality of cancer of CT clustering relies on the precision with which the lung structures are separated from the CT images. A number of scientists have been involved in skull shedding as a required pre-processing procedure. Most of the automated methods built up to now involve initial points or plant begin point. Under human interference the same method cannot be performed effectively on all the obtained images. Selecting target points and human interaction at each slice will contribute to so much computing time. The automated skull stripping process to remove brain cells safely and effectively from both pieces of the various views is the necessity of the day. Lung is the highest single associated field inside the CT. The skull substances are distinguished from the brain regions by specifically obscuring the low density pixels between the regions of the brain and the skull. The meaning of low amplitude is picked from either of the histogram. All pixels beyond this limit value are converted to a single power. Under such, all connection between them could be tested across all isolated areas and these linked regions will be combined into a single linked area. Ultimately the cycle yields brain as the greatest linked area. Unlike other skull stripping architectures, the algorithm continues without any seed collection. While the skull removed picture would only have significance in the cerebral areas, skull grinding may be extended with effectiveness to both convective and axial pictures. The standard distressed image of the skull has three sections of WM, GM, and CSF substances. The skull stripped picture histogram reveals no clear peaks and troughs referring to certain groups. The pixels corresponding to the same area would still appear to differ small. This is because of the imaging device's restricted range and in homogeneity of spectroscopy coils. The contrasting histogram isolates the three highest pixel amounts referring to the three dominant areas. The seed values are derived which relate to the three areas. Awareness regarding the fluctuations of the prefrontal surface pressure values is used in removing these peaks from either of the histogram. WM pixels are lighter in T1 weighted images, CSF pixels are darkest, and GM pixels are aligned on a brighter side. In the proposed study, weighted images T1 are used as the test pictures. The first peak is equivalent to WM, the second peak corresponds to GM, and the last peak corresponds to CSF.

2 Image Database

The Computed tomography of a lung is considered in this work. Processed tomography examine, is like the builtup x-beams, which gives a few pictures or photos of the interior organs of the human. The cross-sectional perspective on pictures, which created in the wake of directing the CT examining, might be designed in an abnormal way as far as various planes, and would thus be able to deliver three-dimensional pictures. These three-dimensional pictures are for the most part be seen on a screen, can be printed further on film put something aside for future reference. In this work additionally, the ordinary lung pictures and a disease influenced lung pictures are taken to portray the malignancy in lung. An example of typical and malignant growth influenced CT pictures are appeared in Fig. 1. The pictures utilized for testing the calculations created are clinical pictures. In this work likewise, the typical lung pictures and a malignancy influenced lung pictures are taken from ten unique people groups to portray the lung disease. The picture information for this exploration work is assembled as ordinary and unusual pictures. The Medical Images are CT Lung pivotal view pictures, CT Lung sagittal view pictures and CT Lung coronel see pictures are taken from ten unique individuals in DICOM format. A test of typical CT lung and malignant growth influenced CT lung pictures are appeared in Figs. 1, 2 and 3.

Figure 3 indicates the solid nodule has changed simply more than two years. If this is a cancer, it is likely to be an adenocarcinoma and may characterize an over diagnosis cancer.

3 Feature Extraction

It is the way toward getting Haralick surface component data of a image, for example, shading, shape, and Texture. Haralick include is one of the significant qualities utilized in distinguishing items or region of enthusiasm for a image. Surface, the example of data or exhibit of the structure set up in a picture, is a noteworthy component of many picture types. From a general perspective, surface alludes to surface attributes and presence of Texture highlights can be removed in a few strategies, utilizing factual, auxiliary, and model-based and change data, in which the most well-known way is utilizing the Gray Level Co event Matrix (GLCM). GLCM contains the second-request factual data of spatial relationship of pixels of a picture [6]. For the most part, the precision of any characterization framework chiefly relies upon the best possible decision of the highlights. Consequently, it is fundamental to locate a decent arrangement of highlights. Essential period of structure in any arrangement framework is the choice of a decent arrangement of highlights which have the capacity of sign division in the component space [7]. A characterization calculation will consistently give an outcome, yet a poor element portrayal will prompt an

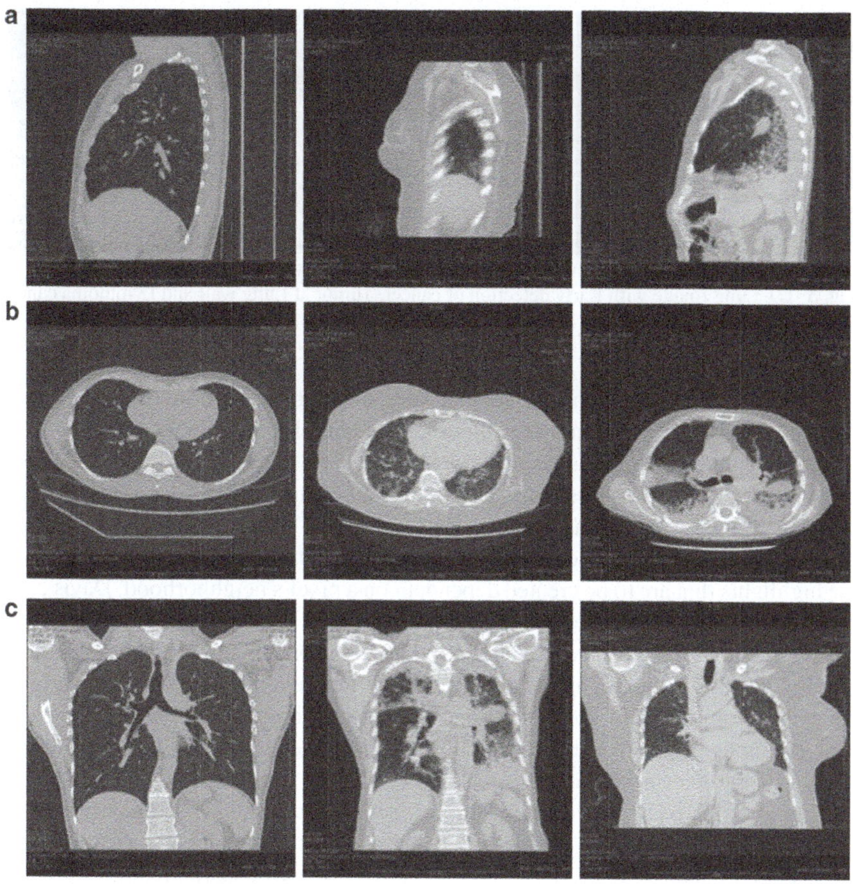

Fig. 1 **a** CT images of lung sagittal views in DICOM. **b** CT images of lung axial views in DICOM. **c** CT images of lung of consolidation views in DICOM

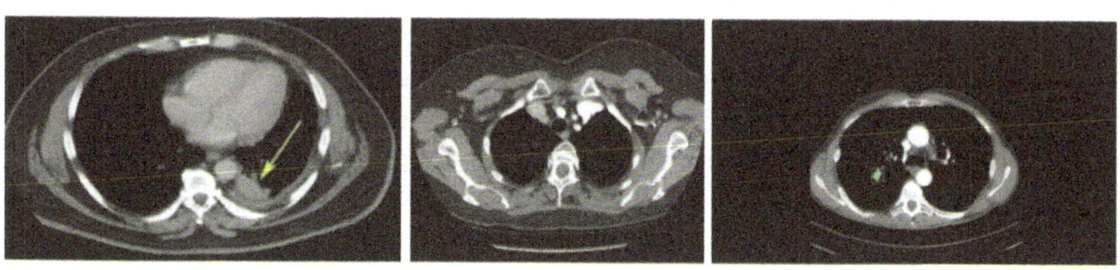

Fig. 2 CT images of lung cancer in DICOm

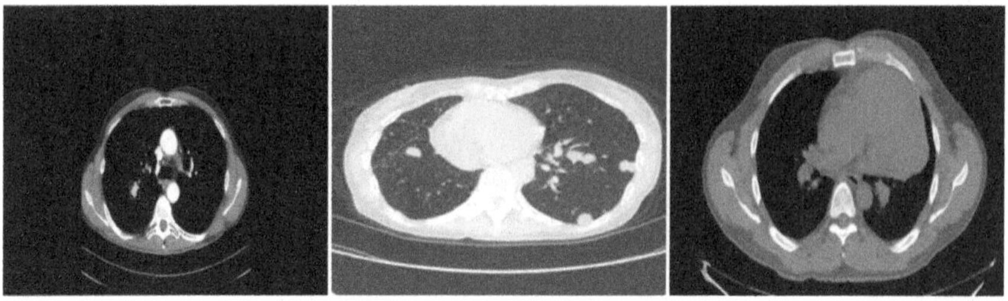

Fig. 3 CT Lung Image with Early detection of cancer, Tumor at Lung wall and Lymthoma cancer Tumors

outcome that doesn't mirror the genuine idea of the basic information. The information ought to be disentangled without loss of data. Finding the best highlights is a troublesome assignment, and it frequently must be practiced through an experimentation procedure. In this work, a dim level co-event matrix (GLCM) is utilized, which is a measurable technique that uses the spatial relationship of pixels. Davis et al. 1979 [8] started the use of dark level co-event matrix (GLCM) so as to discover the highlights that are to be created dependent on a pixel's neighborhood. Davis et al. 1979 proceeded with crafted by "in such a method of the directional circulation of GLCM includes and proposed a lot of polar gram measurements which are rotationally invariant. Haralick et al. [9] 1973 proposed that revolution invariant highlights could be acquired from co-event frameworks by taking the normal and scope of each component type over the four points that is utilized. The dark level distinction insights is another surface portrayal technique, which is firmly identified with GLCM, Doukas et al. 2016 [10]. A co-event lattice, likewise alluded to as co-event appropriation, is characterized over a picture to be the dispersion of co-happening esteems at a given counterbalance. It speaks to the separation and rakish spatial relationship over a picture sub-locale of explicit size. The GLCM is made from a dark scale picture. The GLCM is determined how regularly a pixel with dark level (grayscale power or Tone) esteem I happens either on a level plane, vertically, or corner to corner to adjoining pixels with the worth j. A notable measurable instrument for removing second-request surface data from pictures is the dark level co-event. The GLCM grid is one of the most well-known and compelling wellsprings of highlights in surface investigation. For an area, characterized by a client determined window, GLCM is the lattice of those estimations over all dark level sets. In this technique, highlights are determined dependent on the supreme contrasts between sets of dim levels or normal dark levels rather than unique dim level pixel esteems [11]. This methodology makes the measurements somewhat more powerful to light varieties than on account of GLCM. The dark level co-event network is separated from the previously mentioned pictures. The highlights, separated from the pictures are arranged in Table 1. In this work, the order can be characterized as the ID errand to which a lot of gathering the picture falls, either typical or malignant growth influenced. The dynamic undertakings of characterization can be effortlessly accomplished by the work of neural networks. Haralick highlights outline the relationship in force of pixels that

Table 1 Features of the CT lung images

Features	Normal lung	Cancer lung
Entropy	5.65	1.24
Auto correlation	22.9	12.79
Contrast	0.47	0.21
Correlation	0.96	0.26
Cluster prominence	832.6	134.07
Cluster shade	115	19.21
Dissimilarity	0.2	0.1
Sum of square	23.7	9.84
Sum of average	7.92	3.93
Energy	0.24	0.13
Maximum probability	0.41	0.23
Homogeneity	0.91	0.35
Inverse measure correlation	0.89	0.43
IDM	0.97	0.35

are close to one another in space. Haralick anticipated fourteen textural highlights which are gotten from the co-event network a notable measurable procedure for surface component extraction. It contains data about how picture powers in pixels with a specific situation corresponding to one another happen together. Surface is one of the most fundamental attributes of a picture. In this work fourteen Haralick highlights were utilized to remove important surface data from ordinary and irregular picture of CT lung utilizing the co-event network which is appeared in the Table 1 [12].

4 ANN Based Classification Algorithm

This chapter focuses on the development of Back propagation network and Radial basis network based classifiers that are suitable for determining multiple defects. It gives an outline of the system models, utilized. It likewise shows the advancement of the neural system parameters, for example, neural system design, learning rate, execution work, number of concealed layers and preparing calculations. In this section, execution of the classifiers is additionally examined through order accuracy [13]. One of the generally experienced dynamic errands of human action is order. The order can be characterized as the recognizable proof errand to which a lot of gathering, another perception has a place, based on a preparation set of information containing perceptions [14]. An Artificial Neural Network (ANN), generally called as Neural Network (NN), is a numerical model or computational model that reenacts the structure as well as elements of natural neural systems [15]. It comprises of an interconnected gathering of fake neurons which forms data and produces the important yield. A neural system can be portrayed by the accompanying focuses.

- It is made out of basic components known as neurons. These neurons can work in equal.
- The neural system work is controlled by the associations between its components. The signs are passed between the neurons through these association joins.
- Each association interface has a weight related with it. This weight increases the sign transmitted.
- Each neuron has a related initiation work. This enactment work decides the yield of the neuron.

Neural systems can be utilized as managed arrangement framework and solo characterization framework. Directed learning depends on the framework attempting to foresee results for known models and is an ordinarily utilized preparing strategy. It thinks about its expectations to the objective answer and "learns" from its slip-ups. The information start as contributions to the information layer neurons. The neurons pass the contributions along to the following hubs. As information sources are passed along, the weighting, or association, is applied and when the data sources arrive at the following hub, the weightings are added and either escalated or weakened [16]. This proceeds until the information arrive at the yield layer where the model predicts a result. In a managed learning framework, the anticipated yield is contrasted with the genuine yield for that case. In the event that the anticipated yield is equivalent to the genuine yield, no change is made to the loads in the framework. Be that as it may, if the anticipated yield is higher or lower than the genuine result in the information, the mistake is proliferated back through the framework and the loads are balanced likewise, till the blunder is diminished. This taking care of mistake in reverse through the system is designated "back-proliferation." The activity of a neural system as regulated grouping framework contains the accompanying advances.

- Training of the system
- Testing of the system

During the preparation stage, neural system is prepared to catch the fundamental connection between the picked information sources and yields. In the wake of preparing, the speculation execution of the system is assessed with the assistance of test information. It shows that the prepared ANN can deliver the right yield in any event, for the new information [17]. Subsequent to preparing and testing, the system models can be utilized for characterization of imperfections.

5 Classification of Images

This section centers around Back proliferation arrange based classifiers that are reasonable for deciding illness. One of the normally experienced dynamic undertakings of human movement is order. The order can be characterized as the ID assignment to which a lot of the gathering, another perception has a place, based on preparing a lot of information containing perceptions. In this examination work, the diverse CT pictures are the gatherings and the preparation information incorporate the highlights, which were separated from typical and strange images [18]. In this work, the BPN arrange is utilized for ordering the CT pictures. The highlights are removed from CT pictures of typical lung and malignant growth influenced lung are taken into the investigation. GLCM based highlights are extremely helpful in recognizing infections since the highlights are indicating the wide distinction between the two classes. The Back-Propagation Network (BPN) is utilized to order these pictures. The precision of the system is changed so as to improve the arrangement of the classes dependent on the capacity of created calculation. The inferred highlights, which are tabulated in Table 1, gives a wide contrast between the typical and malignant growth pictures and the proposed pressure calculations don't influence the qualities much. The ideal calculation is picked dependent on the order accuracy [19].

The extracted features consist of two classes. It consists of 14 features. In this, some of the features have similar kind of values. So here only nine features are used to classify the defect of images. The values depend upon the images. This network gives 95.238% classification accuracy (for both normal lung and cancer lung) in identifying cancer disease. Experimental results show that BPN offers better performance measures than other algorithms.

6 Classification Performance

The performances are measured independently for these features. When alluding to the effectiveness of an arrangement organize model, it is basically required to locate the neural system model's capacity to accurately foresee or isolate the classes. In the evaluation of order blunders, a grouping mistake grid is ordinarily shaped. The information about the mistakes arranged by an order model is unmistakably given by the disarray grid. This network is again known as disarray framework or possibility table. The disarray framework genuinely portrays how the recognizable pieces of proof are made utilizing the form. The lines compare to the known radiance of the realities and the section speak to the expectations made through the rendition. The slanting components show the corner to corner parts show the amount of right arrangement made for each class, while the off-askew components demonstrate the mistakes made. At the end of the day, the inclining components on this framework recommend number of examples for which the class outcomes think about the reference measurements. Off askew components in each column give the assortment of tests that have been misclassified by utilizing the classifier, i.e., the classifier is utilizing a name to the ones examples which completely have a place with various marks [8]. In this work, the proposed neural system models, and their exhibitions are estimated utilizing order precision. The precision of arrangement and the deformity savvy characterization exactness are planned from the disarray network. The most extreme over all arrangement precision is chosen dependent on best parameter blend. For all the proposed models, the exactness of arrangement and the deformity astute grouping precision are determined from the comparing disarray lattice for both preparing information and testing data. In the wake of acquiring the disarray lattice, the precision is processed as appeared in Tables 2 and 3 [20]. Precision is that the general rightness of the model and is determined in light of the fact that the aggregate of right groupings isolated by the whole assortment of characterizations (Paul Mather 2010). The characterization exactness is registered by the disarray lattice according to Eq. 1.

$$\text{Overall Classification Accuracy} = \sum_{(i=1)}^{r} x_{ii}/n \tag{1}$$

For all the proposed models of neural system, the grouping exactness for the individual picture type and the general arrangement precision are processed from the disarray grids of the relating systems for both ordinary picture and malignancy picture as referenced above. The order exactness of the Binary classifier finds the proposed pressure calculations don't change the data of pictures and it is holding the nature of images [21, 22].

7 Conclusion

In this work, the algorithm is developed to classify the bio medical images. The features are extracted from CT images of normal Lung and Cancer affected Lung is taken into the study. Even though, each disease type has unique characteristics and patterns, some similarities are also found among these categories that will lead to difficulty in designing a classifier with a correct decision boundary. Hence, the selection of features is a complex problem, which is overcome by careful trial and error process. Moreover, efficient feature selection is still a problem in medical Images and it can be addressed in future, in an effective manner to achieve better results. The classification accuracy of the Binary classifier finds the proposed algorithms suitable for identifying the cancer disease.

Acknowledgements The author wishes to thank Management of Sathyabama Institute of Science and Technology, Chennai, Tamil Nadu, India for the technical support provided by them.

References

1. Osornio rios, R.A.: Identification of positioning system for industrial application using neural network. J. Sci. Ind. India **76**,141–144 (2017)

2. Pandian, R., Vigneswaran, T., Lalitha Kumari, S.: Characterization of CT cancer lung image using image compression algorithms and feature extraction. J. Sci. Ind. Res. Ind. **75**, 747–751 (2016)
3. Pandian, R., Vigneswaran, T.: Adaptive wavelet packet basis selection for zerotree image coding. Int J Sig Imag Sys Eng **9**, 388–392 (2016)
4. Pandian, R.: Evaluation of image compression algorithms. IEEE Und Tech (UT) NIOT, pp. 1–3 (2015)
5. Sheela, K.G., Deepa, S.N.: Selection of number of hidden neurons in renewable energy system. J. Sci. Ind. Res. India **73**, 686–688 (2014)
6. Deng, C., Lin, W., Cai, J.: Content-based image compression for arbitrary-resolution display devices. IEEE Trans. M Media **4**, 1127–1139 (2012)
7. Maglogiannis, I., Kormentzas, G.: Waveleth ROI coding support for mobileaccess to DICOM images over heterogeneous radio networks. Trans. Inform. Technol. Biomed. **13**, 458–466 (2009)
8. Davis, L., Aggarwal, J.: Texture analysis using generalized co-occurrence matrices. IEEE Trans. Pattern Anal. Mach. Intell. PAMI-1 251–259 (1979)
9. Haralick R. M., Shanmugam K., Dinstein I.: Textural Features for Image Classification. IEEE Trans. Syst., Man, Cybern. **3**, 610–621 (1973)
10. Doukas, C., Maglogiannis, I.: Region of Interest Coding Techniques for Medical Image Compression. IEEE Eng. Med. Biol. Mag. **26**, 29–35 (2007)
11. Minh, N.D.: Countourlet transform an efficient directional multi resolutional image representation. IEEE Trans. Image Proc. **14**, 2091–2106 (2005)
12. Lehtinen, J.: Limiting distortion of a wavelet image codec. J. Acta Cyberntica. **14**, 341–356 (1999)
13. Calderbank, A.R., Daubechies, I., Sweldens, W., Yeo, B.L.: Wavelet transforms that map integers to integers. Appl. Comput. Harmon. Anal. **5**, 332–369 (1993)
14. Black, P. E. (ed.): 2008 big-O notation, dictionary of algorithms and data structures. In: U.S. National Institute of Standards and Technolog (1998)
15. Ashraf,M.: Compression strength of stainless steel cross-sections.J. Construct. Steel Res.**62**(1), 105–115 (2006)
16. Bhavani,S. Thanushkodi,K.: A survey on coding algorithms in medical image compression. **2**(5), 1429–1434 (2010)
17. Chen, Y.-Y.: Medical image compression using DCT-based subband decomposition and modified SPIHT data organization. Int. J. Med. Inf. **76**(10), 717–725 (2007)
18. Choong, L.: Cost-effective handling of digital medical images in the telemedicine environment. Int. J. Med. Inf.**76**(9), 646–654 (2007)
19. Cobas Carlos,J.: Compression of high resolution 1D and 2D NMR data sets using JPEG2000. Chemometr. Intell. Lab. Syst. **91**(2),141–150 (2008)
20. Dhawan, S.: A review of image compression and comparison of its algorithms. International Journal of electronics & Communication technology, **2**(1), 22–26 (2011)
21. Dragan, D., Ivetic, D.: An approach to DICOM extension for medical image streaming. DAAAM Int. Sci. Book 25–35
22. Mallick, P. K., Satapathy, B. S., Mohanty, M. N., Saravana Kumar, S.: Intelligent technique for CT brain image segmentation.In: 2015 2nd International Conference on Electronics and Communication Systems (ICECS), pp. 1269–1277. IEEE (2015)

Empirical Study on Different Feature Selection and Classification Algorithms for Prediction of Hepatitis Disease

Niranjan Panda, Sandeep Kumar Satapathy, Shruti Mishra, and Pradeep Kumar Mallick

Abstract Hepatitis is one of the most commonly diagnosed diseases in the world. With the enormous amount of data available in the medical industry, it is difficult to draw important conclusions. With the advent of technology, data mining techniques are used to solve this problem. In this study, we have applied various classifiers namely KNN, Logistic Regression, Naive Bayes, Decision Tree, Support Vector Machine (SVM), and Random Forest on Hepatitis dataset acquired from UCI Machine Learning repository. Two feature selection techniques: Chi-square test and Boruta Algorithm are used to improve the performance of the classifiers. Finally, we analyze which classifier performed the best and classify the patients into live or dead based on various performance measures. It was concluded that Naive Bayes with Chi-Square attribute selection performed better in terms of F1 score value. Overall, Logistic regression, Support Vector Machine, Kernel SVM, and KNN performed equally well with an accuracy of 90.32%.

Keywords Boruta algorithm · Chi-square test · Decision tree · KNN · Logistic regression · Naive bayes · Random forest · SVM

N. Panda (✉)
Department of Computer Science and Engineering, Siksha 'O' Anusandhan, Bhubaneswar, India
e-mail: niranjanpanda@soa.ac.in

S. K. Satapathy
School of Computer Science and Engineering, VIT University, Chennai, India
e-mail: sandeepkumar04@gmail.com

S. Mishra
School of Computer Science and Engineering, VIT-AP University, Amaravati, India
e-mail: shrutim2129@gmail.com

P. K. Mallick
School of Computer Science and Engineering, KIIT Deemed To Be University, Odisha Bhubaneswar, India
e-mail: pradeepmallick84@gmail.com

H. K. Tripathy et al. (eds.), *Technical Advancements of Machine Learning in Healthcare*, Studies in Computational Intelligence 936,
https://doi.org/10.1007/978-981-33-4698-7_4

1 Introduction

We live in the twenty-first century surrounded by heaps of data. We are constantly living through a data exhaust. Overall the fields, information are being gathered and aggregated rapidly. According to International Data Corporation's Digital Universe Study, the amount of data created since the dawn of time up until now is 40,900 exabytes. So, there is a dire need for robust computational methods and techniques to extract useful information from this exponentially growing data. Some new generation tools such as data mining techniques and machine learning algorithms are used to recognize important patterns and extricate valuable details, facts, figures, and trends from large volumes of raw data. Especially in the healthcare industry mining of biomedical data is used to identify medical conditions, increase treatment effectiveness, predict medicines, and ultimately save more lives.

Hepatitis is an inflammatory condition of liver cells, typically caused by a viral infection. There are five unique kinds of viruses categorized as A, B, C, D, E. Consumption of contaminated food or water leads to Hepatitis A and E while Hepatitis B, C, and D commonly occur as a product of parenteral contact with infected body fluids. Causes of non-infectious hepatitis include excessive consumption of alcohol, drugs and other toxins and autoimmune system response. This condition can be self-restricting or can prompt fibrosis, cirrhosis, and liver cancer. As indicated by the World Health Organization, an expected 325 million are living with Hepatitis B and C and for the greater part of the testing and treatment is inaccessible. Common means of transmission for these viruses is through contaminated blood or blood products, use of contaminated equipment and for hepatitis B transmission from infected mother to infant during childbirth, from relatives to kids, and by sexual contact. Acute infection may occur with constrained or no side effects, or may incorporate indications, for example, jaundice, dark-colored urine, fever, loss of appetite, extreme fatigue, nausea, vomiting, and stomach pain.

Diagnosis of acute hepatitis is often easy because of definite symptoms but that of chronic hepatitis can be difficult because of limited to no symptoms. Such patients can remain undiagnosed for years. Mining techniques are widely used on biomedical data to find important correlations and trends for efficient classification and prediction. The objective of this study is to classify the patients to live or dead and predict various performance measures such as accuracy, precision, recall, and F1 score. We apply different classifiers on the Hepatitis dataset obtained from the UCI Machine Learning Repository. Two feature selection techniques are applied to improve the performance of the classifier. Finally the performance parameters are determined to analyze the performance of all the classifiers. Figure 1 shows the entire research process.

The rest of the paper is as follows structured. Section 2 outlines the ACO metaheuristics. Section 3 provides a review with a tabular analysis of different energy aware routing protocols based on ACO. The paper is concluded with future work in Sect. 4.

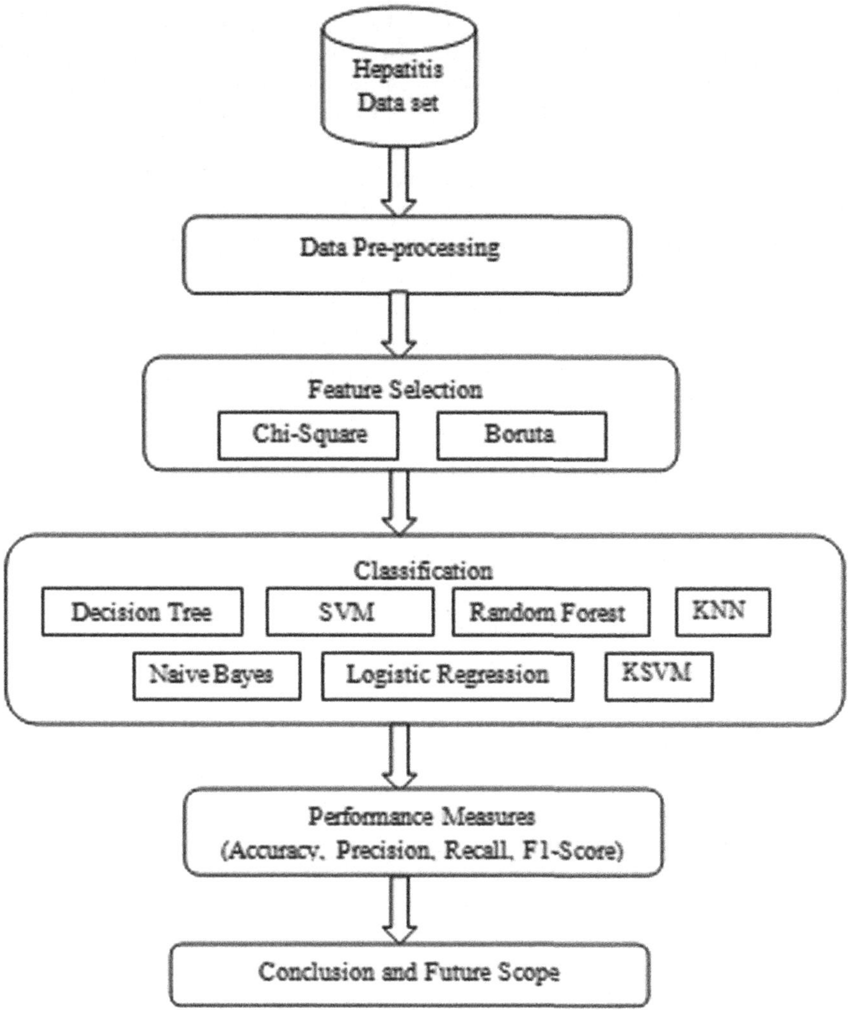

Fig. 1 The flow of the research and the different processes involved in it

2 Literature Review

Previous studies conducted on the diagnosis of hepatitis disease using data mining have used classification algorithms to predict the outcome. S.Pushpalatha and Dr. Jadesh Pandya et al. [5], in their study on the diagnosis of hepatitis, used classification techniques like Naive Bayes and Support Vector Machines. SVM performed better than Naive Bayes on the hepatitis dataset. Varun Kumar.M, Vijaya Sharathi.V, and Gayathri Devi.B.R et al. [6] proposed a predictive model based on optimal feature selection to improve the predictive accuracy for hepatitis. They used SVM and chi-square attribute evaluation for the model. The classification accuracy using SVM significantly increased after feature selection. Karthikeyan, T., and Thangaraju, P. et al. [7], in their study, found Naive Bayes performed better than Decision Tree and Random Forest algorithms.

In this study, we propose the use of classification algorithms like K-Nearest Neighbors, Logistic Regression, Naive Bayes, Support Vector Machines, Random Forest, and Decision Tree for improving the predictive accuracy using Chi-Square Test and Boruta Algorithm for feature selection. Feature selection is an important preprocessing technique as it not only improves the training time of the classifier but also improves the accuracy of the model if the relevant set of attributes is chosen. It simplifies the model and thus makes it easier to interpret.

3 Data Preprocessing

Data preprocessing can improve data quality, and consequently help to improve the accuracy of the subsequent data mining process. It includes data cleaning, integration, data reduction, and data transformation.

3.1 Attribute Identification

The dataset used in this study was collected from the UCI Machine Learning repository [8]. The hepatitis dataset has 155 instances with 19 attributes and a class attribute. The attributes in the dataset are shown in Table 1.

3.2 Data Cleaning

Data cleaning is a data preprocessing technique that is applied to reduce noise, fill in missing values, remove outliers, and correct data inconsistencies. The dataset used had some missing values for several attributes as shown in Fig. 2. Fifteen attributes had 167 missing values represented by "?".

Ignoring all the instances with missing values is not effective as it may reduce the amount of data that could have been useful for the mining process. Assigning a global constant like "0" or "unknown" may interfere with the mining process. In this study, missing values are handled by multivariate imputation via chained equations (MICE). The imputations are performed on a feature by feature basis by defining an imputation model for each feature. MICE use PMM (Predictive mean matching) for quantitative attributes and logistic regression for binary attributes.

Table 1 Attributes in dataset

S.No.	Attribute	Type	Value	No. of missing values
1	Class	Categorical	die (1), live(2)	0
2	Age	Numeric	10, 20, 30, 40, 50, 60, 70, 80	0
3	Sex	Categorical	male (1), female (2)	0
4	Steroid	Categorical	no (1), yes (2)	1
5	Antivirals	Categorical	no (1), yes (2)	1
6	Fatigue	Categorical	no (1), yes (2)	1
7	Malasie	Categorical	no (1), yes (2)	1
8	Anorexia	Categorical	no (1), yes (2)	1
9	Liver Big	Categorical	no (1), yes (2)	1
10	Liver Firm	Categorical	no (1), yes (2)	11
11	Spleen Palpable	Categorical	no (1), yes (2)	5
12	Spiders	Categorical	no (1), yes (2)	5
13	Ascites	Categorical	no (1), yes (2)	5
14	Varices	Numeric	no (1), yes (2)	5
15	Bilirubin	Numeric	0.39, 0.80, 1.20, 2.00, 3.00, 4.00	6
16	Alk Phosphate	Numeric	33, 80, 120, 160, 200, 250	29
17	SGOT	Numeric	13, 100, 200, 300, 400, 500	4
18	Albumin	Numeric	2.1, 3.0, 3.8, 4.5, 5.0, 6.0	16
19	Ptotime	Numeric	10, 20, 30, 40, 50, 60, 70, 80, 90	67
20	Histology	Categorical	no (1), yes (2)	0

3.3 Feature Scaling

Feature scaling is a data transformation technique that involves the normalization of independent variables of data by their Z-scores. The features in the hepatitis dataset were normalized within a particular range so that no variable is dominated by another variable having higher values.

3.4 Feature Selection

Feature selection is a dimensionality reduction technique where only a subset of the features is selected for further processing of data. The features which contribute the most to the response or target variable are kept, and other irrelevant features are discarded. This ensures the reduction of computational cost and may also help in increasing the performance of the model.

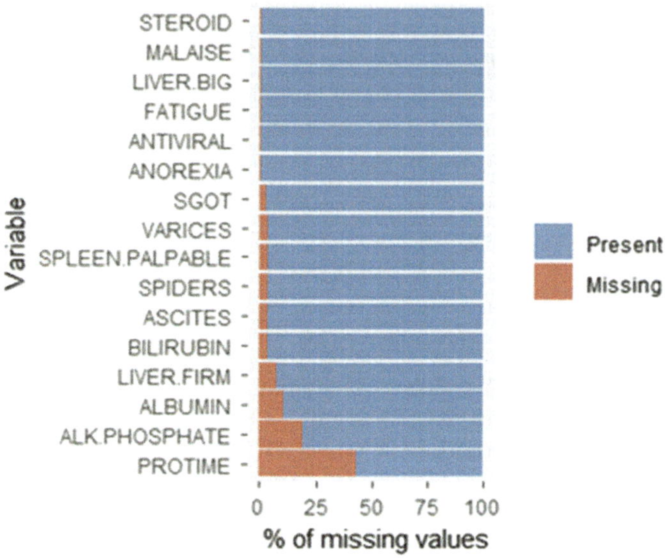

Fig. 2 Percentage of Missing Values. Some attributes have a large number of missing values

3.4.1 Chi-Square Test

The Chi-square test is mostly used for categorical features in a dataset having a categorical target variable. The Chi-square value between each categorical feature and the response variable is calculated, and the features with the optimal chi-square scores are selected.

3.4.2 Boruta Algorithm

Boruta is a wrapper-based feature selection algorithm that works with the Random Forest classifier. It duplicates the dataset and creates shuffled copies of each column that are called shadow features. The data is then trained with the Random Forest algorithm. The Z-score of the original feature is compared with those of its shadow features. Z-score is the number of deviations from the mean value. Original features with higher Z-scores are considered as important by the algorithm, and highly unimportant features get discarded after several iterations.

4 Classification Algorithms

Energy-conscious ACO routing protocols for MANET were discussed in detail in this paper and evaluated on the basis of their working concepts, prospects, and consequences. In our discussion, we concentrated only on energy-conscious as a major concern during the development of the routing protocol, while other considerations such as flexibility, reliability, and QoS can also be considered. Comparison and evaluation of the routing protocols tested has been published, showing that routing protocols based on ACO perform better than traditional routing protocols. Ultimately, it can be concluded that the current MANET scenario requires a multi-path routing algorithm hybrid, reliable, efficient, flexible, safe and energy-conscious to address the disadvantages of existing routing protocols. The content of this paper offers the basic idea of energy-conscious routing strategies based on ACO and can be useful for researchers in the development of new energy-conscious routing protocols.

4.1 Naïve Bayes

Naive Bayes classifier is based on the Bayes' Theorem. It assumes independence among predictors. Every pair of features is independent of each other, and each feature makes an equal contribution to the result. It is a simple classifier that is known to have worked well for real-world situations. A small amount of training data is required, and it is sometimes faster than more sophisticated techniques with the only disadvantage being the assumption it makes.

4.2 Logistic Regression

Logistic regression is a supervised classification algorithm used for binary classification problems. It models the data using the sigmoid function and predicts the probability of the target class based on one or more predictor variables. The outcome is then decided based on a threshold probability.

4.3 Support Vector Machine (SVM)

SVM is a discriminative classifier that creates a decision boundary that can separate two classes of data points. Many hyperplanes can be selected to separate the points. The goal is to locate a hyperplane in an N-dimensional space (where N is the number of attributes) that clearly classifies the data and has the maximum margin.

4.4 Kernel Support Vector Machine (KSVM)

KSVM or Kernel SVM classifier is used to find the decision boundary for non-linearly separable data, where linear SVM cannot operate. Generally, we map the non-linear data to a higher dimension to transform it into a linear form. Several mathematical functions, also defined as a kernel, are used for graphs, images, vectors, texts, and sequence data. There are many types of kernel functions like polynomial, Gaussian, radial basis function (RBF), Laplace RBF, Hyperbolic tangent sigmoid, Bessel function of the first kind, ANOVA radial, and linear spline kernel in one dimension.

4.5 K-Nearest Neighbors (KNN)

The KNN algorithm is a supervised machine learning algorithm that can be used for both classification and regression problems. KNN classifies the data based on their similarity. It assumes that similar data exist nearby, forming clusters. For a test object, the classifier finds K points in the training data that are nearest to the test observation. A distance measure is implemented to find K instances in the training dataset that are most similar to the test observation. The test observation is classified as the class with the majority of nearest neighbors.

4.6 Decision Tree

A decision tree classifier is a supervised learning method where the data is split into partitions iteratively. For a model where the target variable is discrete, the tree is built by binary recursive partitioning. Each internal node of the tree represents a test on an attribute, and each branch of the node indicates its result. Leaf nodes represent the class label. It is easy to interpret due to the simple structuring of decision trees.

4.7 Random Forest

Random forest is an ensemble learning method based on decision trees. This classifier constructs many decision trees from randomly taken subsets of the training set. It combines the outcome from all the decision trees and categorizes the test data based on majority voting. It is a fast algorithm that works accurately on large datasets and handles missing data efficiently.

Table 2 Confusion matrix

Predicated	Actual	
	Positive	Negative
Positive	TP (True Positive)	FP (False Positive)
Negative	FN (False Negative)	TN (True Negative)

5 Performance Measures

Evaluation of the prediction performance of the classifiers is done using accuracy, precision, recall, and F-measure. A confusion matrix summarizes the performance of a classification. For a problem with two classes, the matrix size is 2 × 2 denoting predicted values and actual values [9] (Table 2).

Accuracy is the ratio of correctly predicted observations to the total predictions made.

$$Accuracy = (TP + TN) / (TP + TN + FP + FN) \quad (1)$$

Precision is the ratio of the total number of correctly predicted positives by the total predicted positives.

$$Precision\ TP / (TP + FP) \quad (2)$$

Recall is the ratio of the total number of correctly predicted positives by the total number of positives.

$$Recall = TP/(TP + FN) \quad (3)$$

Accuracy may not be the best performance measure for a classification with an uneven class distribution. In such cases, the F1 score is considered better. F-measure uses both precision and recall.

$$F1\ Score = (2 * Recall * Precision)/(Recall + Precision) \quad (4)$$

6 Experimental Results

EnergyAfter preprocessing of the dataset, several classification algorithms were applied to it. The dataset was first divided into a training dataset and a test dataset. The data was then trained for each classifier, and the test data was classified into live or die. The result of each classification is shown in Table 3. The table shows the performance of all the classifiers without any feature selection techniques as well as with two feature selection techniques. For each classification it was observed that

Table 3 Performance of classifiers

Classifier	Feature seletion	No. of attributes	Accuracy (%)	Precision	Recall	F1-Score
Navie Bayes	Without feature selection	19	86	0.7143	0.7692	0.7407
	Chi-square	12	88	0.7692	0.7692	0.7692
	Boruta	11	86	0.7143	0.7692	0.7407
Logistic Regression	Without feature selection	19	90.32	0.80	0.667	0.7272
	Chi-square	12	90.32	0.80	0.667	0.7272
	Boruta	11	90.32	0.80	0.667	0.7272
SVM	Without feature selection	19	90.32	0.80	0.6667	0.7272
	Chi-square	12	87.09	0.667	0.667	0.667
	Boruta	11	90.32	0.80	0.667	0.7272
KSVM	Without feature selection	19	90.32	0.808	0.667	0.7272
	Chi-square	12	90.32	0.80	0.667	0.7272
	Boruta	11	90.32	0.80	0.667	0.7272
Decision Tree	Without feature selection	19	83.87	0.5714	0.666	0.6153
	Chi-square	12	83.87	0.5714	0.667	0.615
	Boruta	11	87.09	0.667	0.667	0.667
KNN	Without feature selection	19	83.87	1.00	0.16	0.28
	Chi-square	12	87.09	0.667	0.667	0.667
	Boruta	11	90.32	0.80	0.667	0.7272
Random forest	Without feature selection	19	87.09	0.667	0.667	0.667
	Chi-square	12	87.09	0.667	0.667	0.667
	Boruta	11	87.09	0.75	0.50	0.60

after feature selection, the accuracy either increased or remained the same, which means that the classification algorithm performed better and worked more efficiently.

The highest accuracy was observed to be 90.32% for many classifiers. Based on the F-measure, the Naïve Bayes classifier performed the best with the highest F1- score. Boruta performed better as a feature selection method in most of the classifications as it removed more number of irrelevant features and improved the performance of the classifiers. Overall, Logistic regression, SVM, KSVM, and KNN performed equally well with an accuracy of 90.32%.

7 Conclusion and Future Work

According to the results obtained, most of the classification algorithms have performed well after applying feature selection techniques. In some cases, like Logistic Regression and KSVM the accuracy of classification did not improve, but the reduced number of attributes improved the training time of the model and thus provided a faster result. In general, feature selection methods can improve the performance of learning algorithms. The classification accuracy of Naive Bayes increased to 88% from 86% with Chi-Square attribute selection and performed better in terms of F1 score value. Overall, Logistic regression, SVM, KSVM, and KNN performed equally well with an accuracy of 90.32%.

Applying data mining techniques in the field of medical research can lead to a better health care system. It can not only be helpful in the diagnosis of diseases but also in finding out what factors determine them and their symptoms.

In future, a larger dataset may be used. Different classification algorithms can be applied to improve the prediction accuracy and more parameters may be studied for hepatitis diagnosis. Many feature selection algorithms can be implemented to further increase the performance of a classifier.

References

1. Al-Turaiki, I., Alshahrani, M., Almutairi, T.: Building predictive models for MERS-CoV infections using data mining techniques. J. Inf. Public Health **9**(6), 744–748 (2016)
2. USF Health, Morsani College of Medicine. Data mining in healthcare. https://www.usfhealthonline.com/resources/key-concepts/data-mining-in-healthcare, last accessed 2020/08/21
3. World Health Organization."What is hepatitis?: https://www.who.int/news-room/q-a-detail/what-is-hepatitis, last accessed 2020/08/21
4. World Health Organization.: Hepatitis. https://www.who.int/health-topics/hepatitis #tab=tab_1, last accessed 2020/08/21
5. Pushpalatha, S., Pandya, D.: Framework for diagnosing hepatitis disease using classification algorithms. Int. J. Adv. Res. **4**(7), 2189–2195 (2016)
6. Kumar, V., BR, G.D.: Hepatitis prediction model based on data mining algorithm and optimal feature selection to improve predictive accuracy. Int. J. Comput. Appl. **51**(19), 13–16 (2012)

7. Karthikeyan, T., Thangaraju, P.: Analysis of classification algorithms applied to hepatitis patients. Int. J. Comp. Appl. **62**(15), 25–30 (2013)
8. Hepatitis dataset, UCI Machine Learning Repository. https://archive.ics.uci.edu/ml/datasets/ Irvine. CA University of California, School of Information Technology and Computer Science, last accessed 2020/07/18
9. Mallick, Pradeep Kumar, Debahuti Mishra, Srikanta Patnaik, Kailash Shaw: A semi-supervised rough set and random forest approach for pattern classification of gene expression data.Int. J. Rea.-Based Intel. Syst. **8**(3–4), 155–167 (2016)

Metacognitive Neural Network for Emphysema Classification

Shyla Raj, B. S. Mahanand, and D. S. Vinod

Abstract Emphysema is a chronic obstructive lung disorder that causes shortness of breath. Emphysema detection from computed tomography scans is normally done by analysing areas with low attenuation and texture variations in the lungs. To capture both intensity information and texture variations from the lung scans, in this study texture features are extracted using local binary patterns, Gabor filter bank, gray-level co-occurrence matrix and intensity information is extracted from gray-level histogram. The extracted texture and intensity features are inputted to metacognitive neural network to classify as normal, centrilobular emphysema and panlobular emphysema. During the training phase, samples are inputted one-by-one to the metacognitive neural network. The samples are added to the network if it has distinct knowledge otherwise samples are deleted. The study has been conducted on computed tomography scans available from Bruijne and Sorensen benchmark dataset. The performance of metacognitive neural network is compared with commonly used classifiers namely k-nearest neighbour, support vector machine, decision tree and also with similar works on emphysema classification. The comparison results clearly indicate the better performance of the proposed approach for emphysema classification with fewer data samples.

Keywords Emphysema · Metacognitive Neural Network · Texture analysis · Sequential learning · Classification

S. Raj · B. S. Mahanand (✉) · D. S. Vinod
Department of Information Science and Engineering, Sri Jayachamarajendra College of Engineering JSS Science and Technology University, Mysuru, Karnataka, India
e-mail: bsmahanand@sjce.ac.in

S. Raj
e-mail: shylaraj@jssstuniv.in

D. S. Vinod
e-mail: dsvinod@daad-alumni.de

H. K. Tripathy et al. (eds.), *Technical Advancements of Machine Learning in Healthcare*, Studies in Computational Intelligence 936,
https://doi.org/10.1007/978-981-33-4698-7_5

1 Introduction

Chronic Obstructive Pulmonary Diseases (COPD) is a group of airflow obstruction lung disorders with symptoms of breathlessness, wheezing and recurrent cough. COPD is a global health concern and in India, COPD is considered the second most common lung disorder after tuberculosis [1]. COPD is primarily caused due to smoking and other reasons include long time exposure to air pollution, chemical fumes, dust and burning of biomass. Studies have shown that subjects with COPD may also experience cardiac failure, osteoporosis, diabetes, skeletal muscle dysfunction and lung cancer due to airflow obstruction and hyperinflation in the lungs [6]. The common conditions of COPD are emphysema and chronic bronchitis [35]. Emphysema is characterized by degeneration of alveoli and the surrounding lung tissues leading to decreased capacity of the lungs. Detection of emphysema is an important task, because it is the primary cause for shortness of breath and it may be a predictive indicator of lung cancer [30, 45]. The subtypes of emphysema include centrilobular emphysema (CLE), panlobular emphysema (PSE) and paraseptal emphysema. CLE is distinguished by areas of decreased attenuation and affects the upper part of the lungs. CLE is mainly found in tobacco smokers. Paraseptal emphysema is identified by decreased attenuation areas at the periphery of the lungs and lobes. PSE can be found in both non-smokers and smokers and has decreased attenuation patterns localized around the pleura. PSE is found mostly in younger people in comparison to CLE [40].

The primary diagnostic tool for emphysema includes pulmonary function test such as spirometry [35]. Spirometry measures the extent of emphysema by assessing the lung volumes during the inhalation and exhalation process. However, using these tests it may be difficult to detect emphysema and its subtypes in the early stage [13]. Alternatively, imaging modalities such as X-rays and high-resolution computed tomography (HRCT) scans have been employed for the detection of emphysema. HRCT scans are widely used for diagnosis of emphysema as it provides high resolution and high contrast details of the lungs [10, 17]. The visual and quantitative information provided by the HRCT scans closely correlate with the pathological condition of emphysema and thus HRCT aids in early detection of emphysema. The visual assessment of emphysema scans is a challenging task for the radiologist because it is time-consuming task and has large inter-observer variations among the lung patterns [7]. To overcome the shortcomings of manual interpretation, computer-assisted approaches have been reported for emphysema detection [17, 33, 47, 53].

Emphysema is visualized as areas with low attenuation in CT scans close to the Hounsfield Unit (HU) of air, i.e. (-1000). The density mask approach identifies emphysema by counting a number of voxels less than a specified threshold [11, 17]. Muller et al. [24] adopted "density mask" a CT scanner program to identify emphysema by highlighting voxels with low attenuation. Gould et al. [12] reported the lowest fifth percentile method to determine emphysema. Kinsella et al. [17] identified emphysema regions in CT images by using a threshold of -910 HU to indicate emphysema in CT scans. Genevois et al. [11] examined thresholds from the range of −910 to −970 HU to quantify the extent of emphysema and demonstrated that threshold less than −950 HU is the best measure for emphysema quantification. Shaker et al. [41] reported a density-based approach for estimating emphysema in α_1−antitrypsin-deficient subjects. Even though the density mask approach is widely employed for emphysema detection it may not be appropriate for differentiating subtle differences between emphysema subtypes. Alternatively, machine learning approaches have been widely used for accurate and efficient emphysema detection from computed tomography scans.

Supervised machine learning approaches can be largely grouped into batch learning and sequential learning. In a batch learning approach complete set of data samples are used to train the model. Since all the samples are used for training there may be a possibility of over-fitting and also training time increases as the training sample increases. Additionally, when the new samples are added, the model needs to be re-trained once again using complete data samples. On the other hand in the sequential learning approach, data samples are presented one at a time to the model. During the training process, only the samples with distinct knowledge are used. Thereby sequential learning approach use lesser samples and reduces over-fitting [8, 18, 23, 44].

In the literature, machine learning approaches based on texture features have been widely reported for accurate emphysema classification [29, 42, 47]. Emphysema patterns are exhibited as texture changes in the lungs hence texture analysis plays a major role in detecting the disease. One of the early works on emphysema classification based on texture features was reported by Uppaluri et al. [47]. In [47], regional analysis of lungs was performed to determine the absence or presence of emphysema. Texture features were extracted using first-order statistics, gray-level run length (GLRM), gray-level co-occurrence matrix (GLCM) and fractal measures. Using these features on minimum distance classifier, an accuracy of 93% was achieved by Uppaluri et al. [47]. Chabat et al. [7] reported an automated texture-based classification of emphysema subtypes using Bayesian classifier. The texture features were extracted from nth-order statistics, mean values were extracted from GLCM and GLRM. Sensitivity of 73.6% and specificity of 91.2% were reported for classification between healthy, constrictive obliterative bronchiolitis, panlobular emphysema, and centrilobular emphysema. Liang et al. [19] used texture features from the spatial gray-level dependence method, GLRM, and gray-level histogram method to discriminate emphysema in CT scans using backpropagation neural network. Prasad et al. [34] performed automated texture-based multi-level emphysema classification based on co-training and active learning. The texture features were extracted from GLRM, GLCM and gray-level difference method. The results were compared with density mask approach, and it was found that the density mask approach marked more non-emphysematous pixels as emphysematous. In some studies, fractal, shape and global features are used along with the texture features [9, 29, 46, 53]. Xu et al. [53] classified normal lung from emphysema subtypes using 3D texture features extracted from GLRM, GLCM, and fractal measures and Bayesian classifier. It was reported that 3D texture features exhibited better discrimination between normal smoker and non-smoker when compared to 2D texture features. Friman et al. [9] reported a study by employing intensity, shape and global lung features. An accuracy of 89.4% was achieved using backpropagation neural network for classification between true emphysema and image artifacts. Park et al. [29] quantified emphysema using shape features from top-hat transformation and circularity measures and texture features from histogram, gradient, GLCM and GLRM. An accuracy of 77.9% was reported using a support vector machine classifier.

Rotation invariant features such as local binary pattern, Gaussian filter and Gabor filter bank have been employed on emphysema classification [26, 32, 42]. Sorensen et al. [42] used features from the local binary pattern and intensity histogram for emphysema classification using k-nearest neighbour and reported an accuracy of 95.2%. Nava et al. [26] quantified emphysema patterns based on local and global descriptors to represent the texture of patch. The work combined features from the Gabor filter bank and local binary pattern and achieved an F-score of 0.86. Pena et al. [32] employed an automated emphysema detection by using multiple-instance classifier which does not require manual annotations for training. Texture features from GLCM and Gaussian filter banks were employed to classify emphysema in CT scans using a multiple-instance support vector classifier.

Recently some studies have reported emphysema classification using deep learning models [31, 33, 43]. Pei et al. [31] employed convolutional neural network (CNN) for classification of emphysema subtypes with normal lung scans. Features were learned from the raw image by multiple layers of convolutional neural network and a recognition rate of 92.54% was achieved. Peng et al. [33] reported quantification and classification of emphysema by employing a multi-scale deep CNN. Both high-level information and multi-scale information were used to consider the characteristics of different emphysema types and a classification accuracy of 92.68% was reported. Srivastava and Purwar [43] proposed a ImageNet-VGG-CNN model for classification of computed tomography scans. Six features, namely, circularity, solidity, discrete Fourier transform, histogram of oriented gradient, second-order moments of image, and histogram of active contour were used in their CNN model and average recall of 69.56% and precision of 95.26% was obtained.

From the literature, it is found that the majority of the studies have employed batch learning approaches for emphysema classification. However, in most medical classification problems, data is collected in intervals and complete data may not be available at once. In such scenarios, sequential learning approaches are more appropriate and efficient for classification [2, 36, 38, 44, 51]. Recently Metacognitive Neural Network (McNN) classifier based on sequential learning algorithm has been widely used for various classification problems [5, 22, 49].

The main objective of this work is to employ sequential Metacognitive Neural Network classifier for emphysema detection. In McNN, training samples are presented one at the time to the network. If the current training sample has distinct knowledge then the sample is learnt otherwise it is deleted. The network learns by adding neurons or by updating the output weights based on knowledge measures. The advantage of McNN is that it uses fewer samples for training thus avoiding the problem of over-fitting. McNN has been employed for a wide range of medical diagnostic problems [3, 4, 50, 52].

Emphysema detection from computed tomography scans is normally done by analysing areas with low attenuation and texture variations in the lungs. To capture both intensity information and texture variations from the lung scans, in this study texture features are extracted using local binary patterns (LBP), Gabor filter bank, gray-level co-occurrence matrix (GLCM) and intensity information is extracted from gray-level histogram (GLH). The texture and intensity features are inputted to McNN for emphysema classification. To optimally choose the parameters for McNN classifier particle swarm optimization is employed. Performance of the McNN classifier is compared with support vector machine (SVM), k-nearest neighbour (k-NN) and decision tree (DT) classifiers and also with other similar studies on emphysema classification.

The organisation of the paper is as follows. The data used in the work, feature extraction approaches and McNN classifier are described in Sect. 2. The performance results of the McNN classifier is presented in Sect. 3. The major conclusions of the work are summarized in Sect. 4.

2 Materials and Methods

In this work, we propose a classification of emphysema subtypes and normal lung using texture and intensity features and employing McNN classifier. The overall framework of emphysema classification using McNN classifier is illustrated in Fig. 1. The emphysema and healthy lung patches collected from Bruijne and Sorensen benchmark dataset are used in the work. Texture features and intensity information are extracted from these patches using LBP, GLCM, Gabor filter bank and GLH. The combined texture and intensity features are inputted to the McNN classifier. Samples are presented sequentially, one at a time to the cognitive component of the McNN classifier. The metacognitive component uses knowledge measures such as estimated class label, class-wise significance and maximum hinge error for all the training samples. Based on these measures, the sample is either added, deleted or reserved in the network. Finally, McNN classifies the lung images either into normal, CLE or PSE.

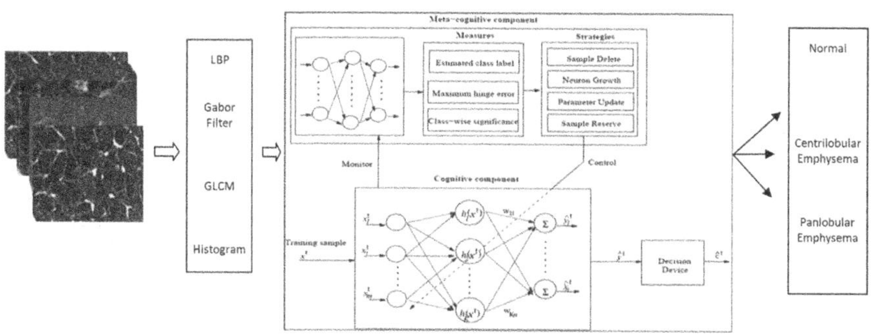

Fig. 1 Framework of emphysema classification using metacognitive neural network classifier

Table 1 The per-class distribution of Bruijne and Sorensen emphysema dataset

Class	Description	Sample-size
Normal	Class with healthy never smokers	59
Centrilobular Emphysema (CLE)	Class with healthy smokers without COPD	50
Panlobular Emphysema (PSE)	Class with smokers with COPD	59

2.1 *Dataset*

In this work, data is used from the publicly available standard Bruijne and Sorensen emphysema dataset [42]. The dataset consists of 168 non-overlapping square patches of size 61 × 61 pixels. The patches are manually annotated from 115 HRCT scans, which are classified into three classes namely normal (NT), CLE and PSE. The HRCT scans are collected from 39 subjects each belonging one of the following categories: (i) 9 healthy subjects who are non-smokers (NT), (ii) 10 healthy who smokers but with no COPD (CLE) and (iii) 20 subjects who are smokers with COPD (PSE). Table 1 provides the description and count of samples of each class in the dataset.

2.2 *Feature Extraction*

Computed tomography scans provide high resolution and high contrast details of lungs which helps in accurate detection and diagnosis of emphysema. Fig. 2 presents computed tomography scans of normal, centrilobular and panlobular emphysema. From Fig. 2, it may be observed that emphysema is visualized with decreased attenuation regions and consists of more homogeneous areas and edges as compared to normal lungs. Lung destruction in CLE is characterized by smaller circular areas and PSE results in low attenuation at sub-pleural areas. To capture texture variations and intensity information from the lungs, in this study both texture and intensity features are extracted. Texture features are extracted using LBP, GLCM, Gabor filter bank and intensity information is extracted from GLH measure.

LBP is a rotation-invariant texture descriptor which analyses the texture variation in local neighbourhood [28]. In LBP, pixel-wise comparison is performed between the center pixel P_c and neighbouring pixels P_i in NXN neighbourhood. LBP analyses the textural alternation in local neighbourhood thus helps in recognizing the normal lung patterns. The multi-resolution representation of lung texture is captured using rotation-invariant Gabor filter bank [14]. The lung textures are analysed in different directions and scales. Gabor filter bank has the highest response in the direction where the texture or the intensity changes, thus recognizing the edges in the emphysema

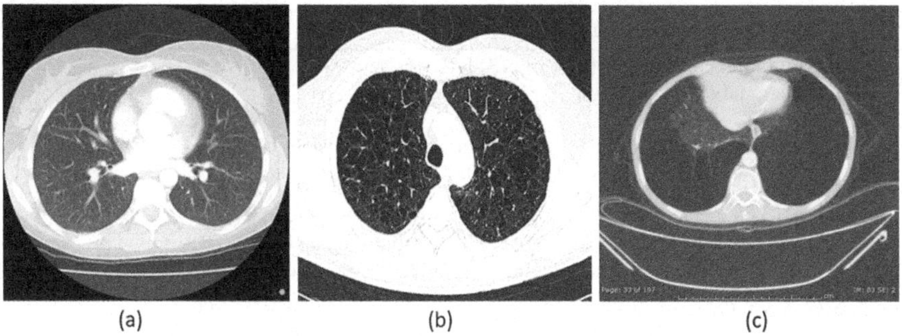

Fig. 2 Computed Tomography scans of **a** Normal **b** Centrilobular Emphysema **c** Panlobular Emphysema

patterns. GLCM analyses the spatial distribution of pixel intensities and yields a count matrix depicting the frequency of different combinations of gray level in a particular direction [15]. Hence GLCM aids in the recognition of homogeneous areas. Measures from gray-level histogram are used to capture the attenuation information in the image. The intensity information is helpful in discriminating between healthy and lungs with low attenuation patterns.

2.3 *Metacognitive Neural Network Classifier*

Metacognitive Neural Network classifier is based on human metacognitive learning principles, namely 'what', 'when' and 'how' to learn. McNN architecture used in this work is the same as [20, 21, 37, 39]. McNN comprises cognitive and metacognitive components. The steps followed in the McNN classifier are explained in Algorithm 1.

Cognitive component Cognitive component is a radial basis feed forward neural network with three layers. The network starts with zero hidden neurons and builds K neurons from $t-1$ training samples. The hidden layer uses Gaussian activation function and output layer uses linear activation function. The estimated output $\widehat{y}_j^t$ for a given input sample $\mathbf{x}^t$ is calculated as

$$\widehat{y}_j^t = \sum_{k=1}^{K} w_{kj} h_k^t, \quad j = 1, \ldots, n \tag{1}$$

where w_{kj} is weight and h_k^t is the hidden neuron response.

Metacognitive component This component consists of estimated class label measure ($\widehat{c}^t$), maximum hinge error (E^t) and class-wise significance measure (ψ_c) along with self-regulated thresholds. Based on these measures for each training sample one of the following strategies is employed.

Algorithm 1: McNN classifier

Data: Train image patches x={x_1,x_2,..., x_t}
Result: Class label c={c_1,c_2,c_3}
repeat
  Step 1: The cognitive component computes estimated class label $\widehat{y}_j^t$ for each training image patch $\mathbf{x}^t$ using eq (1)
  Step 2: The metacognitive component measures knowledge in $\mathbf{x}^t$ using estimated class label ($\widehat{c}^t$), maximum hinge error(E^t) and class-wise significance based on spherical potential(ψ_c).
  Step 3: On the basis of knowledge measure and self-regulated threshold metacognitive component adopts one of the following strategies :
    if patch has similar knowledge then sample is deleted based on eq(2)
    else if patch has significant knowledge to be captured , neurons are added using eq (3) and weights are updated in cognitive component based on eq(4).
    else reserve the sample for future learning
until *For all image patches in training set*;

Sample delete strategy: If the training sample has distinct knowledge then the sample is learnt otherwise the sample is deleted without learning using Eq. (2). The sample deletion strategy reduces computational effort by avoiding over-training of similar training samples.

$$\widehat{c}^t \;==\; c^t \;\textbf{ AND }\; E^t \;\leq\; \beta_d \tag{2}$$

where β_d is the deletion threshold.

Neuron growth strategy If the training sample has distinct knowledge that needs to be learned then new neurons are added to the cognitive component using Eq. (3).

$$\left(\widehat{c}^t \neq c^t \textbf{ OR } E^t \;\geq\; \beta_a\right) \textbf{ AND } \psi_c(\mathbf{x}^t) \;\leq\; \beta_c \tag{3}$$

where β_a is the addition threshold and β_c is the knowledge measure.

Parameters update strategy The output weights of the cognitive component is updated if the estimated class label ($\widehat{c}^t$) is equal to actual class label (c^t) and maximum hinge error (E^t) is greater than update threshold (β_u).

$$\widehat{c}^t \;==\; c^t \;\textbf{ AND }\; E^t \;\geq\; \beta_u \tag{4}$$

Sample reserve strategy The training sample is reserved for future learning if none of the above learning strategies are satisfied.

McNN classifier has several parameters to be initialized such as skip threshold (β_b), adding error threshold (β_a), learning error threshold (β_u), decay factor (δ), overlap factor (K_2), reserve sample limit, spherical potential threshold (ϕ_s), center shifting factor (ζ) and overlap factor for first neuron (K_1). In order to optimally choose the parameters for McNN classifier, particle swarm optimization is employed in the work [16]. For additional information on McNN classifier, one may refer the following work [20, 21, 39].

3 Experimental Results

The classification performance of McNN is evaluated by comparing the results with SVM, k-NN and DT and also with similar works in the literature. The study has been conducted using computed tomography scans available from publicly available Bruijne and Sorensen benchmark dataset [42]. For sake of completeness SVM, k-NN and DT are explained below.

Support vector machines (SVM): SVM differentiates various classes by constructing a hyperplane in multidimensional space. The hyperplane is chosen such that the distance between the hyperplane and the support vectors on each side is maximized [48]. For non-linearly separable data, SVM uses kernel trick and maps them into higher dimension space. Then the data samples are classified by constructing a hyperplane in the high-dimensional space. In this work, SVM with Gaussian kernel is employed for McNN classification.

For given training data $(x_i, y_i) \forall\ 1 \leq \text{i} \leq \text{N}$ where x_i-features y_i-class labels and kernel width $'\sigma'$. The data is mapped into higher dimension space using Gaussian kernel function as shown below:

$$k(x, x_i) = exp(-\|x - x_i\|^2)/2\sigma^2 \qquad for\ \ \sigma > 0 \tag{5}$$

The classifier function f(x) is calculated as :

$$f(x) = \sum_i^N \alpha_i y_i k(x, x_i) + b \tag{6}$$

where α_i - weight, b-bias and k(x,x_i)-support vector

k-nearest neighbour (k-nn): k-nn is based on instance learning or lazy learning. For training data $(x_i, y_i) \forall\ 1 \leq \text{i} \leq \text{N}$ where x_i-features y_i-class labels and k neighbours $ne_k(x)$ =$\{n_1$,n_2,..., $n_k\}$ where k $\geq$ 1. The class label of an unknown sample is determined by computing the distance between the test sample $x_i^{'}$ and each training sample using Euclidean measure as shown below:

$$\sqrt{\sum_{i=1}^n (x_i - x_i^{'})^2} \tag{7}$$

The distance values are sorted in increasing order and top k rows are chosen. The test sample is assigned to the most frequent class in the sorted array. Euclidean is the most commonly used distance measure, other measures include Manhattan, Minkowsky and cosine similarity.

Decision Tree (DT): DT is one of simplest algorithms which classifies data by constructing flowchart like tree structure. The internal node of the decision tree represents the test on the attribute, the branch presents the test's result and the leaf node represents the class label.

The entire training data is first placed at the root node and the best attribute is selected. The training data is continuously split to build the tree with the help of the split criterion. The tree is grown until the subset at a node has the same values or when splitting will no longer add value to the prediction. Given a testing sample, for which class is unknown, the target class is estimated by testing the data against the constructed decision tree. The decision tree can be easily transformed into *if-then-else* classification rules.

The performance of McNN classifier is measured based on sensitivity (recall), specificity, F-score and accuracy. The dataset is randomly divided into 70% training and 30% testing and the experimentation is repeated for ten times to get average classification performance.

$$Sensitivity = \frac{TP}{TP + FN} \tag{8}$$

$$Specificity = \frac{TN}{TN + FP} \tag{9}$$

$$F - score = \frac{2TP}{2TP + FP + FN} \tag{10}$$

$$Accuracy = \frac{TP + TN}{TN + TP + FP + FN} \tag{11}$$

where TP is true positive, TN is true negative, FP is false positive and FN is false negative.

Table 2 presents the class-wise sensitivity, specificity, F-score and accuracy achieved by the McNN for emphysema subtypes and normal lung. From Table 2

Table 2 Classification performance of McNN classifier

Class	Sensitivity	Specificity	F-score	Accuracy
Normal	0.94	0.97	0.94	0.95
Centrilobular Emphysem (CLE)	0.95	0.98	0.95	0.97
Panlobular Emphysema (PSE)	0.90	0.95	0.90	0.94
Mean	**0.93**	**0.97**	**0.93**	**0.95**

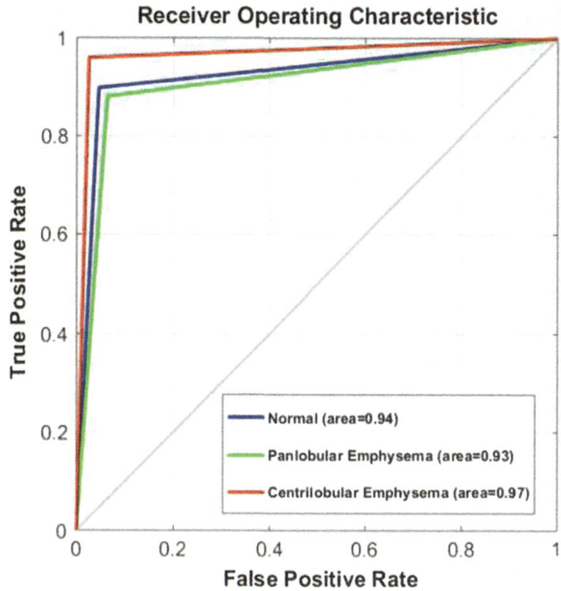

Fig. 3 Classification performance of McNN represented using ROC curve

it is observed that mean sensitivity of 0.93, specificity of 0.97, F-score of 0.93 and accuracy of 0.95 is achieved by McNN classifier. Among different classes, accuracy of 0.97 is observed for CLE, 0.95 for normal lung and 0.94 for PSE. The results clearly indicate that McNN achieves better accuracy with lesser mis-classifications.

Receiver operating characteristic curve (ROC) and its respective area under curve (AUC) have been plotted to graphically represent the trade-off between false positive rate (1-specificity) and true positive rate (sensitivity). The perfect classification is represented by ROC curve passing through the upper left corner. The AUC value ranges from 0.0 to 1.0, AUC < 0.5 means poor classification and AUC value close to 1.0 means excellent classification. From Fig. 3, it is noticed that AUC values for all three classes are above 0.9 which implies the balanced performance in recognition of emphysema subtypes and healthy lungs. Furthermore, the ROC curve of centrilobular emphysema is nearer to upper left corner with AUC of 0.97, followed by the normal pattern with an AUC of 0.94 and panlobular emphysema with an AUC value 0.93. This implies recognition of centrilobular emphysema is superior to normal tissue and panlobular emphysema.

The classification performance of McNN and other commonly used classifiers is tabulated in Table 3. From Table 3 it can be observed that McNN achieves mean sensitivity of 0.93, specificity of 0.97, F-score of 0.93 and accuracy of 0.95. While SVM, k-NN and decision tree produced an accuracy of 0.92, 0.90 and 0.88, respectively. The results clearly indicate that McNN produced an accuracy improvement of 3–7% as compared to other classifiers within fewer training samples. From Table 3, it is observed McNN on an average uses only 86 samples out of 117 for training the

Table 3 Performance evaluation of McNN classifier with other batch learning algorithms

Class	Sensitivity	Specificity	F-score	Accuracy	No. of samples used
McNN	**0.93**	**0.97**	**0.93**	**0.95**	**86**
SVM	0.89	0.94	0.88	0.92	117
k-NN	1.00	0.85	0.88	0.90	117
Decision tree	0.89	0.88	0.84	0.88	117

Table 4 Performance comparison with state-of-the-art technique

Method	Accuracy
McNN	**0.95**
Peng et al. [33]	0.93
Narayanan et al. [25]	0.87
Nava et al. [27]	0.91
Pei et al. [31]	0.93
Sorensen et al. [42]	0.95

model. This indicates that the McNN classifier is trained using only 86 samples with distinct knowledge and the remaining samples are deleted without learning.

The classification performance of our proposed McNN-based approach is compared with similar studies conducted on standard Bruijne and Sorensen dataset as shown in Table 4. Accuracy achieved by the proposed approach is compared with following studies which include novel multi-scale deep convolutional neural networks [33], fuzzy decision tree [25], feature ensemble approach [27], convolutional neural networks [31] and joint LBP-histogram with k-nearest neighbour classifier [42].

From Table 4, it can be observed that our proposed McNN-based emphysema classification produces better mean accuracy than the other works and similar performance is observed between McNN and [42] but most importantly McNN achieves the same accuracy with fewer samples. The results from Tables 3 and 4 reveals that not all training samples are required for the learning process in McNN in contrast to batch learning algorithms where all samples are involved in learning process. When the model is trained with samples with distinct knowledge the problem of over-fitting can be avoided and also better classification accuracy can be obtained as illustrated in this work.

4 Conclusions

In this work, emphysema classification is performed by employing sequential-learning-based metacognitive neural network. To capture the texture appearance of the lungs along with the attenuation information, both texture and intensity features are extracted. Texture features are extracted from local binary pattern, Gabor filter bank, gray-level co-occurrence matrix and intensity information is captured using gray-level histogram. The texture and intensity features are then inputted to metacognitive neural network. To select the optimal parameters for metacognitive neural network classifier, particle swarm optimization is employed. The mean sensitivity of 0.93, specificity of 0.97, F-score of 0.93 and accuracy of 0.95 are obtained and its performance is compared with similar works in the literature. The McNN performance is also compared with commonly used classifiers, namely k-nearest neighbour, support vector machine, decision tree and an accuracy improvement of around 3% to 7% is achieved. The performance comparison clearly indicates that by employing metacognitive neural network better classification results can be achieved with less number of training samples as compared to other machine learning approaches.

References

1. Aggarwal, D., Gupta, A., Janmeja, A., Bhardwaj, M.: Evaluation of tuberculosis-associated chronic obstructive pulmonary disease at a tertiary care hospital: a case-control study. Lung India Off. Organ Indian Chest Soc. **34**(5), 415 (2017)
2. Babu, G.S., Suresh, S.: Meta-cognitive neural network for classification problems in a sequential learning framework. Neurocomputing **81**, 86–96 (2012)
3. Babu, G.S., Suresh, S., Mahanand, B.S.: Alzheimer's disease detection using a projection based learning meta-cognitive rbf network. In: The 2012 International Joint Conference on Neural Networks (IJCNN). pp. 1–8. IEEE (2012)
4. Babu, G.S., Suresh, S., Mahanand, B.S.: A novel pbl-mcrbfn-rfe approach for identification of critical brain regions responsible for parkinson's disease. Expert Syst. Appl. **41**(2), 478–488 (2014)
5. Badrinarayanan, R., Suresh, S., Mahanand, B.S.: Identification of potential biomarkers in the hippocampus region for the diagnosis of ADHD using PBL-McRBFN approach. In: 2014 13th International Conference on Control Automation Robotics & Vision (ICARCV), pp. 17–22. IEEE (2014)
6. Barnes, P., Celli, B.: Systemic manifestations and comorbidities of copd. Eur. Respir. J. **33**(5), 1165–1185 (2009)
7. Chabat, F., Yang, G.Z., Hansell, D.M.: Obstructive lung diseases: texture classification for differentiation at ct. Radiology **228**(3), 871–877 (2003)
8. Dietterich, T.: Machine learning for sequential data: a review structural, syntactic, and statistical pattern recognition, vol. 2396, pp. 15–30 (2002)
9. Friman, O., Borga, M., Lundberg, M., Tylén, U., Knutsson, H.: Recognizing emphysema-a neural network approach. In: Object Recognition Supported by User Interaction for Service Robots, vol. 1, pp. 512–515. IEEE (2002)
10. Galbán, C.J., Han, M.K., Boes, J.L., Chughtai, K.A., Meyer, C.R., Johnson, T.D., Galbán, S., Rehemtulla, A., Kazerooni, E.A., Martinez, F.J., et al.: Computed tomography-based biomarker provides unique signature for diagnosis of copd phenotypes and disease progression. Nat. Med. **18**(11), 1711 (2012)
11. Gevenois, P.A., De Vuyst, P., De Maertelaer, V., Zanen, J., Jacobovitz, D., Cosio, M.G., Yernault, J.C.: Comparison of computed density and microscopic morphometry in pulmonary emphysema. Am. J. Respir. Crit. Care Med. **154**(1), 187–192 (1996)

12. Gould, G., MacNee, W., McLean, A., Warren, P., Redpath, A., Best, J., Lamb, D., Flenley, D.: Ct measurements of lung density in life can quantitate distal airspace enlargement–an essential defining feature of human emphysema. Am. Rev. Respir. Dis. **137**(2), 380–392 (1988)
13. Gurney, J.W.: Pathophysiology of obstructive airways disease. Radiol. Clin. North Am. **36**(1), 15–27 (1998)
14. Han, J., Ma, K.K.: Rotation-invariant and scale-invariant gabor features for texture image retrieval. Image Vis. Comput. **25**(9), 1474–1481 (2007)
15. Haralick, R.M., Shanmugam, K., et al.: Textural features for image classification. IEEE Trans. Syst. Man Cybernet. **6**, 610–621 (1973)
16. Kennedy, J., Eberhart, R.: Particle swarm optimization. In: Proceedings of ICNN'95-International Conference on Neural Networks, vol. 4, pp. 1942–1948. IEEE (1995)
17. Kinsella, M., Müller, N.L., Abboud, R.T., Morrison, N.J., DyBuncio, A.: Quantitation of emphysema by computed tomography using a "density mask" program and correlation with pulmonary function tests. Chest **97**(2), 315–321 (1990)
18. Liang, N.Y., Huang, G.B., Saratchandran, P., Sundararajan, N.: A fast and accurate online sequential learning algorithm for feedforward networks. IEEE Trans. Neural Netw. **17**(6), 1411–1423 (2006)
19. Liang, T.K., Tanaka, T., Nakamura, H., Ishizaka, A.: Automated extraction and diagnosis of lung emphysema from lung ct images using artificial neural network. In: 2006 SICE-ICASE International Joint Conference, pp. 2306–2311. IEEE (2006)
20. Mahanand, B.S., Sateesh Babu, G., Suresh, S.: Meta-cognitive learning neural classifier for Alzheimer's disease detection. In: International Conference on Swarm, Evolutionary, and Memetic Computing, pp. 606–617. Springer (2014)
21. Mahanand, B.S., Sateesh Babu, G., Suresh, S., Sundararajan, N.: Identification of imaging biomarkers responsible for Alzheimer's disease using a McRBFN classifier. In: 2015 International Conference on Cognitive Computing and Information Processing (CCIP), pp. 1–4. IEEE (2015)
22. Mahanand, B.S., Savitha, R., Suresh, S.: Computer aided diagnosis of ADHD using brain magnetic resonance images. In: Australasian Joint Conference on Artificial Intelligence, pp. 386–395. Springer (2013)
23. Mahanand, B.S., Suresh, S., Sundararajan, N., Kumar, M.A.: Alzheimer's disease detection using a Self-adaptive Resource Allocation Network classifier. In: The International Joint Conference on Neural Networks (IJCNN), pp. 1930–1934 (2011)
24. Müller, N.L., Staples, C.A., Miller, R.R., Abboud, R.T.: "density mask": an objective method to quantitate emphysema using computed tomography. Chest **94**(4), 782–787 (1988)
25. Narayanan, S.J., Soundrapandiyan, R., Perumal, B., Baby, C.J.: Emphysema medical image classification using fuzzy decision tree with fuzzy particle swarm optimization clustering. In: Smart Intelligent Computing and Applications, pp. 305–313. Springer (2019)
26. Nava, R., Escalante-Ramírez, B., Cristóbal, G., Estépar, R.S.J.: Extended gabor approach applied to classification of emphysematous patterns in computed tomography. Med. Biol. Eng. Comput. **52**(4), 393–403 (2014)
27. Nava, R., Olveres, J., Kybic, J., Escalante, B., Cristóbal, G.: Feature ensemble for quantitative analysis of emphysema in ct imaging. In: 2015 E-Health and Bioengineering Conference (EHB), pp. 1–4. IEEE (2015)
28. Ojala, T., Pietikainen, M., Maenpaa, T.: Multiresolution gray-scale and rotation invariant texture classification with local binary patterns. IEEE Trans. Pattern Anal. Mach. Intell. **24**(7), 971–987 (2002)
29. Park, Y.S., Seo, J.B., Kim, N., Chae, E.J., Oh, Y.M., Do Lee, S., Lee, Y., Kang, S.H.: Texture-based quantification of pulmonary emphysema on high-resolution computed tomography: comparison with density-based quantification and correlation with pulmonary function test. Investig. Radiol. **43**(6), 395–402 (2008)
30. Pedersen, J.H., Ashraf, H., Dirksen, A., Bach, K., Hansen, H., Toennesen, P., Thorsen, H., Brodersen, J., Skov, B.G., Døssing, M., et al.: The danish randomized lung cancer ct screening trial–overall design and results of the prevalence round. J. Thorac. Oncol. **4**(5), 608–614 (2009)

31. Pei, X.: Emphysema classification using convolutional neural networks. In: International Conference on Intelligent Robotics and Applications, pp. 455–461. Springer (2015)
32. Pena, I.P., Cheplygina, V., Paschaloudi, S., Vuust, M., Carl, J., Weinreich, U.M., Østergaard, L.R., de Bruijne, M.: Automatic emphysema detection using weakly labeled hrct lung images. PloS one **13**(10), (2018)
33. Peng, L., Lin, L., Hu, H., Zhang, Q., Li, H., Chen, Q., Wang, D., Han, X.H., Iwamoto, Y., Chen, Y.W., et al.: Multi-scale deep convolutional neural networks for emphysema classification and quantification. In: Deep Learning in Healthcare, pp. 149–164. Springer (2020)
34. Prasad, M., Sowmya, A., Wilson, P.: Multi-level classification of emphysema in hrct lung images. Pattern Anal. Appl. **12**(1), 9–20 (2009)
35. Rabe, K.F., Hurd, S., Anzueto, A., Barnes, P.J., Buist, S.A., Calverley, P., Fukuchi, Y., Jenkins, C., Rodriguez-Roisin, R., Van Weel, C., et al.: Global strategy for the diagnosis, management, and prevention of chronic obstructive pulmonary disease: Gold executive summary. Am. J. Respir. Crit. Care Med. **176**(6), 532–555 (2007)
36. Runxuan, Z.: Efficient sequential and batch learning artificial neural network methods for classification problems. Singapore **2**, 825–845 (2005)
37. Sateesh Babu, G., Suresh, S.: Meta-cognitive Neural Network for classification problems in a sequential learning framework. Neurocomputing **81**, 86–96 (2012)
38. Sateesh Babu, G., Suresh, S., Mahanand, B.S.: Meta-cognitive q-Gaussian RBF network for binary classification: Application to mild cognitive impairment (MCI). In: The 2013 International Joint Conference on Neural Networks (IJCNN), pp. 1–8. IEEE (2013)
39. Sateesh Babu, G., Suresh, S., Mahanand, B.S.: A novel PBL-McRBFN-RFE approach for identification of critical brain regions responsible for Parkinson's disease. Expert Syst. Appl. **41**(2), 478–488 (2014)
40. Satoh, K., Kobayashi, T., Misao, T., Hitani, Y., Yamamoto, Y., Nishiyama, Y., Ohkawa, M.: Ct assessment of subtypes of pulmonary emphysema in smokers. Chest **120**(3), 725–729 (2001)
41. Shaker, S., Dirksen, A., Laursen, L., Maltbaek, N., Christensen, L., Sander, U., Seersholm, N., Skovgaard, L., Nielsen, L., Kok-Jensen, A.: Short-term reproducibility of computed tomography-based lung density measurements in alpha-1 antitrypsin deficiency and smokers with emphysema. Acta radiologica **45**(4), 424–430 (2004)
42. Sorensen, L., Shaker, S.B., De Bruijne, M.: Quantitative analysis of pulmonary emphysema using local binary patterns. IEEE Trans. Med. Imaging **29**(2), 559–569 (2010)
43. Srivastava, V., Purwar, R.K.: Classification of ct scan images of lungs using deep convolutional neural network with external shape-based features. J. Digit. Imaging, 1–10 (2019)
44. Suresh, S., Dong, K., Kim, H.J.: A sequential learning algorithm for self-adaptive resource allocation network classifier. Neurocomputing **73**(16–18), 3012–3019 (2010)
45. Team, N.L.S.T.R.: Reduced lung-cancer mortality with low-dose computed tomographic screening. New Engl. J. Med. **365**(5), 395–409 (2011)
46. Uppaluri, R., Hoffman, E.A., Sonka, M., Hartley, P.G., Hunninghake, G.W., McLennan, G.: Computer recognition of regional lung disease patterns. Am. J. Respir. Crit. Care Med. **160**(2), 648–654 (1999)
47. Uppaluri, R., Mitsa, T., Hoffman, E.A., McLennan, G., Sonka, M.: Texture analysis of pulmonary parenchyma in normal and emphysematous lung. In: Medical Imaging 1996: Physiology and Function from Multidimensional Images, vol. 2709, pp. 456–467. International Society for Optics and Photonics (1996)
48. Vapnik, V.N.: The Nature of Statistical Learning Theory (1995)
49. Vigneshwaran, S., Mahanand, B.S., Suresh, S., Sundararajan, N.: Using regional homogeneity from functional MRI for diagnosis of ASD among males. In: 2015 International Joint Conference on Neural Networks (IJCNN), pp. 1–8. IEEE (2015)
50. Vigneshwaran, S., Mahanand, B., Suresh, S., Savitha, R.: Autism spectrum disorder detection using projection based learning meta-cognitive rbf network. In: The 2013 International Joint Conference on Neural Networks (IJCNN), pp. 1–8. IEEE (2013)

51. Vigneshwaran, S., Suresh, S., Mahanand, B.S., Sundararajan, N.: ASD detection in males using MRI-an age-group based study. In: 2015 International Joint Conference on Neural Networks (IJCNN), pp. 1–8. IEEE (2015)
52. Vigneshwaran, S., Suresh, S., Sundararajan, N., Mahanand, B.S.: Accurate detection of autism spectrum disorder from structural MRI using extended metacognitive radial basis function network. Expert Syst. Appl. **42**(22), 8775–8790 (2015)
53. Xu, Y., Sonka, M., McLennan, G., Guo, J., Hoffman, E.A.: Mdct-based 3-d texture classification of emphysema and early smoking related lung pathologies. IEEE Trans. Med. Imaging **25**(4), 464–475 (2006)

Analysis of Gaussian and Cauchy Mutations in K-Means Particle Swarm Optimization Algorithm for Data Clustering

Mandakini Priyadarshani Behera, Archana Sarangi, and Debahuti Mishra

Abstract Clustering is an important unsupervised classification process. Some researchers have suggested K-means PSO algorithm to solve clustering problems. But many complex problems require further improvement of the solution. However, in this paper two types of popular mutation techniques are being used with the k-means PSO algorithm for improvement of the clustering problems. In this correspondence Gaussian mutation and Cauchy mutation are two common mutation techniques that are used to mutate the k-means PSO algorithm. The primary objective is to have better convergence as well as accurate results in the solutions of complex problems. The evaluation of the performance of the planned algorithm is done with six datasets and the results have been analyzed well with the existing k-means PSO clustering algorithm. The simulation results showed that both mutation techniques will give better results as compared to the existing k-means PSO clustering algorithm. But Cauchy mutation having stronger ability to escape local optima, effectiveness in results as well as robustness will dominate over Gaussian mutation. This paper verifies that the overall performance of Cauchy mutation operator combining with k-means PSO clustering algorithm is better.

Keywords Particle swarm optimization algorithm · K-means clustering algorithm · K-means PSO clustering algorithm · Gaussian mutation technique · Cauchy mutation technique

1 Introduction

Clustering is a data mining process, in which data is categorized on the basis of similarities and dissimilarities. The main objective of clustering is to arrange the data in groups according to the similarities. Every group is known as a "cluster" that is useful in the decision-making process. Presently, the clustering has become

M. P. Behera · A. Sarangi · D. Mishra (✉)
Department of Computer Science and Engineering, ITER, Siksha 'O' Anusandhan Deemed To Be University, Bhubaneswar, India
e-mail: debahutimishra@soa.ac.in

H. K. Tripathy et al. (eds.), *Technical Advancements of Machine Learning in Healthcare*, Studies in Computational Intelligence 936,
https://doi.org/10.1007/978-981-33-4698-7_6

a popular method used in many fields including statistical data analysis as well as mining, machine learning, pattern recognition, and bioinformatics. Several real-world problems which are generally the problems of optimization are becoming more complicated day by day and traditional optimization algorithms are hard to solve it. However, working on optimization issues in real-world applications has become such a promising research area. In the last few years many researchers have developed many meta-heuristic optimization algorithms focused at problems of clustering. Some authors have explored hybridized algorithm designed by combining PSO with k-means (KM) algorithms [1]. Particle swarm optimization (PSO) is a nature inspired population based meta-heuristic searching algorithm which can be applied to solve various optimization problems. K-means (KM) clustering method is one among the most popular clustering methods which is commonly used. PSO has better global search ability whereas KM is better in local search process. The k-means PSO (KMPSO) algorithm must escape the major drawbacks of vulnerability for the choice of the KM algorithm's initial cluster centers, and is effective in moving from local extreme value and also enhances the rate of convergence of PSO [2]. Nowadays, the KMPSO algorithm is commonly used in the real world. This algorithm because of its programming simplicity and quick operation to find the best possible solution has received considerable attention from researchers and over the previous decades has been widely applied to several optimization problems successfully. But the major drawback of this algorithm is that it presents less accurate solutions. So many modifications have been made in the process of KMPSO clustering algorithm to enhance its performance. In this paper two popular mutation techniques i.e., Gaussian and Cauchy mutation are used to get better the performance of the existing algorithm. Therefore, the modified algorithms are known as Gaussian k-means PSO (GKMPSO) clustering algorithm and Cauchy k-means PSO (CKMPSO) clustering algorithm, respectively. Mutation is a significant technique to extract children from peers and improve the population diversity in describing swarm intelligence. These modifications are proposed only to even further enhancement of the effects of existing KMPSO clustering algorithm. And the outcomes of the suggested clustering algorithm are analyzed properly with the application of datasets. The remaining part of the study is set out as follows. Section 2 describes the detailed literature survey for this study. In Sect. 3 the proposed work is described along with some background study in detail. Section 4 gives the simulation results by using different datasets followed by the conclusion in Sect. 5.

2 Literature Review

Many studies have contributed to the development of the PSO algorithm in order to produce better results, and have combined PSO with other algorithmic approaches. In [1], authors have used clustering methods (KMEAN, PSOKMEAN, and PCAK-MEAN) to boost the cluster outcome according to different parameters (Purity, Random index, and Computational Time) on various datasets retrieved from the UCI

Repository. In [2], researchers have proposed a DMPSO algorithm which will resolve the issues of entanglement into local optima as well as premature convergence while solving complex multimodal problems. In [3], authors have developed a k-means PSO algorithm which addresses the challenge of choosing the initial k-means clustering center and also work on improving the drawbacks of falling easily into the local optima. In [4], authors have presented a comprehensive mapping of recent statistics of swarm-based algorithms that address the clustering problems. They also provided explanation of how well the swarm methods can be implemented with a deep review on present and future scopes in this area. In [5], researchers proposed a hybridized PSO algorithm which employs an adaptive learning process (ALPSO), where a candidate generation process based on self-learning is established. And also, to balance the exploration ability and exploitation ability a tolerance-based search direction adjustment mechanism is designed. In [6], authors have suggested the use of Gaussian mutation and Cauchy mutation techniques in one of the modified versions of very well-known PSO algorithm to get good convergence and fitness outcomes in the solutions of different real-world applications. In [7], researchers have been proposed a competitive swarm optimizer combined along with Cauchy mutation and Gaussian mutation (CGCSO) for huge scale optimization which updates winners' position throughout Cauchy as well as Gaussian mutation for enhancing the capacity of exploitation.

3 Background Study and Computational Techniques

3.1 Particle Swarm Optimization (PSO)

It is a stochastic optimization algorithm based on population. That imitated the individuals' physical movements in the swarm as a method of searching. Every particle is viewed as a point in a D-dimensional searching area, having two attributes, one is the position and another one is the velocity [3]. In this method, position and velocity of every particle of population is being updated by the objective function in order to obtain favorable simulation results. Generally speaking, this algorithm makes use of social interaction between groups [4]. The particles are moving through the search space with a dynamically varying velocity. In each iteration, every particle updates two absolute values: the finest position of the particle so far (personal best) and the finest position in the swarm during that period (global best). The velocity and position of each particle will be updated based on the following Eqs. (1) and (2), respectively.

$$v_{ik}^{(t)} = \omega * v_{ik}^{(t-1)} + c_{pa} * random\left(p_{ik} - x_{ik}^{(t-1)}\right) + c_{ga} * Random\left(p_{gk} - x_{ik}^{(t-1)}\right) \tag{1}$$

$$x_{ik}^{(t)} = x_{ik}^{(t-1)} + v_{ik}^{(t)} \tag{2}$$

where, $v_{ik}^{(t)}$ is taken as the new velocity of the particle, w is considered as the inertia weight, $v_{ik}^{(t-1)}$ is the present velocity of particle, c_{pa} and c_{ga} are personal and global acceleration coefficients, respectively, $random$ and $Random$ are two independent uniformly distributed random variables in a range of [0,1], p_{ik} is the earliest best position of ith particle,$x_{ik}^{(t-1)}$ is the position of particle i in the $t-1$ iteration,p_{gk} is denoted as global best position of the population. $x_{ik}^{(t)}$ is considered as the new position of particle.

3.2 K-Means Clustering Algorithm (KM)

KM is an unsupervised clustering algorithm used for data mining and pattern recognition. The KM algorithm groups the set of data points into a number of predefined clusters in space. For this purpose, the Euclidean distance is widely used as a measure of similarity. The main objective for this algorithm is to combine data points in such a way to reduce the Euclidean distance between data points belonging to each group [4]. The data points on each group cluster are identified by the group centre of mass i.e., cluster centroid. Therefore, the KM algorithm tries to identify the best space points as the centroids of the clusters.

3.3 K-Means PSO Clustering Algorithm (KMPSO)

The KMPSO is an optimization algorithm that combines the PSO along with the KM, can be used for resolving the problems of data clustering. The PSO algorithm is a global searching-based algorithm, with good potential for producing global optimistic results. The rate of convergence of the PSO algorithm closer to the possible solution is extremely slow. In contrast, the KM algorithm converge quickly to a local optimal solution; however its process of obtaining the global solution is slow. The main objective of integrating these methods is to take benefits of both the KM and PSO algorithms. The KMPSO clustering algorithm increases clustering performance, and prevents from being trapped in a local optimal solution [5].

Sequence for the algorithm execution is described in the following way.

Step-1: Initialization of particle position and velocity at random in a d-dimensional problem area and also generate parameters.
Step-2: Compute the fitness for every particle as per clustering criteria.
Step-3: Contrast the currently calculated fitness value with the previously calculated fitness values to choose a better value as the personal best.
Step-4: Update velocity as well as position of the particle based on Eqs. (1) and (2), accordingly.
Step-5: Update personal best and the global best of the particle.
Step-6: Reduce inertia weight.

Step-7: Apply KM clustering algorithm to complete the cluster process of each new-generation particles.
Step-8: Stop if termination condition satisfied and select the best solution; otherwise go to step-2 (Fig. 1).

3.4 Gaussian K-Means PSO Clustering Algorithm (GKMPSO)

Gaussian density function is also known as normal density function. It is described as a result of a random variable calculated by a series of random independent events and the central limit theorem establishes this fact. Gaussian distribution is quite popular as a continuous probability distribution. In statistics, the Gaussian distribution is useful and mostly used in the natural and social sciences to describe randomly generated real variables [6, 7]. The basic necessity of derivation is that the recurrence of the convolution of any finite density function is asymptotically responsible for a Gaussian or regular function [8, 9]. For better clustering results Gaussian mutation operator is integrated along with KMPSO clustering algorithm. Using the Gaussian probability distribution function, the velocity equation can be defined as:

$$v_{ik}^{(t)} = |randomn|\left(p_{ik} - x_{ik}^{(t-1)}\right) + |Randomn|\left(p_{gk} - x_{ik}^{(t-1)}\right) \quad (3)$$

Here, $|randomn|$ and $|Randomn|$ are random generated positive numbers formed based on the absolute value of the Gaussian probability distribution, i.e., $abs[N(0, 1)]$. and $N(0, 1)$ represents a standard deviation of a normal randomly distribution number having zero mean and unit variance.

Sequence for the algorithm execution is described as the following way.

Step-1: Initialization of particle position and velocity at random in a d-dimensional problem area and also generate parameters.
Step-2: Compute the fitness of every particle as per clustering criteria.
Step-3: Contrast the currently calculated fitness value with the previously calculated fitness values to choose a better value as the personal best.
Step-4: Update velocity and position of every particle based on Eqs. (1) and (2), accordingly.
Step-5: Update personal best and global best of the particle.
Step-6: Mutate $v_{ik}^{(t)}$ according to the Eq. (3), now best particle is the current in the Gaussian probability function.
Step-7: Again, by utilizing objective function modify the particle position and determine the global best.
Step-8: Apply the KM clustering algorithm for complete cluster process of each new-generation particles.
Step-9: Stop if termination conditions satisfied select the best solution; otherwise go to step-2 (Fig. 2).

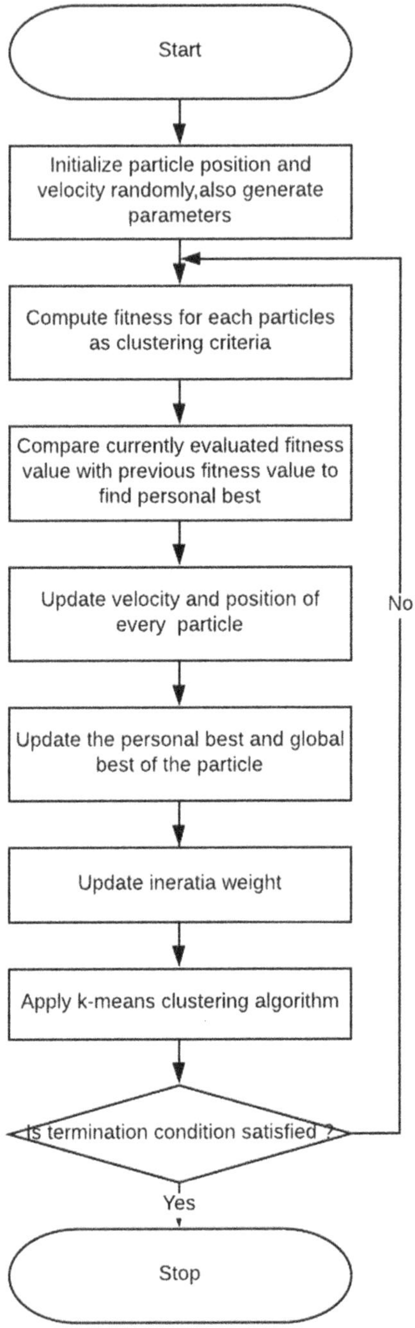

Fig. 1 Flowchart for KMPSO clustering algorithm

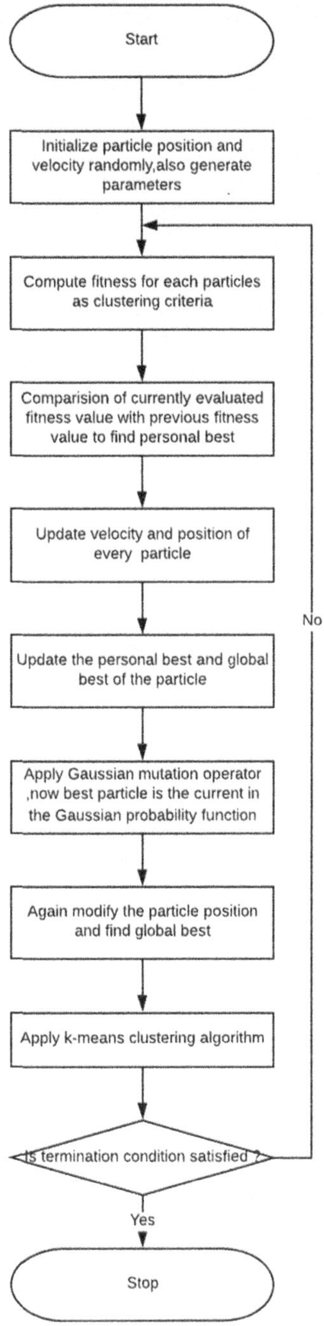

Fig. 2 Flowchart for GKMPSO clustering algorithm

3.5 Cauchy K-Means PSO Clustering Algorithm (CKMPSO)

The utilization of mutation operator in optimization algorithm is not new. Cauchy distribution is assumed to be a continuous distribution of probabilities. Its key objective is to present a minor perturbation in the population from time to time so as to preserve its diversity. Some experimental findings have said that, before convergence, the particle in PSO must switch between the previous best particle and the best global particle observed by each particle. If the search neighbors of the best global particle were included on every iteration, the searching area for the best particle will be extended. This will be beneficial to each particle shifting to the best position. It can be achieved by having a Cauchy mutation operator on the global best particle at each iteration [10]. For better clustering results Cauchy mutation operator is integrated with the KMPSO clustering algorithm.

The Cauchy mutation operator used in this algorithm is described as follows:

$$w(ik) = \left(\sum_{j=1}^{popusize} v[j][i] \right) \Big/ popusize \tag{4}$$

Here, $v[j][i]$ denotes as the ith velocity vector of the jth particle in the population, $popusize$ is considered as the total population, $w(ik)$ is taken as the weight vector in range of $[-w_{\max}, w_{\max}]$, and in this paper $w_{\max} = 1$.

$$p'_{gk}(i) = p_{gk}(i)w(ik) * N(x_{\min}, x_{\max}) \tag{5}$$

and N is a Cauchy distribution function having scaling parameters $t = 1$, $N(x_{\min}, x_{\max})$ is considered as a random number in the range of $[x_{\min}, x_{\max}]$, which acts like a test function domain.

Sequence for the algorithm execution is described as the following way.

Step-1: Initialize the position and velocity of particles randomly in a D-dimensional problem space and also generate parameters.
Step-2: Compute the fitness for every particle as per clustering criteria.
Step-3: Contrast the currently calculated fitness value with the previously calculated fitness values to choose a better value as the personal best.
Step-4: Update velocity and position of every particle based on Eqs. (1) and (2), accordingly.
Step-5: Update the personal best as well as the global best of the particle.
Step-6: Modify the inertia weight based on Eq. (4).
Step-7: Mutate p_{gk} according to Eq. (5).
Step-8: Choose a best particle p_{gk}^{best} from the population. If you have a good fitness value of p_{gk}^{best} than p_{gk} then modify $p_{gk} = p_{gk}^{best}$.

Step-9: Apply the KM clustering algorithm to complete cluster process for all new-generation particles.
Step-10: Stop if termination condition satisfied selects the best solution, otherwise go to step-2 (Fig. 3).

4 Result Analysis

In this section the results obtained of the proposed algorithms have been discussed. The effectiveness of the algorithms i.e., KMPSO clustering algorithm, GKMPSO clustering algorithm, and CKMPSO clustering algorithm has been tested by simulating with six different data sets, including SCADI, EXASENS, IRIS, WDBC, HEART, and WINE, collected from the regular UCI repository. These clustering algorithms are implemented in MATLAB. The parameters setting for KMPSO clustering algorithm, GKMPSO clustering algorithm, and CKMPSO clustering algorithm is described in Table 1. The experimental results obtained are based on the execution time in seconds for six different data sets and are presented in Table 2. Here each data set is described in detail in Table 3. During the experiments, all these discussed algorithms were run with an initial population of random values. The main purpose of the simulation is to reduce the function values and to increase efficiency. For simplicity, the same searching space is taken for all the datasets under simulation. All the experiments have been conducted with a population of 30 particles and 500 iterations. The experimental results obtained by using different data sets are presented in Figs. 4, 5, 6, 7, 8, and 9.

Figures 4 to 9 displays the convergence curve for six different datasets. From these figures it is clearly understood that the convergence curve of CKMPSO clustering algorithm gives better results as compared to both KMPSO clustering algorithm and GKMPSO clustering algorithm. It can also be viewed that the rate of converges of CKMPSO clustering algorithm is higher as compared to both KMPSO clustering algorithms as well as GKMPSO clustering algorithm. The CKMPSO clustering algorithm shows an improvement on performance in comparison to other two algorithms. But on the basis of execution time it is clearly verified that in most of cases the CKMPSO clustering algorithm has highest execution time. This drawback of consuming a very little bit of extra time is manageable as CKPSO clustering algorithm converge faster which leads to a better performance than both KMPSO clustering algorithm and GKMPSO clustering algorithms.

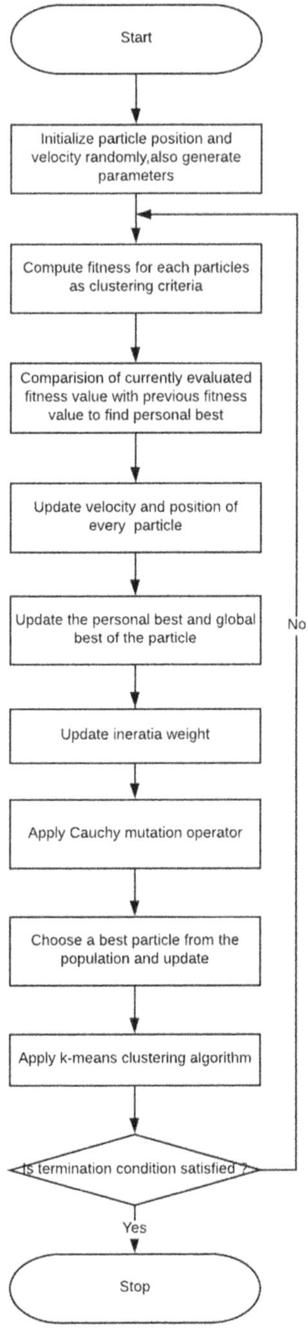

Fig. 3 Flowchart for CKMPSO clustering algorithm

Table 1 Parameters setting for KMPSO, GKMPSO, and CKMPSO clustering algorithms

Parameters	Value
Population	30
Iteration	500
W	1
C1	2
C2	2
W Damp	0.99
K	2

Table 2 Execution time (In Seconds) of different clustering algorithms with used datasets

Datasets used	Algorithms used		
	KMPSO	GKMPSO	CKMPSO
SCADI	8.298	8.343	8.661
EXASENS	9.252	9.297	9.420
IRIS	8.078	8.127	8.211
WDBC	9.448	9.460	9.725
WINE	13.434	13.308	13.581
HEART	8.372	8.413	8.462

Table 3 Data sets design

Datasets	Clustering algorithm used	Instances	Attributes
SCADI	KMPSO	70	206
	GKMPSO		
	CKMPSO		
EXASENS	KMPSO	399	4
	GKMPSO		
	CKMPSO		
IRIS	KMPSO	150	5
	GKMPSO		
	CKMPSO		
WDBC	KMPSO	570	32
	GKMPSO		
	CKMPSO		
WINE	KMPSO	4899	12
	GKMPSO		
	CKMPSO		
HEART	KMPSO	304	14
	GKMPSO		
	CKMPSO		

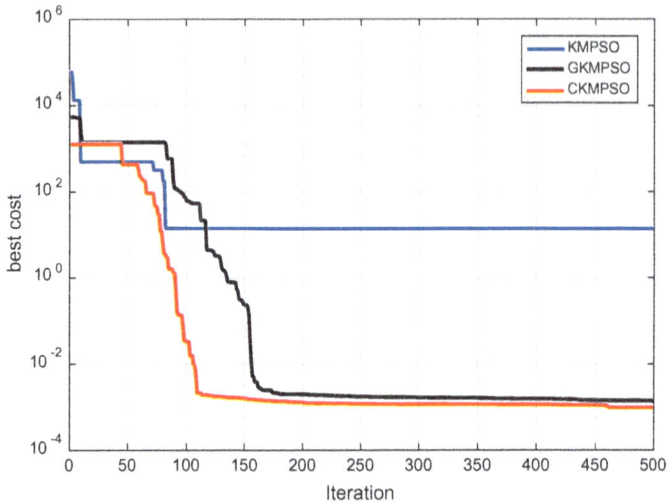

Fig. 4 Convergence curve of SCADI data set

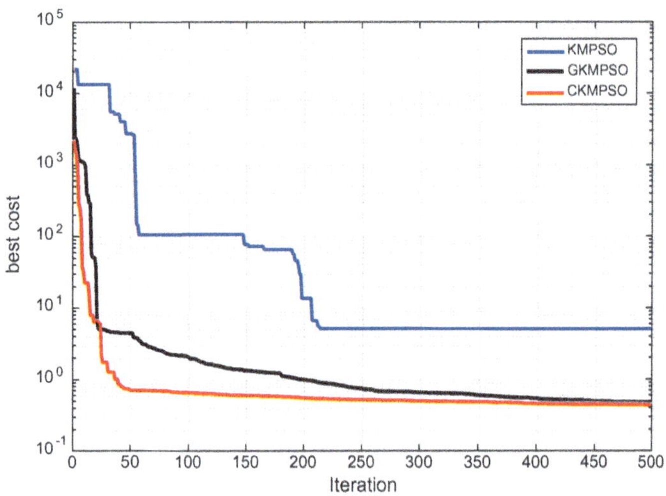

Fig. 5 Convergence curve of EXASENS data set

5 Conclusion

This paper projected two common mutation techniques i.e., Gaussian mutation technique and Cauchy mutation techniques in combination with KMPSO clustering algorithm. Our experimental outcomes show that both the Gaussian and Cauchy mutations are efficient and strong methods for performance development of KMPSO

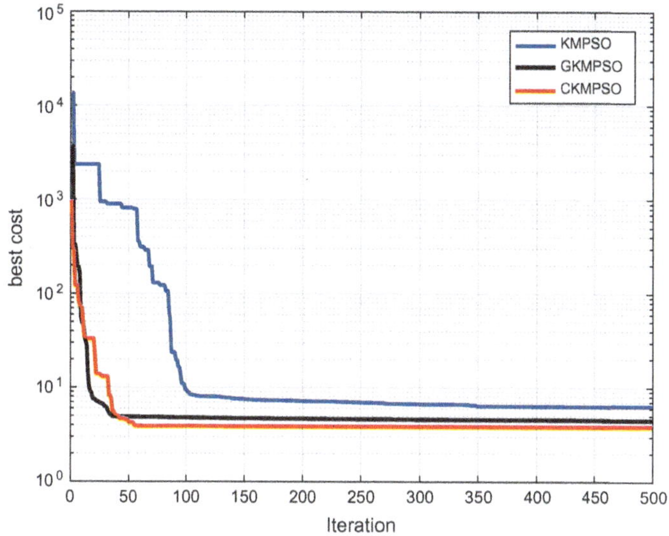

Fig. 6 Convergence curve of IRIS data set

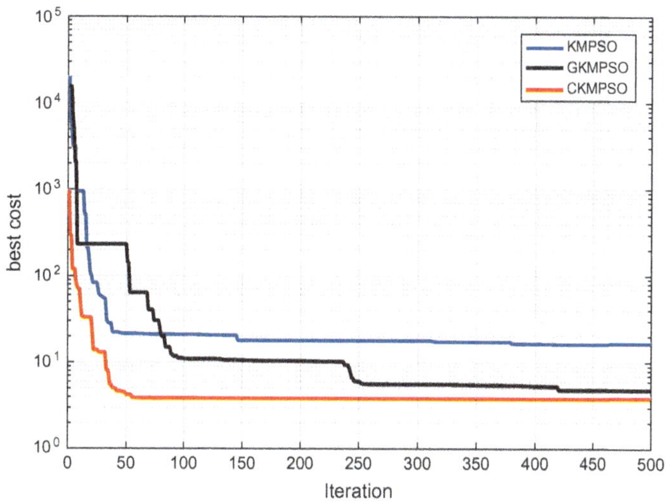

Fig. 7 Convergence curve of WDBC data set

clustering algorithm. In between these two mutation techniques the Cauchy mutation technique has much more strength to escape the local optima and to converge the global optimum and its performance is slight better than the Gaussian mutation technique. In general, the slight extra time consumption during the execution cycle is manageable with higher accuracy result. As both the mutations are easy to implement

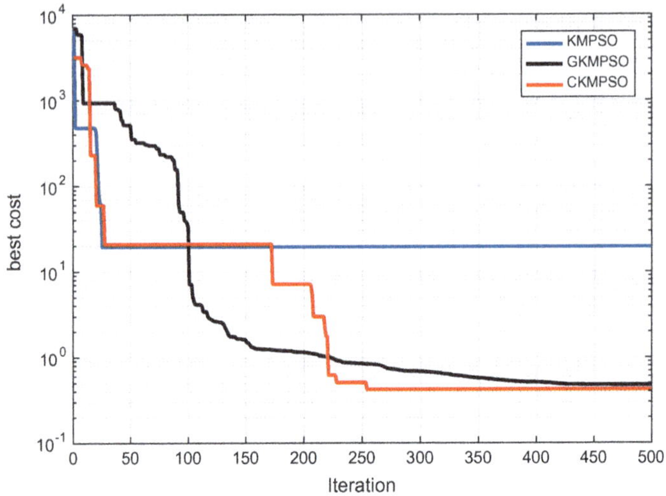

Fig. 8 Convergence curve of WINE data set

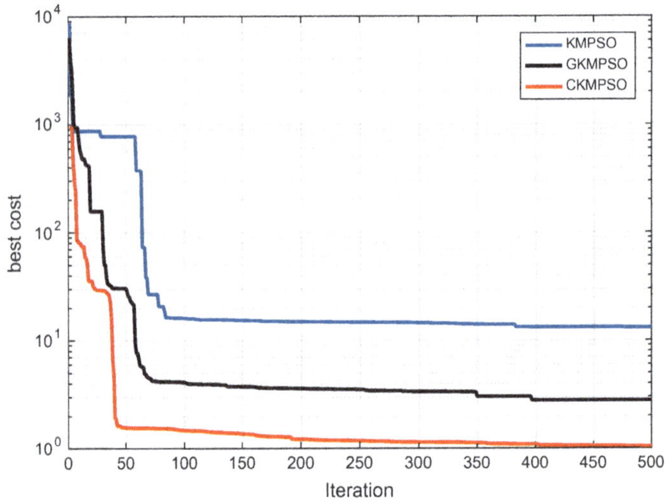

Fig. 9 Convergence curve of HEART data set

and simple to handle any of these two techniques can be applicable for real world optimization problem. But for more accuracy clustering results CKMPSO clustering algorithm can be suggested.

References

1. Malik, H., Laghari, N., Sangrasi, D.M., Dayo, Z.A.:Comparative Analysis of Hybrid Clustering Algorithm on Different Dataset. In: 2018 8th International Conference on Electronics Information and Emergency Communication (ICEIEC), pp. 25–30. Beijing (2018). https://doi.org/10.1109/ICEIEC.2018.8473568
2. Tian, D., Zhao, X., Shi, Z.: DMPSO: diversity-guided multi-mutation particle swarm optimizer. IEEE Access **7**, 124008–124025 (2019). https://doi.org/10.1109/ACCESS.2019.2938063
3. Chen, X., Miao, P., Bu, Q.:Image segmentation algorithm based on particle swarm optimization with k-means optimization. In: 2019 IEEE International Conference on Power, Intelligent Computing and Systems (ICPICS), Shenyang, China, pp. 156–159 (2019). https://doi.org/10.1109/ICPICS47731.2019.8942442
4. Elliackin, F., Macedo, M., Siqueira, H. V., Santana, C. J., Gokhale, A., Bastos-Filho, C. J. A.: Swarm intelligence for clustering—A systematic review with new perspectives on data mining. Eng. Appl. Artif. Intell. **82**, 313–329 (2019) ISSN 0952-1976
5. Wang, F., Zhang, H., Li, K., Lin, Z., Yang, J., Shen, X-L.: A hybrid particle swarm optimization algorithm using adaptive learning strategy. Inf. Sci. **436–437**, 162–177 (2018) ISSN 0020-0255
6. Sarangi, A., Samal, S., Sarangi, S. K.:Analysis of gaussian & cauchy mutations in modified particle swarm optimization algorithm. In: 2019 5th International Conference on Advanced Computing and Communication Systems (ICACCS), Coimbatore, India, pp. 463–467. (2019). https://doi.org/10.1109/ICACCS.2019.8728452
7. Zhang, Q., Cheng, H., Ye, Z., Wang, Z.:A competitive swarm optimizer integrated with Cauchy and Gaussian mutation for large scale optimization. In: 2017 36th Chinese Control Conference (CCC), Dalian, pp. 9829–9834(2017).https://doi.org/10.23919/ChiCC.2017.8028924
8. Krohling, R. A., dos Santos Coelho, L.:Coevolutionary particle swarm optimization using gaussian distribution for solving constrained optimization problems.In: IEEE Transactions on Systems, Man, and Cybernetics, Part B (Cybernetics), vol. 36, no. 6, pp. 1407–1416. (2006). https://doi.org/10.1109/TSMCB.2006.873185
9. Krohling, R. A.:Gaussian swarm: a novel particle swarm optimization algorithm. In: IEEE Conference on Cybernetics and Intelligent Systems, 2004, Singapore, vol. 1, pp. 372–376. (2004). https://doi.org/10.1109/ICCIS.2004.1460443
10. Wang, H., Li, C., Liu, Y., Zeng, S.:A hybrid particle swarm algorithm with cauchy mutation. In: 2007 IEEE Swarm Intelligence Symposium, Honolulu, HI, pp. 356–360. (2007).https://doi.org/10.1109/SIS.2007.367959

Emergence of Drug Discovery in Machine Learning

Subhrojyoti Narayan Roy, Sushruta Mishra, and Shafiz Mohd Yusof

Abstract The discovery of drugs and its pipelines formulation is tough, long, and depend on various factors. Machine Learning comes as a savior to this field and supplies different tools and techniques that are used to drastically improve the discovery as well as the decision-making capabilities for questions that have been well specified and already have an abundant amount of high quality data. There are several possibilities in each and every stage of drug discovery to apply Machine Learning tools and techniques. The applications of Machine Learning have proved from time to time that with some of its approaches generating accurate predictions and insights are very easy. Thus its application has not only been limited to the theoretical part of drug discovery, but has also proven that it can be used in practical conditions too. But there are certain challenges that we need to face that come with Machine Learning. Its inadequacy in terms of interpreting and repeating in its results may sometimes pose as a hindrance to their application in some areas. It also requires consistent and comprehensive high-quality data in almost all areas. There are continuous efforts being put to find a solution for such problems and also growing the reach of machine learning to new fields. Machine Learning can boost data-driven decision-making in this field and has the capability to accelerate the whole process and lessen the failure rates in drug discovery and development.

Keywords Drug discovery · Machine learning · Classification · Supervised learning

S. N. Roy · S. Mishra (✉)
School of Computer Engineering, Kalinga Institute of Industrial Technology, Patia, Bhubaneswar, Odisha, India
e-mail: sushruta.mishrafcs@kiit.ac.in

S. N. Roy
e-mail: ssubhrojyotiroy@gmail.com

S. M. Yusof
Faculty of Engineering and Information Sciences, University of Wollongong, Dubai, UAE
e-mail: ShafizMohdYusof@uowdubai.ac.ae

H. K. Tripathy et al. (eds.), *Technical Advancements of Machine Learning in Healthcare*, Studies in Computational Intelligence 936,
https://doi.org/10.1007/978-981-33-4698-7_7

1 Introduction

Various machine learning techniques have revolutionized several fields related to artificial intelligence, for example, fields like computer vision, natural language processing have taken huge leaps in development in recent years. Non-artificial intelligence fields like B2B sales and marketing have also hugely benefited from the introduction of machine learning techniques in their respective fields. There is still one question that remains unanswered and that is, will it be able to transform the fields of medicine the same way it did to other fields?

Each day we give rise to a massive amount of unstructured and noisy data. One of the biggest advantages of using deep neural nets is their unique ability to develop complex and appropriate features without the need to code them by hand explicitly. There has been a lot of progress that has been made, and strong and compelling ideas have been proposed and are being developed currently. Figure 1 gives a pictorial view of the combination of drug and technology and how technology can help us with the whole process of drug discovery.

There is a lot of excitement that comes from the general population and academic community whenever there is new drug discovery, especially if it cures an incurable disease. Drug discovery is a crucial element for healthcare development and human well being. We all know drug discovery can be a very expensive business. It can take years sometimes to find the correct cure for a pandemic. On average it is estimated that a single pharmaceutical company spends about 10–15 years in making a drug and close to $4 billion to bring the new drug to the market. That's a huge amount of time, money, and risk to put into something when other pharmaceutical companies are

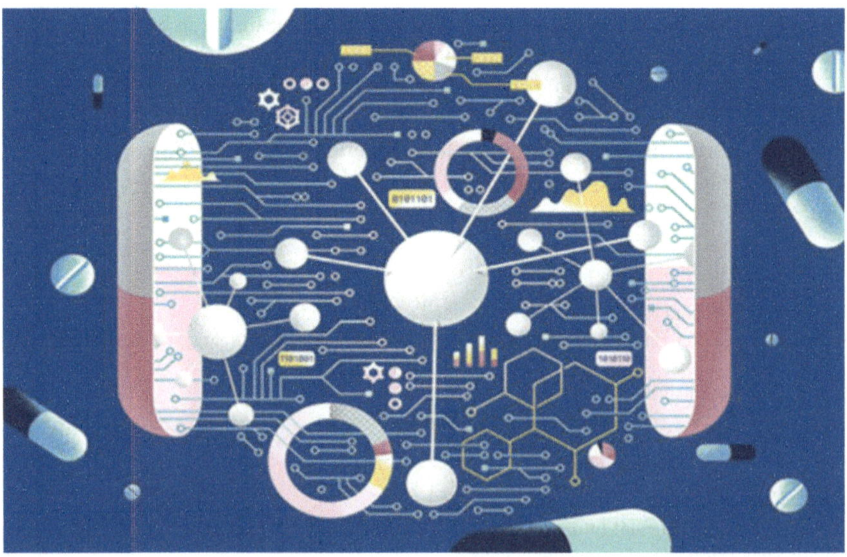

Fig. 1 Amalgamation of drug & technology

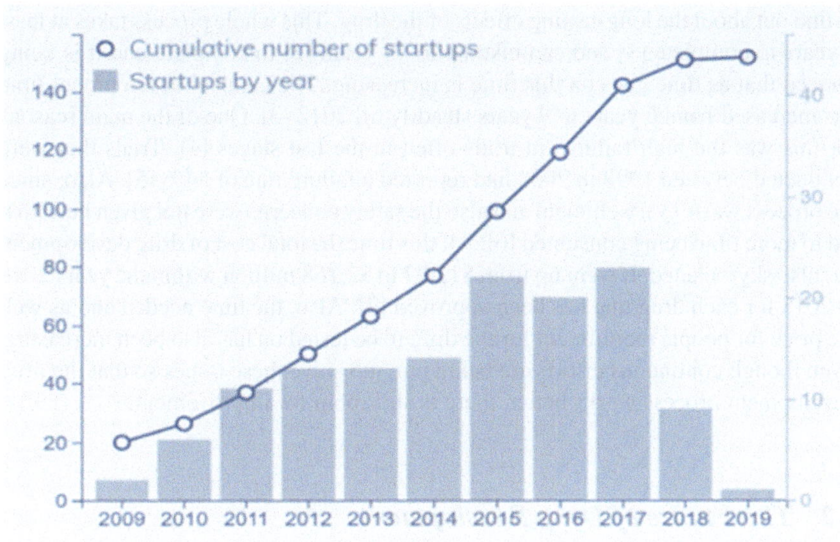

Fig. 2 Growth in AI start-ups in the field of drug discovery

also competing to sell their version of that drug on the market. Once the medicine is created, it's time for the testing phase. The clinical trial is very important as it decides the effectiveness of a medicine. For that, pharmaceutical companies require a lot of volunteers who are ready to bear everything that comes with the cure which is very risky for the people involved in the trial as well as the company. This process can put a pharmaceutical company's existence in jeopardy as it is so risky and unsafe. On top of that, the companies need to provide insurance to these volunteers before performing any experiments on them, given if something goes wrong. This only adds up to the overall expenditure of developing a drug, let alone the costs of bringing it to the market. With all these risks in hand, the number of A.I. enabled start-ups for Drug discoveries is growing at a steady rate as shown in Fig. 2. The year 2017 saw the biggest rise in A.I. enabled start-ups as shown in the Figure below.

1.1 Current Context in Drug Development

Drug Discovery has always been a long and high expenditure process. This is mainly to ensure the patients' health safety and also to boost the effectiveness of the drug. The whole process of drug development is divided into many different phases. The first phase is called Phase 0 and this consists of basic research and tests. This stage mainly aims at finding out how effective and how efficient the drug is and also how the body reacts to it. The other three stages are used for clinical trials (Phase I, Phase II, and Phase III). Sometimes, there is another phase called Phase IV, which is used to find out about the long-lasting effects of the drug. This whole process takes at least 5 years to complete [1] and can take up to 15 years [2] to complete and it is being noticed that as time goes on this time is increasing. The Clinical development time has increased from 6 years to 9 years steadily till 2012 [3]. One of the main reasons for this was the high failures in trials often in the last stages [4]. Trials that were conducted between 1998 to 2008 had reported a failure rate of 54% [5]. Also, since the process wasn't very efficient and also the safety concerns were not given heed to it led to more time being consumed [6]. All this time the total cost of drug development has also skyrocketed. It went up from $1,477 to $2,168 million within the years 2010 to 2018 for each drug that has been approved [7]. Also, the time needed and as well the price for people recruitment for the drug to be tested on has also been increasing. Even though continuous efforts are being put into solve these issues so that the drug development process works better, there is still room for improvement.

1.2 The Future of Drug Development

Most of the pharmaceutical companies are trying to focus on diseases that will be profitable for them, as the whole process of development takes a long time and is very costly, although a few efforts have been made to promote research for diseases that are not very profitable [8]. There has been an increase in the number of drug development processes for cancer therapy as well as for anti-infective drugs. The most popular and studied drug development pipeline has been breast cancer, lung cancer, and Alzheimer's disease. But this also means that the numbers of patients also affect the drug discovery process and diseases with a limited number of people may get drugs developed after a long period of time. Till now we have understood that drug discovery is a long process and also an expensive one. One way of tackling both of these problems is by automating some of the tasks which require a lot of workforce as well as resources. For this reason, there has been a huge increase in the association of ML and AI companies with pharmaceutical labs and research centers. These companies are contributing hugely to the field of bioinformatics. Machine learning [9], Artificial Intelligence and robotics [10] are being used hugely to automate certain parts of the drug development process. This allows the drug development processes to get faster and also saves time and money by not making mistakes that generally humans make. It is estimated that [11] their usage could indeed shorten up the drug candidate identification phase from a few months to one year. Although we should be cautious and not completely be dependent on these methods to solve the failure rate problem [12]. But, with the help of ML in drug development we can not only decrease the cost of drug development [13] but, also make the therapies more oriented toward the patient [14, 15].

1.3 Toward an Automated Search for Therapies

To fully understand the research that is being done in drug development it is suggested to read the introductory parts of the referenced papers [13, 16–18]. Although a fully automated process for drug development may seem like a dream now [16], with continuous efforts from fields like biology, mathematics, computer science there is a great chance of it happening within our lifetimes. Efforts from the mentioned fields may not have completely automated the drug development process, but it has certainly helped in fastening and also lowering the costs in the entire drug development processes. The use of ML methods is useful only when there is a large quantity of high-quality data present about the drugs and their therapeutic indications, their interactions within the body of the patient, factors affecting those drugs, etc.

2 Use of Machine Learning in Drug Discovery

Developing a new drug usually generates a vast amount of data. In these areas whether data generation is so high, machine learning provides a huge opportunity to process this data and predict outcomes that can make the process of drug development much easier and better. All the data that has been created and stored over the years can be processed by using the tools and techniques provided by machine learning. Machine learning helps us in making much more decisions with greater confidence. Research firms like McKinsey state that, there can be a generation of around $300 billion in revenue every year in the healthcare sector if we can utilize Big Data and Machine learning to its full potential. Machine learning could aid hugely with predictive modeling of biological processes as suggested by many experts. Figure 3 gives us a pictorial representation of machine learning helping in increasing drug discovery capabilities such as target identification. Time taken to develop medications will be much less if these technologies are incorporated earlier into the processes of drug discovery.

Opportunities for the biochemical and pharmaceutical industries have been increased hugely with the introduction of machine learning to their development processes. It allows a better understanding of the vast amounts of data that are being produced. This can potentially improve a lot of the processes and outcomes in the pharmaceutical industries. The combination of big data with machine learning is contributing massively to helping with the expenditure and deadlines of developing a drug. New molecules that have shown promise and are highly potential can be identified by predictive modeling of biological processes and drugs and developed with a high probability of success. Computer-processing power has developed exponentially over the past two decades. Combine this with the present availability of big data sets and the development of much more complex as well as efficient algorithms. All these developments have brought major improvements to the field of machine learning. AI now can focus on much more specific tasks rather than more generalized

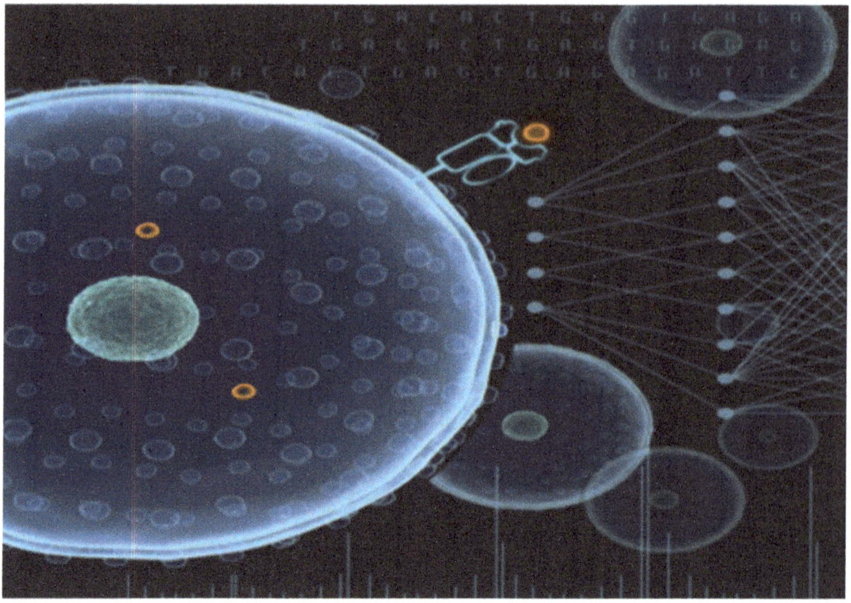

Fig. 3 Incorporating AI with drug discovery

tasks that were done in the early days. AI has hugely improved in terms of analyzing, understanding the data. Techniques like natural language processing and artificial neural networks have become hugely popular as they are designed in a way to mimic the way our human brain works. Below Fig. 4 represents small molecules for drug discovery. The use of ML in such fields also results in very good results and will be discussed in brief as the chapter goes on. All this progress has also started a new wave of start-ups that are focused on AI for drug discovery, with many of them using it to find hidden patterns in the vast volumes of chemical data.

2.1 Helping Cancer Patients Through AI: BERG

The Boston based company Berg, Massachusetts, mainly deals in the sector of biotechnology. The company has developed a model that is able to find out new mechanisms of cancer that were previously unknown. This was achieved by performing several tests on both cancerous and healthy human cell samples. The company has created an AI platform that it uses to analyze the biological data that comes from the patients to understand better the difference between a normal cell that is healthy and a cell that is diseased. The Company's key focus is to develop treatments for diseases based on the biological origin of the diseases. The company doesn't focus on the traditional trial and error approach, rather it believes in using data generated from the patients and their respective biology to come up with better and more-predictive

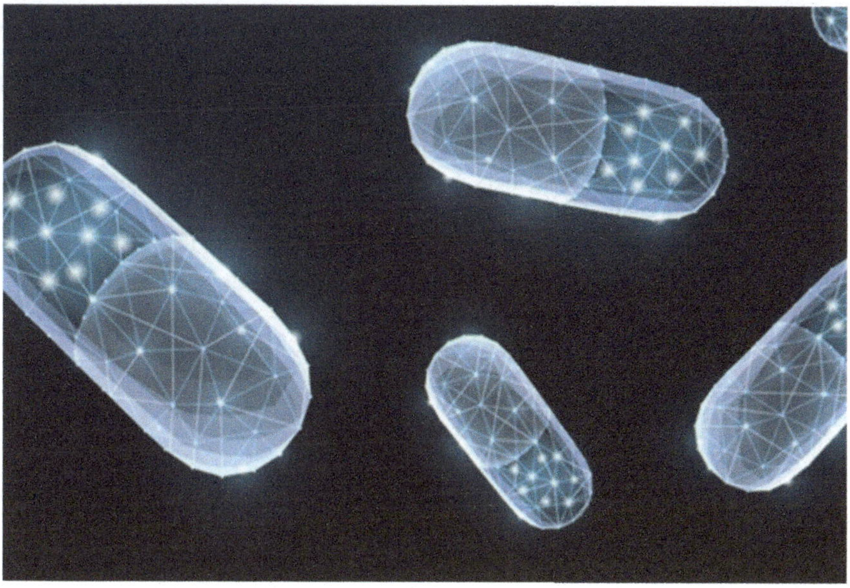

Fig. 4 Small molecules for drug discovery

hypotheses. With this unique approach, they have been able to understand the presence of certain molecules which occur naturally in cancer metabolism. Researchers there have now understood how new cancer drugs work and have also shown some uses in the healing of the disease. The company is also working on diabetes and Parkinson's disease and is looking for therapies for these diseases as well.

2.2 *AI Taking the Charge Here: BenevolentBio*

BenevolentBio is a London-based start-up firm that also has its own AI platform. It is run by Jackie Hunter, CEO, Director, BenevolentBio. She has expressed her feelings about the use of AI in drug discovery and recommends adopting AI as soon as possible when it comes to pharmaceutical companies that want to be successful. They feed this AI platform with data from sources such as research papers, patents, clinical trials, and patient records, etc. Their AI platform then forms a representation. This representation includes more than one billion known and deduced relationships between biological entities such as genes, symptoms, diseases, proteins, and tissues, etc. The AI platform that the company uses has the ability to perform like a search engine and thus it can be queried like one. It is generally used to create 'knowledge graphs'. It creates 'knowledge graphs' of a different medical condition and the genes that are associated with the medical condition. It can also show the compounds that seem to affect it. The company uses ML techniques like natural language processing to recognize entities and understand their relationships to other things as most of the entities the AI platform receives isn't well annotated. The company queried their AI platform that they developed to suggest new ways to treat amyotrophic lateral sclerosis (ALS), also known as motor neuron disease (MND). The AI platform then found out around 100 already existing compounds as having potential. Among the 100 existing compounds, researchers at BenevolentBio selected five compounds to undergo tests using patient-derived cells at the Sheffield Institute of Translational Neuroscience, UK. It was also found after further research out of the five compounds selected that four of these compounds had promise in them, and one of them was shown to delay neurological symptoms in mice.

2.3 *Robots for Drug Discovery?*

On June 12, 2007, a robot called Adam discovered the function of a yeast gene. With this discovery human beings' dominance over the discovery of scientific knowledge would end. Adam did this by exploring various public databases, and then came upon hypotheses about the particular genes code for enzymes that catalyze reactions in the yeast named Saccharomyces cerevisiae. Adam also physically tested its predictions using robotics in a lab. These results were then cross-checked by researchers and it was found out of the 19 genes on which Adam's hypotheses were checked, nine were new and correct and only one was wrong. Eve was created in January by the same team that had developed Adam. It was considered that Eve was Adam's more advanced robot colleague. Soon Eve was put into work and it discovered triclosan, a common ingredient in toothpaste, which had the potential to treat drug-resistant malaria parasites.

3 Stages of Drug Development

To understand better how Machine Learning is used in Drug Discovery, it would be wise to understand first the stages of drug development as seen in Fig. 5. The different stages of drug development are as follows.

3.1 *Successful Applications in Drug Discovery*

Target selection and validation: History suggests that research in the pharmaceutical sector started from observing medical effects. The new world of drug designing is based on analyzing the biological paths and therefore making it easier to identify 'druggable' targets.

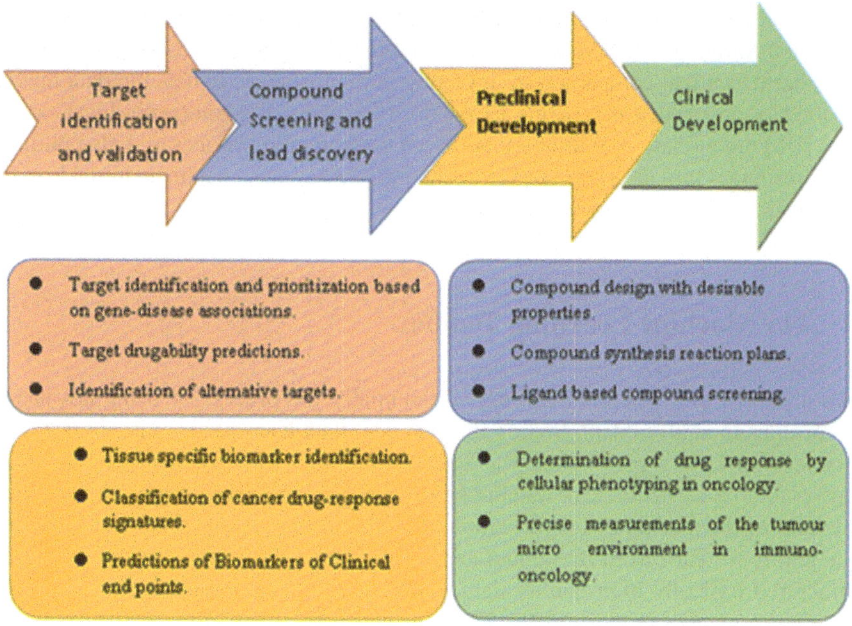

Fig. 5 Drug discovery life cycle and its successful applications

Hit discovery: Library compounds are scanned in vast quantities, as much as possible to reveal new activities. It might sound like a very big task, but the fact is that a million compounds is actually a very tiny proportion of the whole chemical world. The screening depends mostly on the robotics and automation present in the laboratory. There is also something called virtual. This process aims at almost the same type of screening but using software instead only.

Hit to lead: Here, we restrict the optimization of possible hits to increase the affinity. The data for (V) HTS is vast but it has very low accuracy. So, any potential hits have to be confirmed before. This is generally done by using multiple independent types of assays.

Lead optimization: Here the process starts to generate feasible candidates for the drug by further optimization of the drug candidates. There are various other factors than target affinity that contribute in deciding whether a compound can be a practically viable medicine. Some other factors include pharmaceutical codynamics—which refers to the biochemical and physical effects of drugs on the living organism) and pharmaceutical co kinetics.

Machine Learning is applicable to each and every stage of drug discovery and its development. All the stages should be on board with utilizing the advanced ML algorithms we have today combined with high computational power and the availability of large data sets in today's world. This will help us in easily finding more novel targets. This incorporation of ML will also better prove for associations between the target and the disease, modify the small-molecule compound design and optimization for the good, develop new biomarkers for prognosis, etc. Already most of the pharmaceutical companies are investing in the resources to develop data that is needed to support research in this area of drug discovery. Big companies like Google and IBM are already providing cloud-based computation services and also putting their resources into the pharmaceutical and healthcare space to gain an initial lead in this field as it has shown great promise.

4 The Machine Learning Toolbox

We all know that machine learning is essentially the process of using advanced algorithms to analyze data, finding insights, and then learning from it and last but, not least making a prediction. Machine learning generally gives a computer the power to do a particular task without being explicitly trained to do so. This is done by training the machine with vast amounts of data on top of algorithms that provide the ability to learn from these data and perform the job. As the amount of clean, structured basically high-quality data increases, the ML models tend to improve their performances proportionally. Thus, the best uses of ML are in areas where the problem at hand has already huge amounts of data present and the only unknown part is the formula relating this data. Machine learning broadly can be divided into two types: Supervised and Unsupervised learning as seen in Fig. 6. Supervised learning is useful in areas where the output values are data categories or continuous variables; whereas unsupervised learning is useful in places where exploratory data analysis is required. Different types of machine learning algorithms are required for different scenarios. Sometimes the problem at hand might be a classification problem, where we need to divide the data into different labels or sometimes it may be a regression problem where the output value is actually a continuous value or sometimes we may not have labeled data at all and might have to depend upon unsupervised machine learning techniques like clustering as shown in Fig. 7. These associations help us to

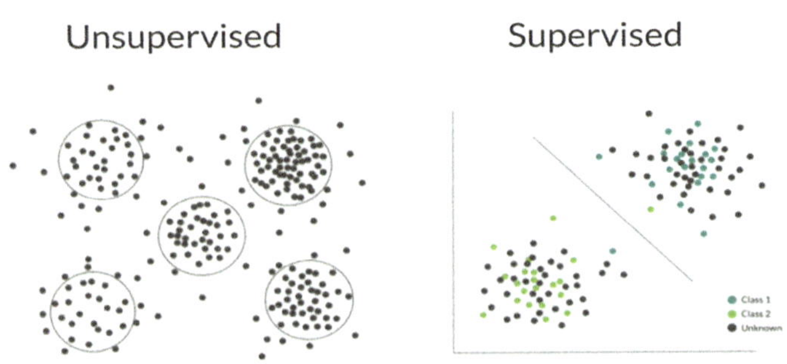

Fig. 6 Supervised versus unsupervised learning

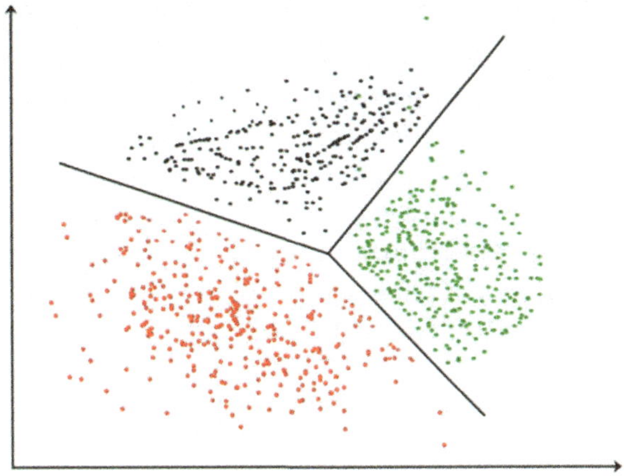

Fig. 7 Clustering in machine learning

find out patterns in the data to get better insights from it and thus understand the data better.

In Supervised learning, the model is trained upon known input and output data relationships so that it can be useful in predicting outcomes for new inputs in the future. In unsupervised learning, the algorithms try to find hidden patterns in the input data and then cluster this data in purposeful ways to find some good insights about the data [19, 20].

5 Model Selection Concepts

The job of a good ML model is to perform well is to generalize the training data that it has been trained upon, to the test data that we have at hand. Generalization basically refers to the concept of how well the model has been trained, and how well the concepts present in the data were learned by the model apply to the new data that the model was not trained upon during training. Each technique has its methods. These vary from prediction accuracy, time taken to train the amount of variables they can handle. Algorithms should be used and chosen on the type of problem statement we have at hand while keeping the factors of amount and the type of data we have in our minds. Figure 8 depicts the different types of machine learning techniques that are most popularly used in today's world. It also shows which algorithms are generally used for different drug discovery, biological related fields.

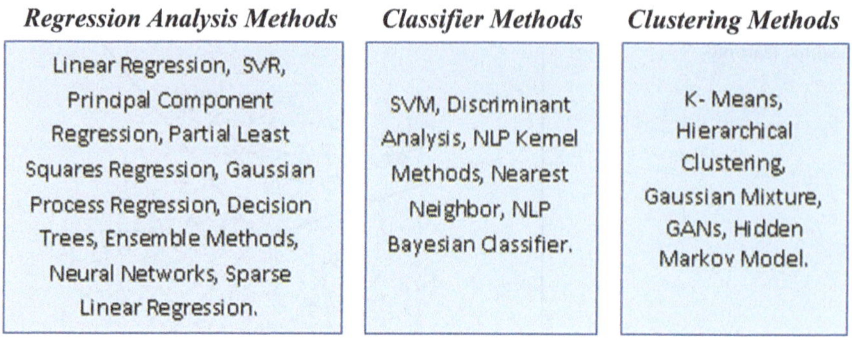

Fig. 8 Different machine learning algorithms used in drug discovery

5.1 Generalized ML Concepts

The figure shown above describes the various machine learning techniques that are currently being used in today's world to accelerate the processes of drug discovery. Supervised learning techniques here are more focused on answering questions related to the fields of prediction of data labels and continuous values; whereas unsupervised learning is more focused on finding patterns in the data present and allow clustering of the data. But with these techniques comes its own range of problems too. One such problem would be Model Over-fitting. This problem occurs when the model starts to learn the noise as well as the signals present in the training data. When this model is brought to the real world it results in bad results, which impact the performance of the whole model. The model performs very poorly on the new data that is being poured into it in the real world. This over-fitting problem results in great training accuracy, but bad testing accuracy. Another big problem that comes with training models is under-fitting and it is actually the situation when the model can neither provide good results on the training data nor on new data. Here the model fails to catch the signals present in the data and thus fails in providing a good training or testing accuracy [21].

There are many methods to prevent over-fitting in our models, like to use resampling methods or to keep a part of the data set separated from the start and use it later as a validation data set. Validation set is used generally to tune the model hyper-parameters. Regularized regression methods such as Ridge regression (L1), LASSO regression (L2) or elastic nets, are also used in the Figure against over-fitting. These models add penalties to the parameters of the model, forcing it not to create a complex model and rather generalize the data. This results in much better predictions. The below picture depicts the regularization term that penalizes the model, resulting in a much more generalized simple model performing better in the real world.

Another popular method for avoiding over-fitting is the dropout method. This method just randomly removes some units present in the hidden layer. But how do we actually test whether our models are working or not? For that, we have various evaluation metrics such as the area under the curve (AUC) which is used to evaluate classification models, classification accuracy, and logarithmic loss—used to evaluate classification models example. From the confusion matrix, we can further derive metrics such as recall (sensitivity), precision, accuracy, etc. These metrics can be used to understand the performances of different classification models.

In recent years the availability of better quality data sets has surged massively and as we know better quality data sets results in better model fitting which is truly priceless in making high and efficient performing models. With the rise of machine learning, several software libraries have also come up to perform the difficult mathematical computation associated with this field. These computations are done on a collection of platforms like tensor processing units (TPUs), Graphical processing units (GPUs), and central processing units (CPUs). In recent years, GPUs have proven themselves to very useful in the case of training large models. The parallel processing power of the GPUs highly accelerates the process of training the models. ML has a big advantage in almost each and every field as most of its commonly used frameworks are open-sourced. This leads to a larger community of people contributing to the growth of this technology and thus widening its reach. Popular frameworks like Tensor flow, PyTorch, Keras, and Scikit-learn have already been made open-sourced and are helping in running in several open-sourced applications every day.

5.2 Deep Neural Network Architectures

Deep Learning is generally based on the ANNs (Artificial Neural Network) and is a part of the AI ecosystem. It uses multiple deep neural networks as seen in Fig. 9 simultaneously to create models that are capable of detecting features from large amounts of data be it labeled or unlabeled.

Deep Learning and artificial neural networks generally differ in the areas of scale as well as the complexity of the networks that are used in them, respectively. Neural Networks are generally very easy to understand, we have an input layer through which we feed the data into the model. This data is then taken by the hidden layers present after the input layer. Here, non-linear transformations are done on the features and then it is passed on to the output layer where the predictions are generated. Deep Learning needs to have a higher number of hidden layers because the computational power required by it is much higher than traditional neural networks. Generally, traditional neural networks use one or two hidden layers. This is because of the lack of high computational power present back in the day and the use of hardware was limited. There have also been advancements in the algorithms that Deep Learning uses. Deep learning may consist of numerous amount of hidden layers to process the data received from the input layer. Deep learning requires much more powerful hardware platforms than general CPUs. That is why with the rise of Deep learning, the rise of using GPUs for it has also risen. Traditionally neural networks had only 1 or 2 hidden layers as the hardware was not able to support any more computation

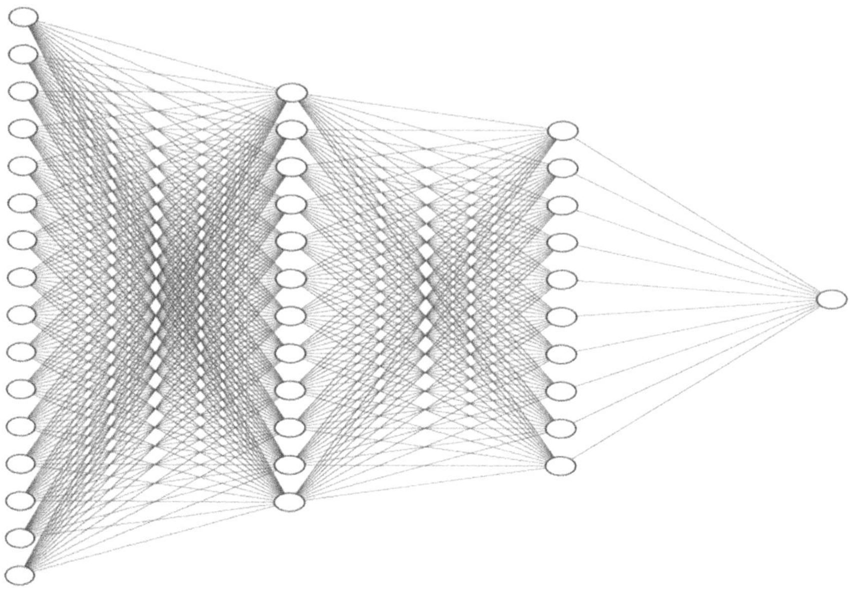

Fig. 9 A general deep neural network

in those days. Deep Learning has led to huge developments in fields like Computer Vision and Natural Language Processing.

Since its inception Deep learning has led to applications in various fields and the field of drug discovery isn't a stranger to it. Some of its biggest application includes biological-image analysis, molecular design, synthesis prediction, and bio-activity prediction, etc. Deep learning is also not restricted to specific problems only thus having several different architectures that can be used for different purposes. CNNs (Convolution Neural Networks) were one such architecture that has proved its worth time and again as seen in Fig. 10. They are best used for speech and image recognition. There are also different types of CNNs. As an example, Graph convolution networks where graphs or networks are applied to the data.

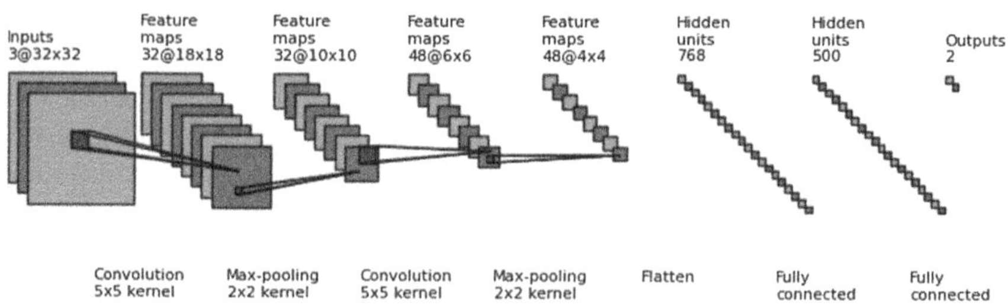

Fig. 10 Working of a CNN

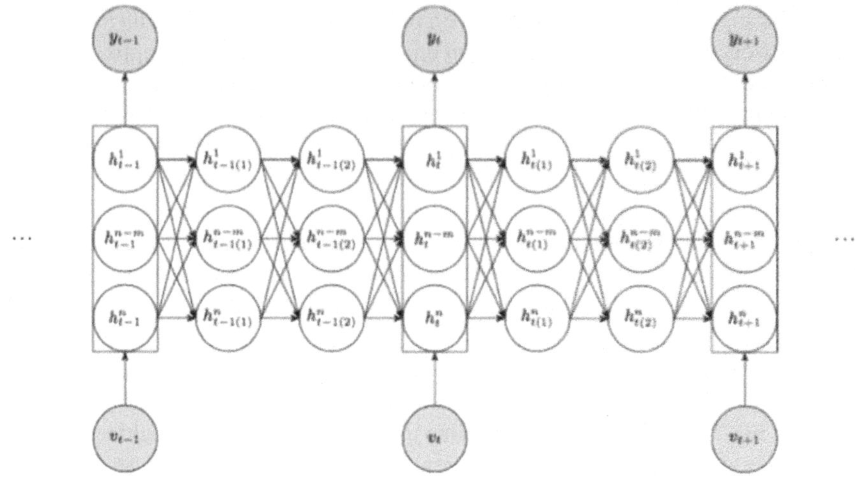

Fig. 11 A simple RNN

Recurrent neural network (RNN) represents another interesting form of deep neural networks. It is like a chain of repeating modules in a neural network. RNNs as shown in Fig. 11 are generally used for the analysis of dynamic changes over time. It is generally used in places where everlasting information is required. Long short-term memory neural networks are also a type of RNN; these networks are mostly focused on understanding dependencies which are long term.

Generative adversarial networks generally constitute two arbitrary networks. Usually, the combination of feed-forward neural networks and CNNs is the most prominent. In GANs one of the network's duties is to produce content and the other network's job is to classify that content.

6 Applications of ML in Drug Discovery

6.1 Target Identification and Validation

Drug discovery begins with the approach of developing drugs that will have its affect on the disease state. We start the process with target identification that has a viable therapeutic hypothesis. This process of selecting the target on the basis of evidence that we have gathered is called as target identification and prioritization. Then, we come to validating the role of the chosen target. This is done by using physiologically relevant ex vivo and in vivo models (target validation). These early target validations are very important for successful drug discovery projects. Later these drugs also go through clinical trials, but this target validation helps in narrowing the efforts to the projects which huge amount of data is being generated every day. This includes modern biological data as well. Today, we have the ability to store these huge data sets and later work on them by opening them up to public databases. This provides new opportunities in the stage of target identification and validation. However, these data sets are multidimensional and need proper analysis to build models that are valid and can make proper predictions for target identification. This is where ML comes to the scene. Since most of the experiments now are data-driven, machine learning can be used in all those experiments. The first step in drug discovery is target identification. Here we establish a relationship between the target and the disease. Establishing causality requires demonstration that modulation of a target affects disease from either naturally occurring (genetic) variation or cautiously designed experimental intervention. However, ML can be used here to analyze large data sets with data on the function of a putative target to make predictions about potential causality, driven, for instance, by the properties of known true targets. Correct ML models can reduce the cost, time, and effort demanded by other experiments. A type of machine learning algorithms called supervised machine learning has provided some very good results in drug target prediction and in the prediction of drug target interactions.

6.2 Small-Molecule Design and Optimization

The whole process of finding a drug candidate that can affect (block o activate) a target protein is very extensive. It includes very high virtual and experimental throughput screening of large compound libraries. Deep learning has been applied to a lot of work in this field. Multitask neural networks, to ligand based virtual screening; deep learning has been providing great resources for this field. Deep neural networks have continuously been used in finding the properties of small molecules for their high predictive power. To find better routes for chemical synthesis, deep neural networks and tree algorithms are also being used. There have been many debates in the field of small-molecule design and how to best represent it in the chemical structure Fig. 12. There are a lot of representations that exist as seen in Fig. 13. Some representations work well for some problems while for others it doesn't. Hopefully, with the rise of ML in almost every field, the field of cheminformatics also gets better and we can get a better guidance on which representation to use for a given molecule.

6.3 Predictive Biomarkers

Machine learning has also changed the discovery of biomarkers. It has helped in creating much better drug sensitivity predictive models. These improvements have led to much better successful clinical rates and have made it easier to understand the mechanisms of action of drug. Now with these improvements, choosing the right drugs for the right patients has also become easier. The later clinical trials that take place are very expensive as well as time consuming. Thus, bringing in machine

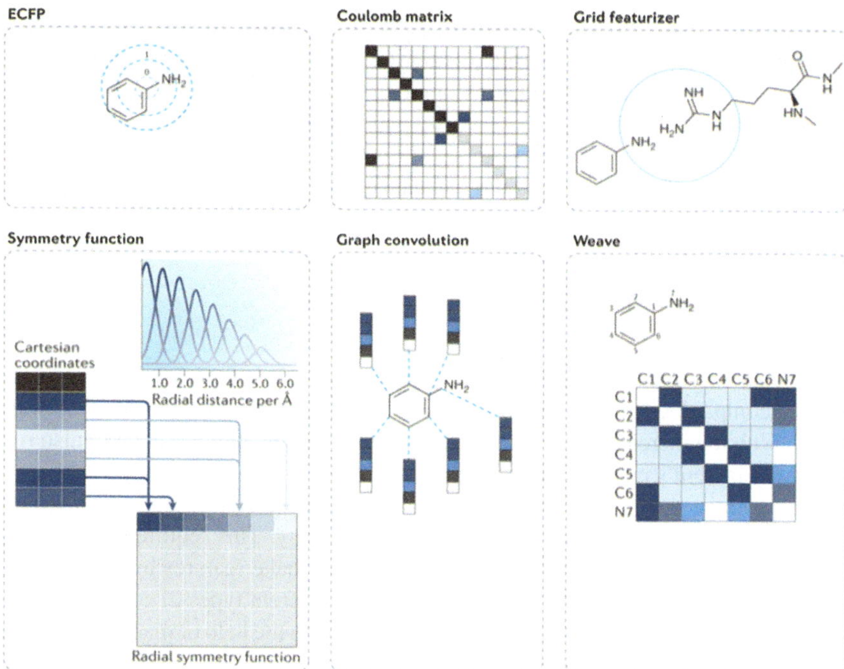

Fig. 12 Compound structure representation in machine learning models

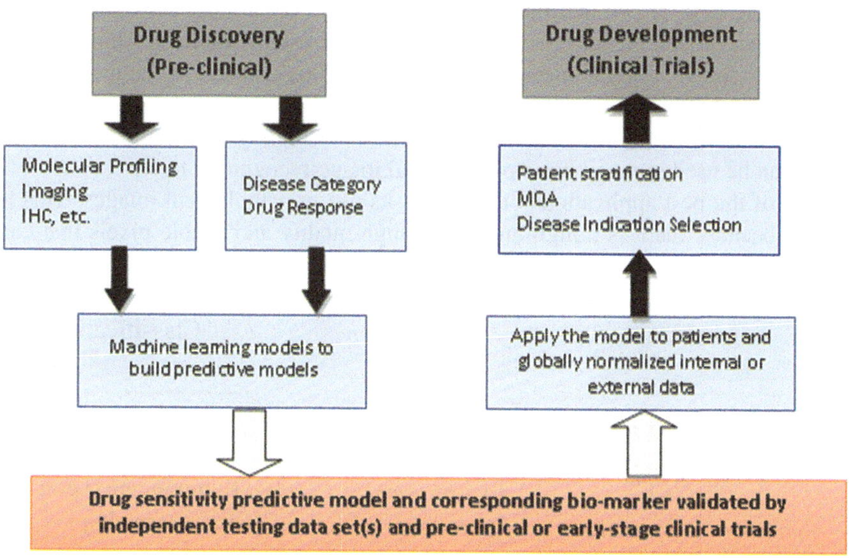

Fig. 13 Use of predictive biomarkers to support drug discovery and development

learning here would be very helpful as it would be better to build a ML model than can it's apply prediction earlier, using the pre-clinical trial data. Translational biomarker can be easily predicted by ML models that are trained pre-clinical data sets. These models can also be applied to stratify patients after being validated using other independent data sets. The model can also be applied to find potential indications in patients and can also recommend the mechanisms of a drug as depicted in Fig. 13.

6.4 Computational Pathology

Drug treatments sometimes affect certain tissues and cells in the body. Thus pharmaceutical companies need to test a lot of drugs before selecting the one that they want to use. With the increase in clinical trials, the need for new biomarkers will also rise to identify patient's response to different therapies.

Earlier to the rise of machine learning, most of the algorithms that were used for tissue image processing were more inspired by biology. This required a combination of pathologists and some computer scientists to make features by hand. These features were then given to a computer to classify different types of cells or tissues. In particular cases such as immune-oncology, Here with the help of machine learning we can generate a large number of features that has the ability to explain the spatial relationships for the cells. This makes the work of the pathologists much easier and removes the burden of deriving features by hand. There also have been huge leaps taken in the field of cell and tissue detection via Deep learning. This allows us to measure with much higher precision the tumors micro-environment. Thus features that can establish the relationship between cells and tissue can now be measured at a scale as highlighted in Fig. 14.

Deep learning frameworks can perform the job of finding the features on its own and it can be used in many basic pathological image-recognition tasks.

One of the best applications of CNNs is its use in pathological images. This is mainly because there is a high amount of high quality and usable pixels that can

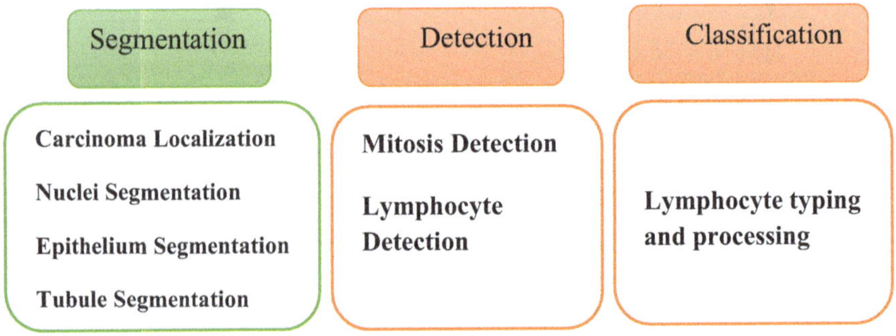

Fig. 14 Computational pathology tasks for machine learning applications

use in the image training process. If a DL network is provided with a good amount of well-curated examples, the algorithm can learn features automatically for a wide variety of classification tasks. For example, a multi-scale convolution neural network (M-CNN) was used in a supervised learning approach for phenotyping high-content cellular images in a solo step as opposed to several, independent customized steps. CNNs can work very well with the pathological images. This is mainly because of the availability of large no. of pixels that are viable for use being present, which can be used for training.

7 Conclusion and Future Scope

It can be said with confidence that machine learning has boosted many of the processes of drug discovery and with the recent developments on deep learning there are many more opportunities yet to open. With the increase in the amount of data produced every day, and taking into factor that most processes today are data-driven. It can be said that the influence of machine learning is going to be even bigger in the coming days. All this has been clearly represented in this chapter. We have talked about applications of machine learning in all stages of drug development such as target identification and validation, drug design and development, and biomarker identification and pathology for disease diagnosis and therapy prognosis in the clinic. Today in each and every step of drug discovery and its development ML approaches are being fitted into the pipeline. But with all this, we also need to train our researchers to understand the science behind pharmaceutical as well as computer science, computational statistics and statistical ML for the actual implementation of ML in drug discovery.

References

1. Eliopoulos, H., Giranda, V., Carr, R., Tiehen, R., Leahy, T., Gordon, G.: Phase 0 trials: an industry perspective. Clin. Cancer Res. **14**(12), 3683–3688 (2008)
2. Xue, H., Li, J., Xie, H., Wang, Y.: Review of drug repositioning approaches and resources. Int. J. Biol. Sci. **14**(10), 1232 (2018)
3. Schuhmacher, A., Gassmann, O., Hinder, M.: Changing R&D models in research based pharmaceutical companies. J. Trans. Med. **14**(1), 105 (2016)
4. Khanna, I.: Drug discovery in pharmaceutical industry: productivity challenges and trends. Drug Discovery Today **17**(19–20), 1088–1102 (2012)
5. Hwang, T.J., Carpenter, D., Lauffenburger, J.C., Wang, B., Franklin, J.M., Kesselheim, A.S.: Failure of investigational drugs in late-stage clinical development and publication of trial results. JAMA Int. Med. **176**(12), 1826–1833 (2016)
6. Lowe D.: The latest on drug failure and approval rates. blogs.sciencemag.org/pipeline/archives/2019/05/09/the-latest-on-drugfailure-and-approval-rates. Accessed 16 Sept 2019
7. Deloitte Centre for Health Solutions. Embracing the future of work to unlock R&D productivity. deloitte.com/content/dam/Deloitte/uk/Documents/life-sciences-health-care/deloitte-uk-measuring-roi-pharma.pdf. Accessed 25 Dec 2018

8. Meekings, K.N., Williams, C.S., Arrowsmith, J.E.: Orphan drug development: an economically viable strategy for biopharma R&D. Drug Disco. Today **17**(13–14), 660–664 (2012)
9. Walker, J.: Machine learning drug discovery applications—pfizer, Roche, GSK, and more. emerj.com/ai-sector-overviews/machine-learningdrug-discovery-applications-pfizer-roche-gsk. Accessed 16 Sept 2019
10. Meath, P.: How the AI revolution is speeding up drug discovery. jpmorgan.com/commercial-banking/insights/ai-revolution-drug-discovery
11. Chan, H.S., Shan, H., Dahoun, T., Vogel, H., Yuan, S.: Advancing drug discovery via artificial intelligence. Trends Pharmacol. Sci. (2019). Accessed 16 Sept 2019
12. Armstrong, M.: Big pharma piles into machine learning, but what will it get out of it? (2018). evaluate.com/vantage/articles/analysis/vantagepoints/big-pharma-piles-machine-learning-what-will-it-get-out-it. Accessed 16 Sept 2019
13. Dutton, G.: Automation cuts drug development to 5 years. lifescienceleader.com/doc/automation-cuts-drug-development-to-years-0001. Accessed 16 Sept 2019
14. Dugger, S.A., Platt, A., Goldstein, D.B.: Drug development in the era of precision medicine. Nat. Rev. Drug Discov. **17**(3), 183 (2018)
15. West, M., Ginsburg, G.S., Huang, A.T., Nevins, J.R.: Embracing the complexity of genomic data for personalized medicine. Genome Res. **16**(5), 559–566 (2006)
16. Ekins, S., Puhl, A.C., Zorn, K.M., Lane, T.R., Russo, D.P., Klein, J.J., et al.: Exploiting machine learning for end-to-end drug discovery and development. Nat. Mater. **18**(5), 435 (2019)
17. Hodos, R.A., Kidd, B.A., Khader, S., Readhead, B.P., Dudley, J.T.: Computational approaches to drug repurposing and pharmacology. Wiley Interdiscip. RevSyst. Biol. Med. **8**(3), 186 (2016)
18. Pope, A.: The evolution of automation for pharmaceutical lead discovery (2010). case2010.org/Automation%20for%20Pharmaceutical%20Lead%20Discovery.pdf. Accessed 16 Sept 2019
19. Mishra, S., Tripathy, H.K., Mallick, P.K., Bhoi, A.K., Barsocchi, P.: EAGA-MLP—an enhanced and adaptive hybrid classification model for diabetes diagnosis. Sensors **20**, 4036 (2020)
20. Mishra, S., Mallick, P.K., Jena, L., Chae, G.S.: Optimization of skewed data using sampling-based preprocessing approach. Front Public Health. 8:274 (2020). Published 2020 Jul 16. https://doi.org/10.3389/fpubh.2020.00274
21. Mallick, P.K., Mishra, D., Patnaik, S., Shaw, K.: A semi-supervised rough set and random forest approach for pattern classification of gene expression data. Int. J. Reasoning-Based Intell. Syst. **8**(3–4), 155–167 (2016)

Deep Learning Frameworks in Healthcare Systems

Anuttam Dash and Chinmaya Dehury

Abstract Consider we are living in a remote place which is far away from any near-by hospitals or we don't have enough time to take a leave from the work to visit a hospital or we can't afford the rapidly increasing medical services costs. This is one of the few scenarios where we can relate to the fact that computer systems and algorithms if they may help in detection or diagnosis of the diseases can be revolutionary and life changing. Over the last decade there has been an increase in the study of how computers, particularly through the disruptive technologies like deep learning, can help in the pervasive sensing for health and well-being. Several researchers have proposed numerous works to detect diseases such as Cancer, RA, heart or lung diseases, Diabetic Retinopathy, Parkinson's Disease, etc. Deep learning techniques enable computers to adapt and self-learn from the information fed into the systems by continuously recognizing the structures and patterns in them. This helps the computers to detect and diagnose a particular disease. This paper focuses on the recent studies in the field of deep learning which can be used for the disease detection and diagnosis. They have been discussed in correlation with the benefits of deep learning in the healthcare sector and their future scope in the same. We have proposed three case studies to highlight the significance of deep learning in healthcare sector by highlighting relevant use cases in each of them. First case study assess the age-related macular degeneration from fundus images by using DNN screening technique. Second case study uses CNN model for the exudate detection of diabetic retinopathy. Third case study uses Deep learning technique to classify cataract fundus images. Finally, the observations made in each of the case studies have been compared and analyzed.

Keywords Deep learning · Evolution algorithm · Artificial neural network · Convolutional neural network

---

A. Dash (✉)
Kalinga Institute of Industrial Technology, Bhubaneswar, Odisha, India
e-mail: anuttam.dash@gmail.com

C. Dehury
University of Tartu, Tartu, Estonia
e-mail: chinmaya.dehury@ut.ee

H. K. Tripathy et al. (eds.), *Technical Advancements of Machine Learning in Healthcare*, Studies in Computational Intelligence 936,
https://doi.org/10.1007/978-981-33-4698-7_8

1 Introduction

Artificial Intelligence is used in finding increased prominence in healthcare organizations of varied sizes, types and specialities because of its ability to provide better care for patients by the improvement in the efficacy and the reduction of costs. In a small span of period, the advancement in AI has impacted the market; providing payers, providers and stakeholders with a zillion of gears and tools to select from. At the same time, organizations are finding it difficult to acquaint themselves with the lingo and understand the elusive alterations between dynamic terms such as AI, Deep Learning and semantic computing.

Healthcare organisation's need to have an understanding of different flavours of AI and how it can be applied in different scenarios, in order to efficiently and effectively identify the tools that would best suit their need, or to hire the right kind of talent (data science professionals) to develop in-house solutions. They have to have an understanding about the kind of data that is fed into the system and the accuracy and reliability of the data that comes out as output, so that they can take their investment decisions accordingly.

Deep learning is one of the branches of AI that has been able to bring transformative changes in the healthcare sector. It has the ability to analyze and process data with rapidity and exactness never seen before.

2 Literature Survey

A dynamic and fast growing sector in the medical industry involves the use of disease detection and diagnosis through computer systems and algorithms. Machine learning shows a really impressive scope for disease detection and diagnosis. Computers are self-capable of learning insights from the health data that can be used for the diagnosis of the disease. Datasets can be classified using many machine learning techniques [1, 2]. Some of them are unsupervised, supervised, semi-supervised, reinforcement, deep learning techniques [3] and evolutionary learning.

Supervised learning on one hand deals with labelled data [4] while on the other unsupervised learning techniques deal with unlabelled data. In unsupervised learning techniques the pattern or structures within the data is estimated through the phenomenon of density estimation [5]. Semi-supervised techniques are somewhat a combination of supervised and unsupervised learning techniques. It comprises of both the labelled and unlabelled data, but the quantity of unlabelled data in the dataset is more than the labelled data [6]. Reinforcement learning is a sequence of systematic well-defined approaches which leads to the optimality in achieving a solution. In other words, here, the system knows when the answer is wrong but does not know how to correct it. It uses probabilities to solutions to get to the correct answer [7]. Evolutionary algorithms take inspiration from the nature to seek optimal or near-optimal solution to a problem at a reasonable computational cost. It is based on the natural phenomenon of natural selection, reproduction and survival of the fittest [8]. In deep learning techniques the optimal parameters are gradually learnt by the neural network through back-propagation techniques [8]. The self learning ability of the neural networks help them to draw insights from the data and self train themselves to recognise patterns in the data [9].

Disease progression can be quantified by continuous evaluation of bio-markers during the treatment [10, 11]. Disease can only be affectively controlled by the increase in the efficiency of medical treatments in terms of sensitivity and reliability.

In the system presented by Huo [12], the space width of finger joint of the patients suffering from the early stage of rheumatoid arthritis is efficiently quantified. Almost 96% of the joints are identified. Suma [13] worked in the direction of safe and cost-effective diagnosis of RA by the use of thermal image segmentation techniques like k-means image segmentation. The system claims an accuracy of 93%. Langs [14] developed a system for the detection of erosions and joint space narrowing in RA patients through the use of active space models of local topography and shape of bone. The system showed an accuracy of 92%. Multivariate statistical model proposed by Jhajharia which used PCA extracted features to detect the possibility of breast cancer showed an accuracy of 96%. Jhajharia [15] has made use of a neural network trained on the PCA features for predicting the possibility of breast cancer. Zheng [16] used a combination of AI techniques along with the DWT feature extraction technique to detect the masses in the mammograms with an accuracy of 97.3%. Wang [17] proposed a 12 level CNN architecture for detection of breast cancer by distinguishing the BAC from non-BAC to detect BAC patch wise. The coefficient of determination in the linear regression graph of calcium mass quantification obtained 96.24%. Khobragade [18] proposed an ANN model for the detection of lung diseases like pneumonia, TB, lung cancer by using an intensity-based method. The accuracy obtained was 86%. Otoomet, al developed a system for analysis and detection of coronary artery disease by the use of Bayes Net, SVM, Functional Trees [19] which thus obtained accuracies of 85.5%, 85.1%, 84.5%, respectively. Vembandasamy et al. [20] used Naïve Bayes to detect the possibility of heart disease with an accuracy of 86.42%. Authors in [21] presented a dimensional reduction approach for effective classification of diabetes disorders. It served as an optimisation model for machine learning classification task. Mishra et al. [22] presented a sampling-based approach that helped in optimisation of data skewing in healthcare datasets. This sampling approach proved to be an efficient model for dimensionality reduction.

3 Deep Learning in Overview

Deep learning uses forms of machine learning algorithm that uses coated structure to process and analyze data.

Data successively passes through multiple layers, the output of every layer being fed as input for the next layer. The accuracy of Deep Learning algorithms can be improved by providing them with more and more data. As the models process more data, the model learns from previous results and is able to make connections and associations.

Deep learning is lightly founded on how neurons in a human brain process information. Alike to how electrical signals travel across cells of living creatures, each subsequent layer is activated upon receiving stimuli from the neighbouring neurons.

In ANNs (Artificial Neural Network) data travels back and forth across multiple layers to refine and produce optimal output.

The hidden layers perform mathematical translations on the raw data to convert it into machine understandable output (Fig. 1).

According to an article published in 2015 under the flagship of Nature which was written by technocrats from Facebook, Google, the University of Toronto, Université de Montréal, deep learning techniques are like the methods of representation-learning having multiple representation levels produced by combining simple and non-linear modules that each convert one-level representation (with raw input) to higher abstraction level representation.

This implies multifaceted functions can be learned with enough of such representations. Higher representation layers intensify input layer features that are significant for discernment and overpower immaterial variations.

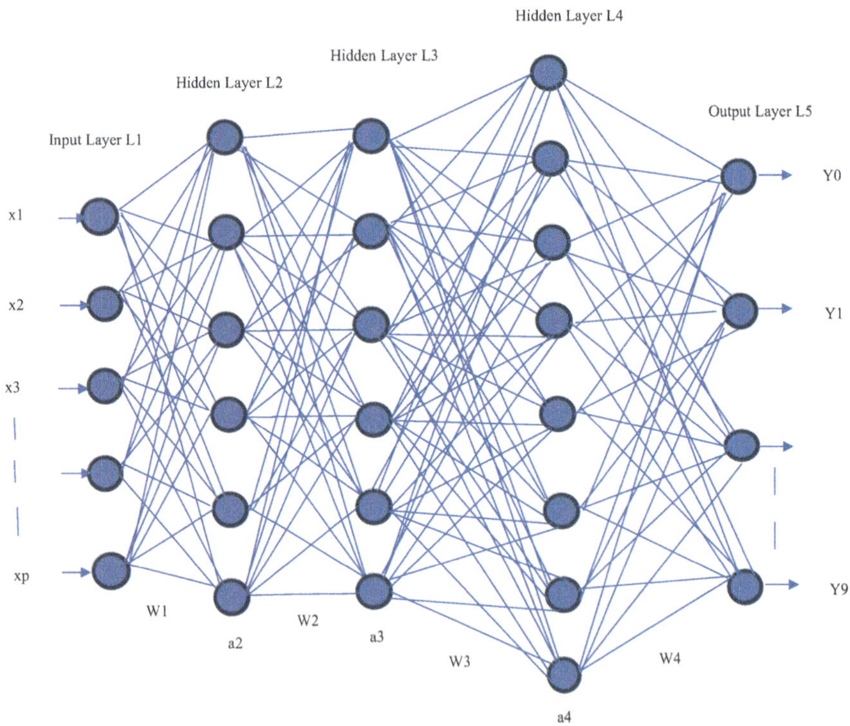

Fig. 1 Illustration of a deep neural network

The multi-layered structure helps model of deep learning to perform classification jobs such as pointing out elusive irregularities in medical images, grouping patients with a like physiognomies into risk-based groups, or high point relations between outcomes and symptoms within vast amounts of unstructured data.

In contrast to other machine learning algorithms, Deep learning requires less human involvement.

Unlike other basic machine learning models, it does not require a programmer to check the correctness of the conclusion. Due to its layered structure, it is able to measure the accuracy of its answers.

On top of that, it requires less pre-processing of information. The filtration and normalization tasks that should have been completed by the programmers before feeding data into the network are actually taken care of by the network itself.

However, Deep Learning models are self-capable of identifying the depictions needed for classification or regression problems. Thus, decreasing the supervision time and in turn speeding the process up to derive relevant insights from selected dataset.

Naturally, the mathematics that goes into building deep learning estimators are extremely complex and there exists different sub-strategies that can be deployed to build different variations of network.

Deep learning is evolving very fast and thus approving better computing capabilities in the world across different industries thereby providing substantial value to user experience and supporting reasonable decision making.

4 Benefits of Deep Learning

Deep learning solves few of the complex problems that were unsolvable by machine learning algorithms. It uses neural networks to increase computing efficiency and get accurate results. The applications of Deep Learning techniques are Natural Language Processing, face recognition, speech recognition, for example, when a facebook user uploads a picture, facebook automatically suggests the names of other friends in the picture by means of deep learning methods. Deep learning models also have the capability of understanding human audio and to convert it into text data. In the future, Deep Learning combined with IoT may bring about tons of revolutionary innovations.

The presence of huge amounts of data in big data ecosystem makes it an advantage. With the coming of Big Data Era availability of huge amounts of data will provide ample opportunities for innovations in Deep Learning. According to **Andrew Ng**, the chief researcher of Baidu (Most Popular Search Engine in China) and Google Brain Project's leader, deep learning models can be compared to a rocket engine and the large quantity of data that we provide to such algorithms can be compared to the rocket fuel.

Deep Learning models are powerful engines capable of producing actionable results in a plethora of applications including big data for discovery of knowledge, application of knowledge and prediction using that knowledge. Identifying patterns and regularities lies at the heart of scientific and technological progress across the world. Deep learning can be used to draw new valuable insights from the data we already have.

Deep Learning models can also be used to draw insights about consumer data from CRM applications, social media websites and other open domain data to better customer segmentation, to predict churn rate, for detection of fraud. Finance Industry is increasingly relying on deep learning techniques to make stock predictions and execute right time trades. In the healthcare sector, deep learning models are being tested to repurpose already available drugs used for treating new diseases so that it can be made available to the general public in shorter time span.

By using satellite imagery, Governmental organizations are also using to deep learning models to fetch real time understandings for production of food, energy infrastructure, etc.

The list of applications of Deep learning can go on and on. However, one thing is for sure, given the wide variety of applications that deep learning can be deployed into, there is enthusiasm for deep learning. In the future, we can suppose huge investments being made in this technology to solve complex challenges across different industries.

5 Deep Learning in Healthcare Sector

DL (Deep Learning) has been of great assistance to healthcare professionals and scientist to draw concealed insights from data and thus assisting the medical industry better. Deep learning helps to provide accurate analysis of diseases. The doctors are able to take better decisions and treat the patients better.

- **Drug Discovery**: Deep learning has been helpful in the discovery and development of medicines. The technology can suggest medications to the patient by looking at the past medical history, the medicines the patient was consuming in the past, the patients symptoms, tests, etc.
- **DL (Deep Learning) for Medical Imaging**: Automated imaging of medical images is another vital application of Deep learning that is vital to modern medicine. Interpreting diseases by understanding medical images can be extremely idiosyncratic. Computerized Diagnosis can help deliver an impartial valuation of implicit disease procedures. In order to build models for disease progression such as multiple sclerosis, Alzheimer's and stroke, detailed maps of different regions of brain and brain images relating to multimodal data are required. CNN has outstanding performance in computer imaging, thus it is being increasingly used by medical imagery research community. The fact that CNN can be used aggressively in computer imaging has been emphasized in a study of CNN methodologies in segmentation of brain pathology and in one journal of deep learning techniques in computerised segmentation, detection and shape analysis.

- **Persistent Detection for Well-Being and Health**: Persistent sensors allows to continuously monitor health and well-being. Examples of persistent sensors are implantable, wearable and ambient sensors. For example, an appropriate tracking of the food consumed by an individual in a day and his/her energy expenditure can help in reducing obesity and recover the personal well-being of an individual. For chronic disease patients, implantable and wearable devices can help to efficiently monitor their health, thus enabling them to live independently. Wearable and implantable sensors (supplemented with human activity recognition feature) can also be used to take better care of patients with disabilities. It can also be used to monitor and analyze vitals like respiration rate, blood pressure and body temperature for patients undergoing critical care.
- **Medical Informatics**: Medical Informatics uses huge amount of data in clinical setting to improve Clinical Decision Support System both in terms of quality and medical services accessibility. Electronic health records (EHR) is an information well of patients which contains patient details such as exams of diagnosis, diagnoses, treatment and medication directions, allergies, records of immunization, multivariate times series from sensors (like EEG from intensive care sections), images of radiology, test results from laboratory. Efficient mining of Electronic health records (EHR) will provide valuable insights to improve healthcare system.
- **Public Health**: Deep Learning can be used in applications such as lifestyle diseases modelling (ex. Obesity), air quality prediction and monitoring, surveillance, drug safety surveillance, etc. Existing predictive models are capable of modelling accurately evolution of diseases or air pollution spread. Though, they have some limitations. They are unable to incorporate real time data that is essential to control the spread of a pandemic or recognize the opposing effects of newly accepted drug (medicine). Deep Learning models have good generalization capability. They optimize the cost function sequentially as more and more training data is made available. Stochastic Gradient Descent is used as an optimisation function in Deep Neural Networks. For such reasons, Deep Learning joined with recommendation systems and network analysis are recommended as vital approaches to use in Public Health studies.

6 Use Cases of Deep Learning in Health Care Industry

In Majority of the industries deep learning models are in research phase or pilot phase in the pre-commercial phase. However, Deep Learning is gradually improving in several applications in the medical field. Few of the prominent examples include ground-breaking applications for patient-facing, devising plans for improving user experience for health IT domain.

6.1 Imaging Analytics And Diagnostics

CNNs (Convolutional Neural Networks) is the neural networks that can be used for interpreting images like x-ray images and MRI images. Conferring to Computer Science specialists at the Stanford University, CNNs are designed to process images. Thus, they are able to operate efficiently even with huge images. Hence, CNNs are outstanding the accuracy of human diagnosticians in classifying some of image diagnostic studies features.

As per a June 2018 study in the *Annals of Oncology, a CNN that was developed to identify images of dermatology identified images with 10% more precision than human classifiers. Both CNN and human classifiers were provided with info about patients'* sex, age and the suspect feature body site. Even then, CNNs outclassed the human clinicians by 7%.

A number of German academic institutions have said that *CNN can help dermatologists in detection of melanoma irrespective of their individual training level and experience. Few researchers from* Mount Sinai Icahn School of Medicine have designed a deep neural network that is proficient of detecting critical nerve conditions like stroke and brain haemorrhage 150 times quicker than human radiologists. It just takes 1.2 s for the tool to analyze the image and give the findings to the doctor. According to Joshua Bederson, MD, Professor and System Chair Department of Neurosurgery at Mount Sinai Health System and Neurosurgery Simulation Core Clinical Director, since time is a crucial factor in treating these acute neurological conditions, any tool that is able to reduce the time to diagnose this condition will help in better patient treatment outcomes.

Generative Adversarial Networks (GAN) is another type of Deep Learning approach that can be used to make impressively truthful medical images from scratch.

The models real scanned images to learn and generate MRI or CT images synthetic versions. This gives researchers access to endlessly diverse without any concern for patient privacy. The models are so precise that they can be used to train deep learning models in future to diagnose clinical results.

It is challenging to train deep learning models for Medical imaging as pathologic findings are generally rare. GANs can be used to generate abnormal MRI images with brain tumours. Thus offering a low-cost, automatable source of diverse data supplementing the already available huge corpus of data. For example, using GAN, we can systematically change the size of a tumour, its place in brain to generate desired image. Such a strategy would be useful in reducing AI's some of the biggest pain points, i.e. a lack of reliable shareable high-volume dataset and necessity to validate the dataset.

6.2 ANN in Healthcare

Unlike traditional computing, Artificial Neural networks closely resembles the structure and operation of the human brain. ANNs are parallel distributed systems in which the elements are interconnected and function parallelly. Neural networks don't haves central controls as all the elements are interconnected and changes in them happen as and when information is passed through them or based on some evolving rules. One objective of neural networks is to be able to comprehend the functioning of the human brain while it does functions such as sensorial concept categorization, perception, learning, concept association. However, nowadays, a lot of effort is being put on training the deep learning models for recognizing patterns and their classification, compressing data and optimization.

A generic ANN can be thought of as a computational network with a set of interrelated neurons that operate in response to an external stimulus. Like its biological complement, artificial neurons are assured together. This ensures flow of information throughout the network. Artificial neural networks mimic integration of signal and firing of threshold behaviour of organic neurons by mathematical equations. Stimuli are passed from one neuron to the other by means of interconnections or synapses. A Stimulus can be inhibitory or excitatory. If the input signal is excitatory, the neuron will propagate excitatory signals to the other connected neurons. Similarly, if the input is inhibitory signal, the neuron will propagate inhibitory signals to the other neurons connected to it (Fig. 2).

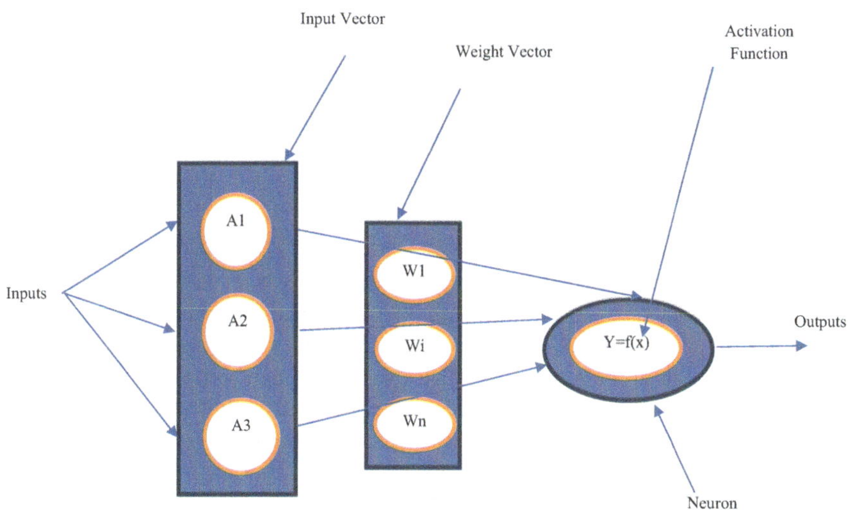

Fig. 2 Basic model of a single neuron

6.2.1 Modes of Behaviour

In an ANN, the network is trained first and then tested before actually using any model for practical purposes. During the training phase, the network is fed with a variety of examples and the network guesses the output of each of these examples. After feeding the network with multiple such examples, the network reaches a stability state wherein it has been able to learn enough to be able to generate a satisfactory output. In the learning phase, the weights of each of the interconnected neurons are continuously updated to provide best possible output to a set of input. There are two ways in which networks can acquire: Unsupervised technique or Supervised technique.

(a) **Supervised learning**: The network is served with a set of input–output pairs. The objective is to impart the network to be able to generate desired output for the respective inputs. For example, the network is fed with a input and it generates an output. This generated output is compared with the wanted output. The network then rectifies this error in output by adjusting the weights of its neurons until the network reaches an output approximately same to wanted output or until the time the network is not further able to make improvement in the performance.
(b) **Unsupervised learning**: The network is served with input signals and the network arranges itself to generate an output reliable with a stimulus or a group of stimulus. The inputs usually form a cluster and each element of the cluster corresponds to some feature in the real world. In both the cases, once the training stage is over, the weights associated with each of the neurons are frozen and cannot be changed any further. In the testing stage, the network is fed with unseen output. If the network has been trained appropriately, it would generalize input and be able to generate output that is close enough to the desired output.

6.2.2 Structure of ANNs

A neural network has a layered structure wherein each layer has a set of neurons. The neurons across the different layers are interconnected. Information flows though each of the layers in an input–output format, i.e. each layer receives input, operates it and then sends it to the next layer. MLP (Multilayer perceptron) is one common example of an ANN network. Multilayer perceptrons usually have three layers to process information including one hidden layer. However, there is no restriction how many hidden layers that an MLP can have. The input layer receives the signal and transmits it to the next layer. The hidden layer obtains the weighted sum of the input layer signals, passes it through an activation function and sends the output to the next layer. The next layer might be either a hidden or an output layer. Examples of activation functions are sigmoid, unit step, saturation and hyperbolic tangent activation functions. The neurons in the output layer process the weighted hidden layer

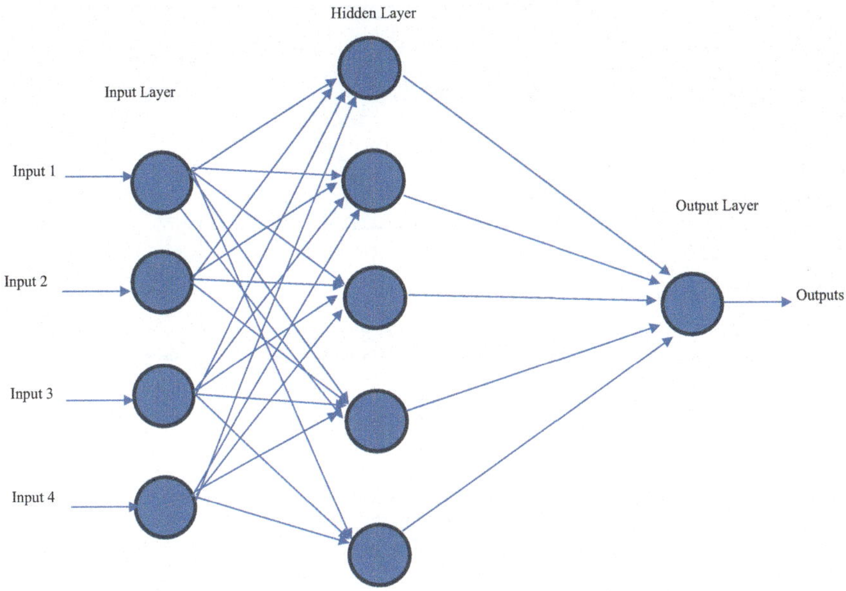

Fig. 3 Basic Diagram of a Multilayer Perceptron

signals using an activation function and generates an output. Information keeps on propagating through the network until an output is produced (Fig. 3).

6.3 Revolutionary CNN Model Overview

Convolutional neural networks are different from the usual neural networks. In addition to the neurons, the input–output and hidden layers, it has a filter. The filter is able to identify certain types of patterns in images. It is like a flashlight. It can be used to flash on different parts of a picture and identify the different features present in the picture. The features can then be jotted down onto a feature map. Layers at the start are usually used to identify relatively simpler things like edge detection. As we progress through the layers, the latter layers can be used to identify relatively complex features like eyes, nose, fingers, etc. All these features are put in a list at the end of the network. This list can be finally used to classify an image. Apart from convolutional layers, CNN's also contain pooling and classification layers (Fig. 4).

Pooling layers help to ensure that the training of neural networks is done much quickly. It is done by the reduction of the images in their dimensions. It is very similar to a convolutional layer, where image is passed over by a filter, excluding now, the data is passed over the filter, the most important information is extracted and put into matrix of smaller dimensions. In this way it becomes easier for the computer for

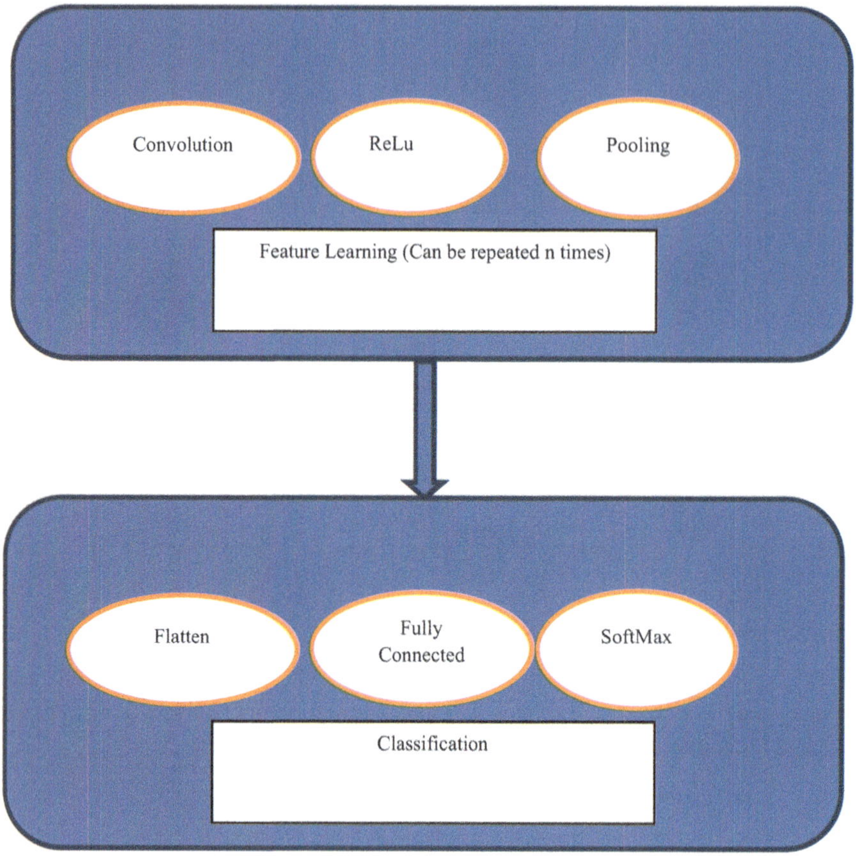

Fig. 4 Standard architecture of a CNN

further computations. All these layers are then joined together to produce a **soft-max** function (classification layer) that outputs the result of final classification.

7 Future of Deep Learning in the Healthcare Sector

Enthusiasm and curiosity for deep learning is everywhere, taking the fancies of rule makers and regulators, care providers, private companies and also patients. The office of the National Coordinator (ONC) keeps a very high hope for deep learning and some developers are already applauded for obtaining ground-breaking results. In a new study about the role of AI in healthcare domain, the agency distinguished that few deep learning algorithms have already created ground-breaking results. The study said that there have been significant demonstrations made by some algorithms of Deep Learning about their efficiency in Health Care. The quality of the training sets is directly proportional to the medical expertise, and the applications of the deep learning algorithms help in providing better results. The Study emphasized initial achievements in DR (Diabetic Retinal) detections and the grouping of skin cancer as two fields where deep learning might be varying the status quo. In the future analytics can be an area of focus because of the fact that deep learning already has been applied in many high-valued applications.

To be precise clinical applications will make up a very small part of future deep learning applications in the healthcare domain.

The technology is essential to various consumer friendly technologies, applications on mHealth, chatbots and virtual assistants like Google Assistant., Alexa, Siri.

These tools can entirely change the conventional way of how patients relate with healthcare applications by providing home-based monitoring of chronic disease, 24/7 contact to plain triage and latest habits to whole administrative tasks.

Customer communication and support are two initial applications. With Market disrupters like Amazon going to launch new user friendly health choices to users, it might be only a dependent of time before when interacting with Alexa will become as normal as talking to a medical professional.

Several analytics and voice recognition on the basis of deep learning also have the potential to deliver some assistance to nurses and physicians stressed with EHRs.

Google is involved in taking medical discussions data from clinic and utilizing deep learning techniques to decrease loads on healthcare professionals.

Several research studies have showed the latent of NLP and deep learning to comprehend casual chat in a noisy surrounding, leading to the option of using an intelligent, ambient transcriber to help in documentation.

Google is working with data scientists from Stanford University and the physicians to better refine the system to such an extent that it can be used in real clinical environment.

EHR vendors are also investigating the efficiency of machine learning algorithms to provide relevant data in the systems by avoiding irrelevant conversations and interactions.

To learn habits of users and understand their needs and according to the analysis display correct information in appropriate time by avoiding irrelevant information is what artificial intelligence helps in and is what the top priority of the major IT providers for healthcare domain.

Artificial Intelligence has evolved a lot over the years through continuous research and development and is thus ready to deliver better consumer specific applications to both the healthcare professionals and the patients.

James Golden (Senior Managing Director for PwC's Healthcare Advisory Group) said that we now have enough physical computational resources to develop better AI applications.

The increase in the interest for progressive approaches, enhanced computational power and mounting interest in ground-breaking approaches of preventing, predicting and lowering healthcare cost will create a new field for deep learning in Healthcare.

Over the years there have been a growth in the number of advanced use cases, investment from bigger IT companies in industry, huge flow of data to fuel data analytics algorithms. This in turn implies that deep learning will be playing a major role in meeting the consumer friendly application needs of consumers in the years to come.

8 Implementation of Deep Learning in the Real World Health Scenario

There have been several research studies already conducted in the past to analyze, mitigate and deal with various problem domains of healthcare sector in the real world. Some of the real world case studies highlighting the importance of deep neural networks in the healthcare sector have been mentioned in this section.

8.1 Assessing the Fundus Images-Based Macular Degeneration by Using Deep Neural Network

A study of deep CNN has been provided in this case study to find the feasibility of utilizing method of transfer learning to test if an individual in suffering from AMD (Age Related Macular Degeneration). AREDS (Age related eye disease study) dataset containing 150,000 samples of images has been used to which also contains qualitative grading results suggested by ophthalmologists and expert graders. A VGG16 batch normalized neural network implementation at the final fully connected layer has been proposed. For study, two experiments were held. Firstly, the images are categorized into two classes-based on some clinical measures: Advanced and No or Early AMD. Secondly, the images were divided into 4 classes: Advanced AMD, No AMD, Intermediate AMD, Early AMD. An accuracy of 92.5% was achieved for the binary class problem using VGG16 model having approximately more than 100,000 images. Thus, the variation in the accuracy from 83 to 92.5% implies that for the purpose of AMD screening it is better approach to use a deep CNN model with sufficiently large amount of images than using pre-trained neural network. Also it was found that for such studies VGG16 Model is much better than other shallow models like AlexNet, etc.

8.1.1 Dataset Overview

The AREDS dataset has been used here for study. The National Eye Institute sponsored a major clinical test for AMD and this is what we say AREDS. Patients having an age range of 55–80 years having no illness condition that can trigger difficulties for long-period follow and acquiescence with study medications. The images were classified by CRC (Central Reading Centre), ophthalmologic tests and corrected visual insight. After grading about 4,757 volunteers were registered in one of many categories of AMD, counting individuals with no AMD. 1,2,3 (a & b), 4 (a & b) are the categories to which the images in AREDS have been categorized. This categorization is done on the basis of eye size and amount of druse in eye, visual acuity and other manifestations of AMD.

Fundus pictures at every call have been evaluated and graded by AREDS, covering the facts about the type, existence and drusen extent, subretinal hemorrhages, existence/degree of RPE depigmentation, geographic atrophy and sub retinal fibrosis including AMD category, simple scale of AMD, AMD severity. Two arrays of evaluations were done such as, (1) binary classification- Early or NO AMD and Advanced or Intermediate AMD. Basing the adequate amount of information in AREDS 116,875 images collected from 4140 volunteers were used (Fig. 5).

The dataset was scanned through to eliminate low quality and hazy images. Every image was pre-processed and cropped to focus on centre of the macula and encompassing it to just the temporal disk margin. For grading AMD particularly this portion in the eye is very important. In order to match every images of varying sizes to the reference image it they were resized to attain a resolution similar to that of the reference image. To achieve this a mask (retinal portion in the image) needs to be found out using a threshold value. In order to rescale the images a best fit circle was determined where the radius of the moving images was the same as that of the reference image. The physical distance between two images is the distance from a pixel to a neighbouring pixel. Figure 6a depicts the original image before pre-processing and Fig. 6b shows the cropped image focusing on the macular centre. Finally, the result of additional pre-processing of images for the classification domain was studied. Greyscale images as illustrated in Fig. 6c are created by taking green channel intensities. The reason for choosing green channel is because it provides best fundus images contrast as is evident from many studies. The final data is called green only data (Table 1).

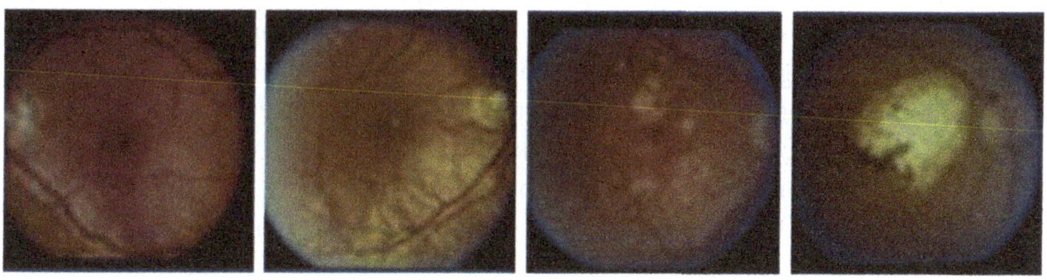

Fig. 5 From left No AMD, Early stage, Intermediate stage and Advanced AMD

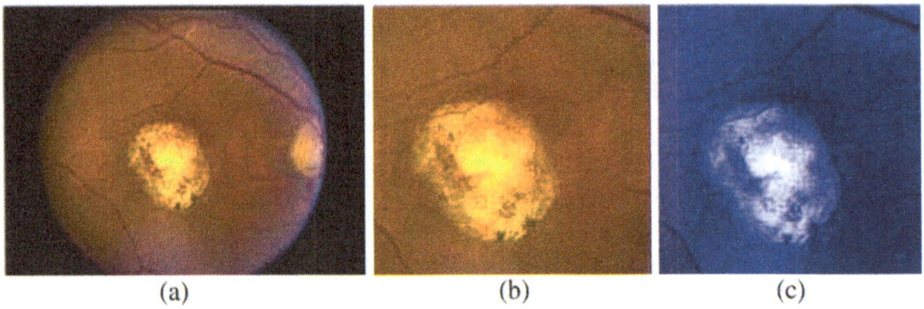

Fig. 6 **a** Original image **b** cropped macula **c** green channel only

Table 1 Number of images in each class

Class	Number of images
No AMD	36,135
Early stage	28,495
Intermediate	36,392
Advanced AMD	15,853

8.1.2 Model Used

There have been numerous progresses in image analysis field and computer visions using deep learning. Thus the feasibility of using these networks for the classification of AMD in fundus images was studies. A combination of 3 models deep learning was used for this purpose. At first the efficiency of transfer learning methodology using the pre-trained ResNetmodel (usage of ImageNet Dataset) was used and then a neural network was explicitly trained on AREDS dataset containing fundus images. VGG16 which is a 16 layered neural network (winner of ILSVRC-2014) was used for this purpose. In order to improve the generalization, batch normalization technique was used in the final fully connected layer. For the comparison the ResNet has been used. ResNet used in this study consists of 50 layered ResNet (Implemented in Keras) proposed by Kaiming in ILSVR-2015. In transfer learning the image features are taken from the trained models on comparatively bigger datasets for the purpose of classification. VGG consists of a very naive architecture where only 3×3 or 2×2 pooling layers are utilized throughout the entire architecture. About 2500 images from each class ($2500 \times 4 = 10{,}000$) were kept aside for the purpose of testing. The remaining of the dataset was divided in 80:20 ratio for validation purpose and training purpose. Same approach was applied for GO images. For training the batch size was set to 100 having images of size 224×224. Epoch limit was set to 1000 but with a constraint of stopping the training if there happens no performance improvement in 50 consecutive epochs. The final model obtained was tested then.

8.1.3 Results

An accuracy of 92.5% was obtained in traditional model without using transfer learning. All the accuracies have been illustrated in Table 2. In pre-trained network the accuracies obtained for AMD detection problems were 78.1% and 86.5% for 4-class and 2-class, respectively and 83% and 92.5%, respectively when VGG16 was used without pre-trained network. The results for 2-class problem stands out to be better than same class problems in other studies. The accuracy got by using VGG16 without transfer learning for identifying No/Early and Intermediate/Advanced AMD was 92.5% which is significantly better than the previously claimed 91.6% as shown in Table 3. The naming conventions used have been mentioned in the following lines. 1. No AMD, 2. Early AMD, 3. Intermediate AMD, 4. Advanced AMD, VwTL, VGG16 with Transfer Learning, Vw/oTL—VGG16 without Transfer Learning, RN-ResNet50 (Table 4).

Referring to the Figures from previous studies on this field we conclude that the results got in this study is comparable to human grading. Thus, this study opens up the gateway for the usage of automatic grading systems in bioinformatics and

Table 2 **a** Accuracies obtained by all three models when all the four classes are considered. **b** Accuracies obtained by all three models when all the two classes are considered

a

Dataset	Four classes				
Metric	Overall accuracy	1	2	3	4
VwTL	77.6	83.1	72	74.4	80.9
Vw/oTL	83	86.4	81.5	79.1	85
RN	79.1	84	76.6	74.6	81.2

b

Dataset	Two classes		
Metric	Overall accuracy	1+2	3+4
VwTL	85.2	87.3	83.1
Vw/oTL	92.5	94	91
RN	88.5	91.2	86.3

Table 3 Comparative analysis of the obtained best model with the previous models on the dataset of similar size

Study	2-class accuracy (%)
VGG 16-layer	92.50
AlexNet 8-layer	91.60

Table 4 GO AMD classification results

Pre-processing/classes	2-class	4-class
GO (%)	92.4	83.2

telemedicine which can ultimately help in reducing the time, and cost incurred and the need for expert grading personnel.

8.2 *CNN Model for Identification of Diabetic Retinopathy*

In order to monitor the DR progress exudate detection of diabetic retinopathy through computer aid techniques can be really helpful. Here the technique of pixel-wise identification of exudate through deep CNN has been adopted. Expert labelled images of exudate were used to train the deep CNN model after which it was saved to be used as offline classifier. Reducing computational time along with leveraging pixel level accuracy was achieved by extracting potential images of exudate by means of morphological ultimate opening algorithm. Finally, the trained CNN model is fed with the local region (64 × 64) surrounding the candidate pixels. The final results come up to be a 91.92% for pixel-wise accuracy, 88.85% for sensitivity, 96% for specificity by using the proposed CNN architecture.

8.2.1 Methodology

Figure 7 illustrates the framework used for exudate detection. For training the CNN Model, 64 × 64 patches mined from the radiance modified green channel images were used and the model was then saved. In order to go further with the retinal image

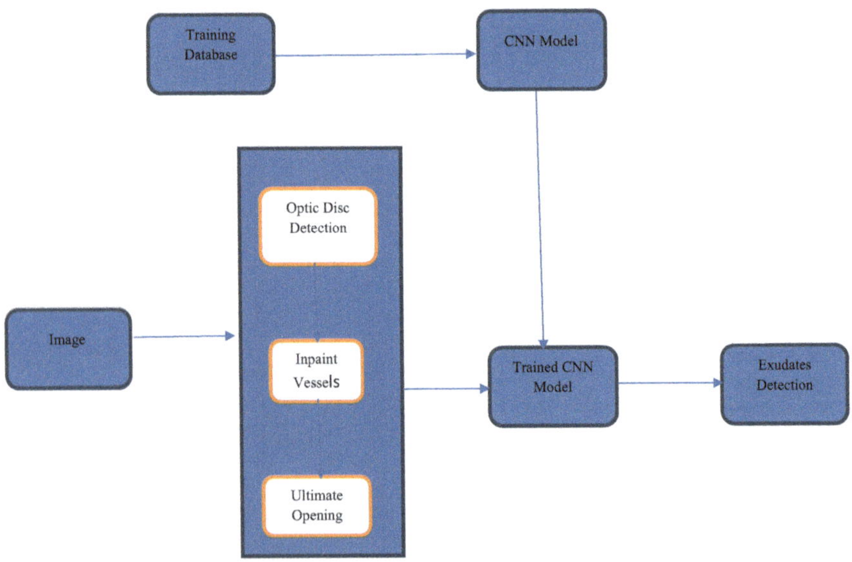

Fig. 7 Framework for exudate detection with deep learning

processing the blood vessels and optic nerve was first removed. Then the seed points (potential exudate images) are then obtained by using the opening algorithm. In order to detect whether the native patches that surround the seed points are exudates or not they are passed to the CNN model. Pixel level identification can only be achieved through a CNN model if every pixel is applied with the CNN model, but this can be really time consuming when it comes to calculating all the pixels in the fundus images. Hence, we use ultimate opening algorithm which removes all the unnecessary points in the background of potential exudate candidate. Ultimate opening method can remove 1–20% of the total pixels in the images conditional to symptoms of exudates in the images. This helps in speeding up the process (Fig. 7).

8.2.2 Optic Disc Detection Removal

Before detecting the exudates there is a need to remove optic disc after its detection because both exudates and optic disc are bright objects and are of same colour. Local phase symmetry algorithm was adopted for detecting the optic disc. It is non-dimensional expanse of the mark of symmetry of the feature in native zone. The centre of the optic disc helps to give a strong response as the optic disc appears as a bright elliptical or circular section. In order to obtain the entire optic disc zone, the growing zone is used and this is done by the help of extreme response of the local phase symmetry. Radius of Optic disc can be defined as the smallest radius of the circle encompassing the region growing.

8.2.3 Separation of Retinal Vessels

Vessel segmentation and in painting the vessel based on the results of the segmentation are used for the retinal vessels removal. However, the drawback of this method is we cannot use this method for the removal of fine vessels. According to Zhang et al. usage of supremum operation after operation of opening and morphological closing can help to in paint dark structures such as haemorrhages, microaneurysms, vessels. This methodology has been adopted in the study because it is efficient in fine vessels removal and other types of dark lesions keeping intact the bright lesions. Figure 8a illustrates the green channel retinal image and Fig. 8b illustrates it's in painting result.

8.2.4 Ultimate Opening Strategy

Ultimate opening is used to extract the exudate suitable points after small dark lesions and retinal vessel are removed. A temporary result is obtained which is nothing but the maximum residue obtained by applying the image with the opening operations with the cumulative structure element size. The previous step is looped till the maximum of given size of structure is reached. Figure 8a after passing through ultimate opening

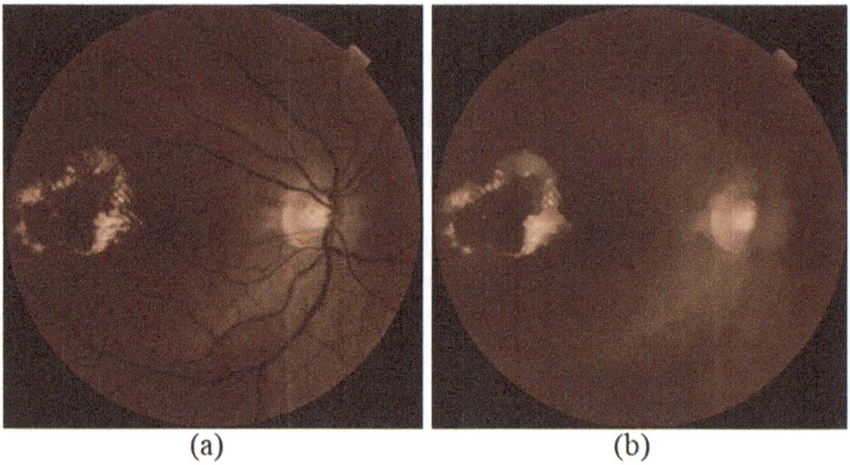

Fig. 8 Illustrates the dark lesions and retinal vessels being removed. **a** green channel image; **b** final image after removing dark lesions and retinal vessels

becomes Fig. 9a. For the purpose of calculating a suitable threshold encompassing a structuring element covering a local zone, Otsu algorithm is applied and Fig. 9b illustrates the result. But if observed carefully Fig. 9a is not representing all the exudate candidate points as is getting reflected in Fig. 8a. Some of the zones are larger than or smaller than the actual zones in Fig. 8a. Therefore, refining Fig. 9b is essential and to do the needful Fig. 9b is inpainted with the green channel image as illustrated in Fig. 8b and the difference between the inpainted and the original image is obtained which is illustrated in Fig. 9c. The difference image (Fig. 9c) is segmented to obtain a better candidate image.

8.2.5 Convolutional Neural Networks

When compared to the models like SVM and random forest CNN is a much better model where the features are automatically detected from the input image unlike to the manually fed features in SVM and random forest. CNN models are very effective in image analysis for its classification and recognition. Normally a CNN model has a convolutional layer, activation layer, pooling layer. These three were stacked up to form a fully connected layer.

Table 5 shows the CNN Model architecture used. The model is fed with the 64 $\times$ 64 patches extracted out from the light modified green channel images. The CNN model is trained using the modified green channel images and expert comments. CNN model training is done by using limited algorithms of image processing excluding for illumination modification to eliminate the variation in brightness. Once the training of CNN Model is done it is then used as a classifier.

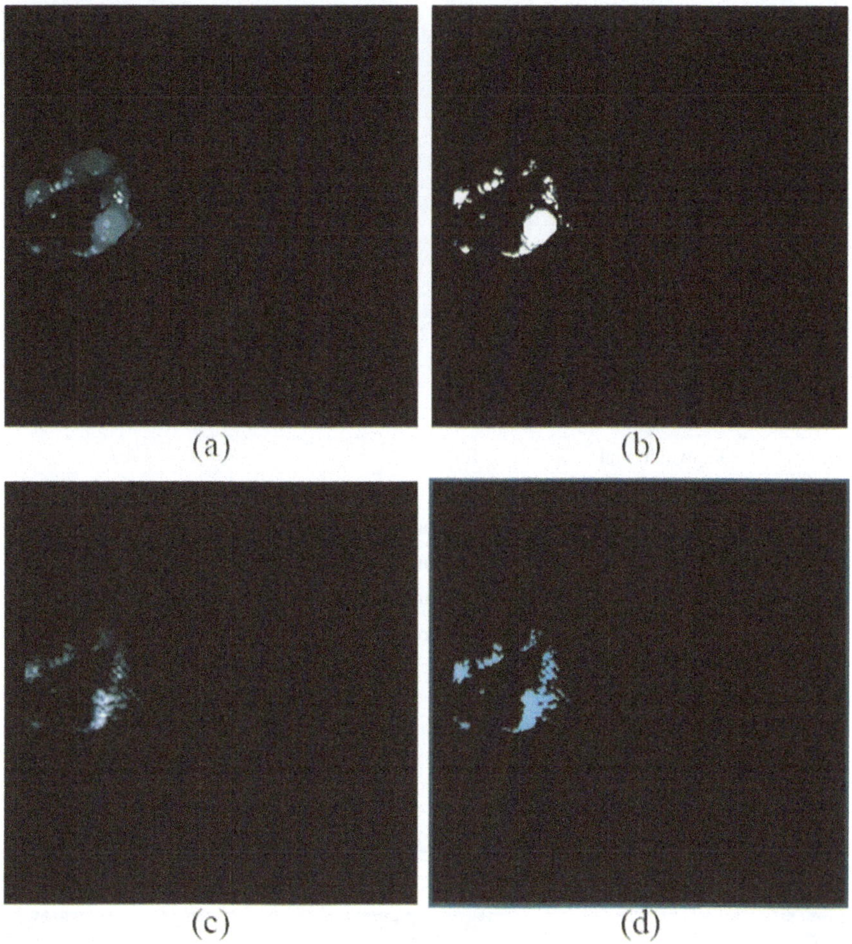

Fig. 9 Opening algorithm used to obtain candidate points. **a** result of opening algorithm; **b** result of segmented opening algorithm using otsu thresholds; **c** shows the residual image obtained by the difference in green channel image and inpainted image; **d** potential exudate images of candidates

8.2.6 Results

In this section the performance of the CNN model architecture has been compared in both the training as well as test set based on the parameters like accuracy, sensitivity, specificity, F-score. All the relevant values are mentioned in Table 6. Just below that the pictorial representation of exudate identification method is also mentioned (Fig. 10).

Table 5 Architecture of the CNN model

No.	LayerType	Maps	Size	KerSize
0	Input layer	1	64	–
1	Convolutional	32	62	3 fi 3
2	Convolutional	32	60	3 fi 3
3	MaxPool	32	30	2 fi 2
4	Convolutional	64	28	3 fi 3
5	Convolutional	64	26	3 fi 3
6	MaxPool	64	13	2 fi 2
7	Convolutional	96	11	3 fi 3
8	Convolutional	96	9	3 fi 3
9	MaxPool	96	4	2 fi 2
10	Convolutional	128	2	3 fi 3
11	MaxPool	128	1	2 fi 2
12	Fully Connected	64 Neurons		
13	DropOut	64 Neurons		
14	Fully Connected	64 Neurons		
	Output Layer	2 Neurons		

Table 6 Proposed CNN model architecture performance analysis

	Training set (%)	Test set (%)
Accuracy	96.21	91.92
Sensitivity	94.28	88.85
Specificity	98.06	96.00
F-Score	96.05	92.61

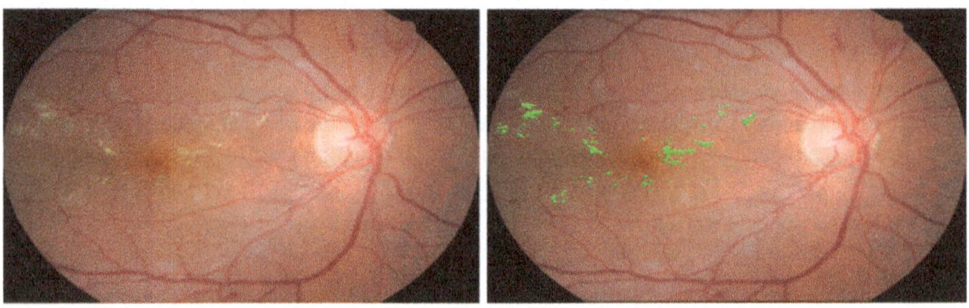

(a) (b)

Fig. 10 Result of exudate identification by using the mentioned method. **a** Image with exudate; **b** the exudates obtained by the algorithm has been illustrated in green colour

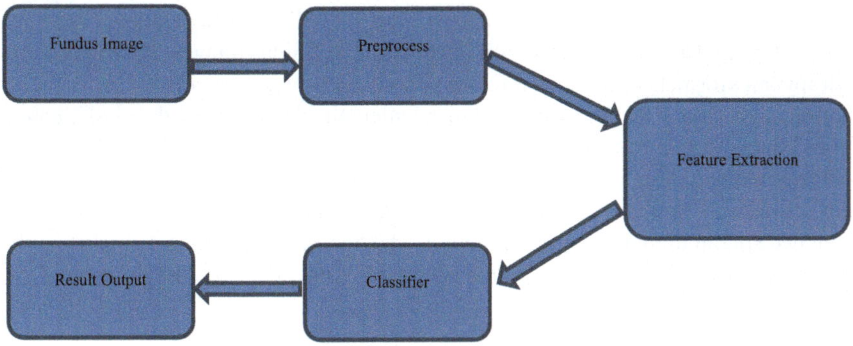

Fig. 11 The flow chart of cataract classification

8.3 Cataract Fundus Image Mitigation Using Deep Learning Approach

The situation of milky layer formation on the eye lens is called cataract. Cataract may even lead to permanent eye blindness. Therefore, considering the range up to which cataract can affect eyesight, it is essential to use the computer science to detect cataract earlier by using the methodology of classification of retinal image. In this step mainly the features of the retinal image are extracted. The images of fundus are first pre-processed using the maximum entropy technique. Further, more features of the images of the fundus are extracted by using deep learning model. Then several algorithms for classification domain are utilized to identify the features that are extracted. Then Softmax and SVM model are incorporated to classify the cataract by utilizing the features extracted through deep learning methods and extracted wavelet features from RV (retinal vascular). The classes to images are categorized are normal, slight, medium or severe. Better results of classification are obtained when deep learning is used to extract the features followed by using Softmax for classification. The results thus obtained show that this study done on deep learning is operative and has real world value.

8.3.1 Methodology

See Fig. 11.

8.3.2 Pre-processing

Image pre-processing is required because of the varying quality of images used here. The most important step of fundus image pre-processing is image enhancement. Earlier histogram equalization method was used to enhance the quality of the image but specifically for this study it won't be fruitful as it will leave huge amount of image information and also the blood vessel information of fundus images. Here maximum entropy transformation is selected foe pre-processing. In maximum entropy transformation, the iterative technique is used to calculate the threshold for the classification of gray images followed by the utilization of transform function for the local gray image transformation. The separation point is found out by taking the gray images edges followed by the threshold value calculation on both sides and non-linearly stretched spatial domain improve function. This method improves the quality of the image retaining the information of the original fundus image to a larger extent.

8.3.3 Deep Learning

Figure 12 illustrates the model of the convolution layer used. The kernel size of the conv layer is set to be 11, number of output to be 96 and stride being 4. In order to extract the local features each input layer neuron is linked to the previous local receptive field layer.

After the local features are found out the location of the relationship between them and other features is found out too. Local features and the features sharing weight make parameter calculation in the convolution much easier. Here the activation function used is ReLU. The ReLU function introduces non-linear properties to the neural network which enables it to do non-linear mappings from input to the outputs. Also the neural networks using the backpropagation. Non-linear features are fully extracted by this method. The pooling layer is used to compress the size of the input image matrix.

Feature map compression helps to reduce the computational time of the network and also to extract the main features. In pooling a window of size 3 and a stride of 2 was taken. The input zone of the image was normalized by using a Norm layer. It can help in reducing the probability of overfitting by increasing the learning rate. The features extracted become more standardized.

The input image of size 3048×2432 gets reduce to $256 \times 6\times 6$ as feature maps after passing through the layers of convolution and pooling. Figure 13 shows the 3rd, 4th, 5th of the deep learning network, namely fc3, fc4, fc5, respectively.

Machine learning system can be built under the supervision of experts for designing feature extractors and production of feature vectors from the raw data.

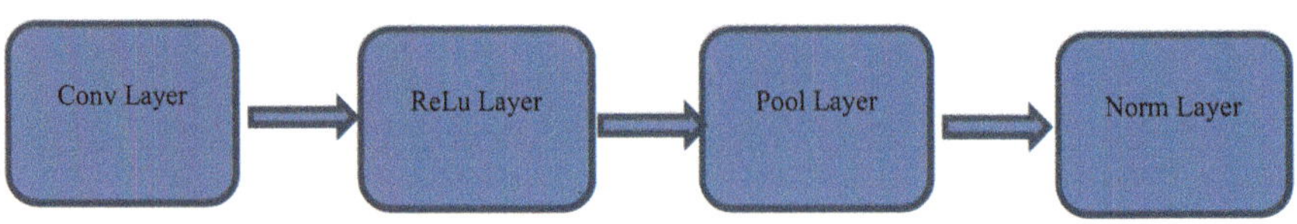

Fig. 12 CNN layer model

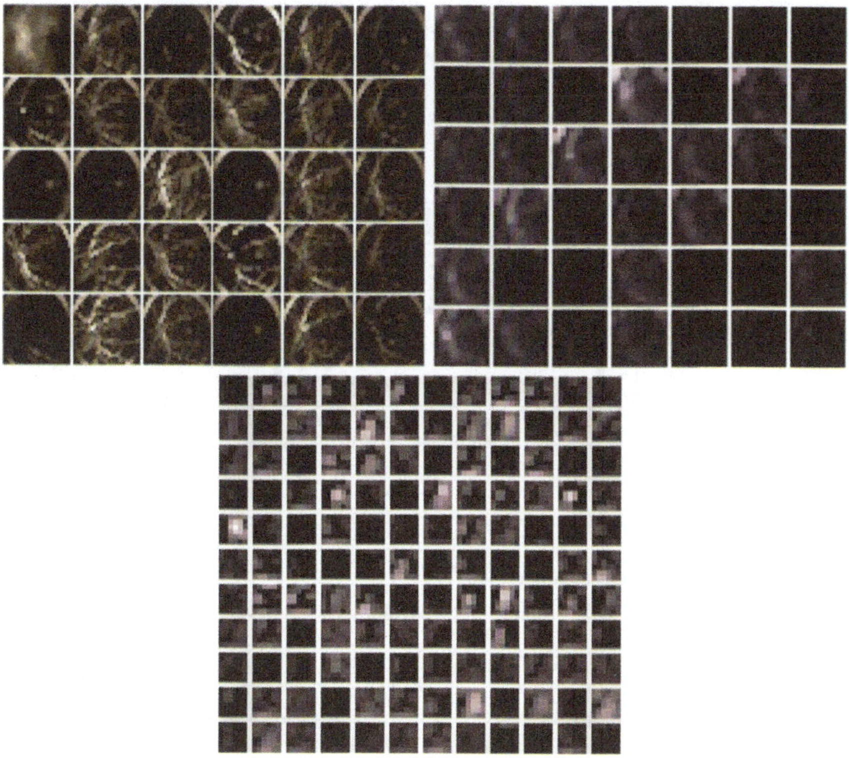

Fig. 13 fc3, fc4, fc5 extracted image

There is no need for the deep learning systems to extract the artificial design characteristics. The method proposed has remarkable robustness and generalization standards. All the features tasks for classification in the following stage are derived from the fc5 data layer. However, the matrix generated in the fc5 layer has a big size and there is no knowledge about the numbers in the matrix. The feature map distribution curve has been illustrated in Fig. 14.

8.3.4 Results

Below results shows the classification results for the given dataset for different scenarios. Feature B moves ahead in the game with an accuracy of 84.7% in svm classification results (4) while feature A takes the lead in classification results (2). However, feature A has better accuracies in both soft-max classification results (2) & (4) with accuracies 94.07% and 90.82%, respectively (Tables 7, 8, 9 and 10).

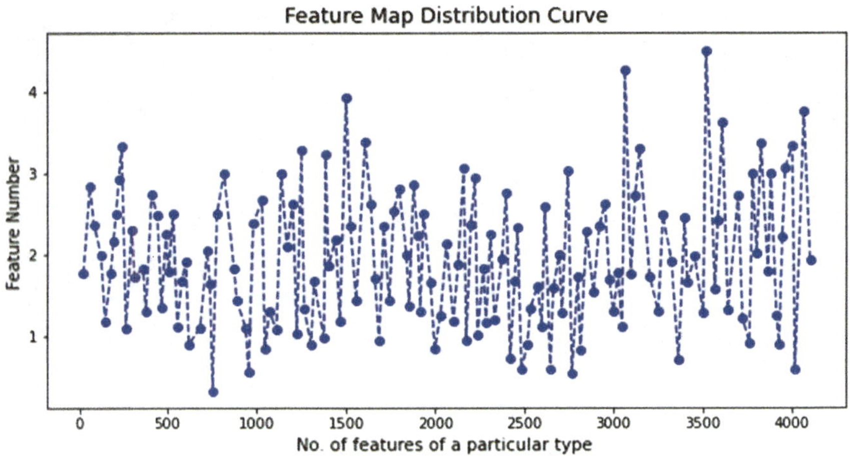

Fig. 14 Feature map distribution

Table 7 SVM classifier classification results (4)

Features	Normal	Slight	Medium	Severe	Accuracy
A	88.92	80.22	87.2	81.63	82.94
B	90.91	76.81	90.47	55.3	84.7

Table 8 The SVM classification results (2)

Features	Normal	Non-Normal	Accuracy
A	87.82	91.06	89.83
B	91.95	83.88	86

Table 9 The soft max classification results (4)

Features,	Normal	Slight	Medium	Severe	Accuracy
A	95.63	83.23	91.04	82.61	90.82
B	87.99	90.12	77.82	68.75	84.17

Table 10 The soft max classification results (2)

Features	Normal	Non-normal	Accuracy
A	93.95	95.84	94.07
B	82.07	80.85	81.91

9 Observations

Based on the studies discussed and examined in the Sects. 8.1, 8.2, 8.3 we obtained few observations that were worth discussing. Some of the drawbacks in the model along with the distinguishing features have been mentioned below.

9.1 Study

- Grading and detection of AMD in eye retina can be efficiently done by making use of deep learning models.
- The accuracy of the models can be improved by pre-processing the images of fundus to eliminate the lens glare and non-uniform illumination.
- When compared with pre-trained models the models trained explicitly with fundus images produces much better results. Moreover, deeper models classify the fundus images more effectively. The cost incurred for analysis and screening of fundus images can be lessened by using the automated grading through deep learning models.

9.2 Study

- For both training and testing set the accuracy obtained for pixel-wise classification was high.
- With the upsurge in the amount of training data and variation the model will show better accuracy and performance which is evident from the nature of machine learning.

9.3 Study

- The five layer conv layer approach to the traditional CNN Model helped in separating numerous non-linear combinations characteristics of images of fundus through a multi-layered non-linear mapping.
- The features extracted using the deep learning when compared to the previous experiment features helped to distinguish the cataract lesions degree in the training set up to a greater extent.
- The number of images for study purpose was very less still by using the proposed architecture the classification accuracy was greatly improved (Table 11).

Table 11 Comparative analysis of the studies in 10.1, 10.2, 10.3 on the basis of few parameters

	Study 8.1	Study 8.2	Study 8.3
Domain of work	Analysis of fundus-based macular degeneration using DNN	Diabetic Retinopathy identification using CNN	Cataract fundus image study using deep learning
Dataset used	AREDS Dataset	E-Ophtha EX	DRISHTI-GS1
Preprocessing technique	Rescalling + Quality scanning	Ultimate Opening + Optic Disc Detection + Impaint Vessels	Maximum entropy transformation
Technology used	VGG16 + CNN	CNN	CNN
Results obtained	Accuracy of 92.5% in VGG16 and 88.5% in CNN	Accuracy of 91.92%	Wavelet feature classification accuracy of 84.7%

10 Conclusion

The study focuses a light on the recent developments and works in the field of AI techniques, particularly in the field of deep learning that can be used for the detection of various kinds of diseases. These techniques help the doctor to make decision in clinical environment by analyzing the relevant data points and medical imagery of the patient. Deep learning techniques acts as an interface between the image data that is archived and the clinical image flow. Moreover, the use of deep learning in disease detection and diagnosis can leverage the speed of decision making by reducing the false positive rates. Also it can be observed from the study that different deep learning techniques have showed really impressive results in detecting and diagnosing various diseases. With continuous discoveries and advancements in AI by leveraging the use of deep learning techniques, we can be able to surpass the human accuracies of disease diagnosis.

References

1. Shie, C.K., Chuang, C.H., Chou, C.N., Wu, M.H., Chang, E.Y.: Transfer representation learning for medical image analysis. In: IEEE Engineering in Medicine and Biology Society, pp. 711–714 (2015)
2. Meherwar, F., Maruf, P.: Survey of machine learning algorithms for disease diagnostic. J. Intell. Learn. Syst. Appl., 1–16 (2017)
3. Yu, D., Deng, L.: Deep learning and its applications to signal and information processing. IEEE Signal Process. Mag. **28**(1), 145–154 (2011)
4. Shi, J., Malik, J.: Normalized cuts and image segmentation. IEEE Trans. Pattern Anal. Mach. Intell. **22**(8), 888–905 (2000)
5. Kumar, A., Kim, J., Cai, W., Feng, D.: Content-based medical image retrieval: a survey of applications to multidimensional and multimodality data. J Digit Imaging **26**(6), 1025–1039 (2013)

6. Tajbakhsh, N., Shin, J.Y., Gurudu, S.R., Hurst, R.T., Kendall, C.B., Gotway, M.B., Liang, J.: Convolutional neural networks for medical image analysis: full training or fine tuning? IEEE T Med Imaging **35**(5), 1299–1312 (2016)
7. Albu, A., Stanciu, L.: Benefits of using artificial intelligence in medical predictions. In: 1EEE, E-Health and Bioengineering Conference (EHB) (2016)
8. Abedini, M., Codella, N.C.F., Connell, J.H., Garnavi, R., Merler, M., Pankanti, S., Smith, J.R., Syeda-Mahmood, T.: A generalized framework for medical image classification and recognition. IBM J. Res. Dev. **59**(2/3), 1:1–1:18 (2015)
9. Bishop, C.: Pattern Recognition and Machine Learning. Springer, New York (2006)
10. Gelenbe, E., Yin, Y.: Deep learning with random neural networks. In: Neural Networks (IJCNN), 2016 International Joint Conference (2016)
11. LeCun, Y., Bengio, Y., Hinton, G.: Deep learning. Nature **521**(7553), 436–444 (2015)
12. Huo, Y., Vincken, K.L., Lafeber, F.P., Viergever, M.A.: Automatic quantification of radiographic finger joint space width of patients with early rheumatoid arthritis. IEEE J. Magaz. **63**(10), 2177 – 2186 (2016)
13. Suma, A.B., Snekhalatha, U., Rajalakshmi, T.: Automated thermal image segmentation of knee rheumatoid arthritis. In: IEEE International conference on Communication and Signal Processing (ICCSP) (2016)
14. Langs, G., Peloschek, P., Bischof, H., Kainberger, F.: Automatic quantification of joint space narrowing and erosions in rheumatoid arthritis. IEEE Trans. Med. Imaging **28**(1) (2009)
15. Jhajharia, S., Varshney, H.K., Verma, S., Kumar, R.: A neural network based breast cancer prognosis model with PCA processed features. In: IEEE, International Conference on Advances in Computing, Communications and Informatics (ICACCI) (2016)
16. Zheng, L., Chan, A.K.: An artificial intelligent algorithm for tumor detection in screening mammogram. IEEE Trans. Med. Imaging **20**(7), 559–567 (2001)
17. Wang, J., Ding, H., Bidgoli, F.A., Zhou, B., Iribarren, C., Molloi, S., Baldi, P.: Detecting Cardiovascular Disease from Mammograms With Deep Learning. IEEE Trans. Med. Imaging **36**(5), 1172–1181 (2017)
18. Khobragade, S., Tiwari, A., Patil, C.Y., Narke, V.: Automatic detection of major lung diseases using Chest Radiographs and classification by feed-forward artificial neural network. In: IEEE, International Conference on Power Electronics, Intelligent Control and Energy Systems (ICPEICES) (2017)
19. Otoom, A.F., Abdallah, E.E., Kilani, Y., Kefaye, A., Ashour, M.: Effective diagnosis and monitoring of heart disease. Int. J. Softw. Eng. Appl. **9**, 143–156 (2015)
20. Vembandasamy, K., Sasipriya, R., Deepa, E.: Heart diseases detection using Naive Bayes Algorithm. IJISET Int. J. Innovat. Sci. Eng. Technol. **2**, 441–444 (2015)
21. Mishra, S., Tripathy, H.K., Mallick, P.K., Bhoi, A.K., Barsocchi, P.: EAGA-MLP—an enhanced and adaptive hybrid classification model for diabetes diagnosis. Sensors **20**, 4036 (2020)
22. Mishra, S., Mallick, P.K., Jena, L., Chae, G.S.: Optimization of skewed data using sampling-based preprocessing approach. Front Public Health. **8**, 274 (2020). Published 2020 Jul 16. https://doi.org/10.3389/fpubh.2020.00274

Deep Learning Neural Network and CNN-Based Diagnosis of Heart Diseases

Adyasha Rath, Debahuti Mishra, and Ganapati Panda

Abstract This chapter deals with a critical review of articles on Deep learning Neural Network (DLNN) and Convolutional neural network (CNN)-based diagnosis of heart disease (HD) published in journals between 2017–2020. The review of these articles highlights the source of HD data, the problem statement, the methodology used, types of features extraction, and features selection or features reduction employed in HD detection. In addition, it presents the contribution, key results obtained as well as the limitations and possible further extensions of the research work. It is believed that the presentation in the chapter will provide useful guidance to the new researchers to further their research work using DLNN and CNN-based approaches in the area of health care.

Keywords Diagnosis of heart diseases · Coronary heart disease · Deep learning · CNN · Classification of heart disease

1 Introduction

According to WHO, the cardiovascular disease (CVD) is the major cause of global mortality. As reported by Indian Heart Association, 50% of Indian heart patients are less than 50 years and 25% are less than 40 years of age. The CVD includes cardiomyopathy (heart muscle disease), arrhythmia (irregular heartbeats), and coronary artery disease (issues relating to blood vessels). Heart failure and the heart

A. Rath · D. Mishra (✉)
Department of Computer Science and Engineering, Siksha 'O' Anusandhan (Deemed To Be) University, Bhubaneswar, Odisha, India
e-mail: debahutimishra@soa.ac.in

A. Rath
e-mail: adyasharath1996@gmail.com

G. Panda
Department of Electronics and Tele Communication, C V Raman Global University, Bhubaneswar, Odisha, India
e-mail: ganapati.panda@gmail.com

H. K. Tripathy et al. (eds.), *Technical Advancements of Machine Learning in Healthcare*, Studies in Computational Intelligence 936,
https://doi.org/10.1007/978-981-33-4698-7_9

attacks are two forms of the heart disease (HD). When one of the arteries leading to the heart is blocked, the blood flow is cut off. This gives rise to most of the heart attacks. On the other hand, heart failure develops gradually. In this case, the heart muscle becomes weaker and hence the pumping of the blood becomes difficult to nourish the cell. Diabetes, hypertension, atherogenic dyslipidemia, central obesity, smoking, and physical inactivity are some of the factors which are responsible for alarming rise of coronary heart disease (CHD). It is reported that nearly 50% Americans suffer from some type of HD. The HD is mostly contributed by blood clot, high cholesterol, plaque build up, blood pressure, and obesity. Healthy lifestyle and proper diet can prevent many of these conditions. Some representative examples of warning sign for assessing the heart condition are shortness of breath, numb, chest pain, and fatigue. Few initial tests to diagnose HD are stress test, blood test, electrocardiogram, recording, X-ray, ultrasound, MRI, and CT-scan.

In India, the chance of suffering of urban people from HD is three times more than that of people living in villages. According to American heart association 2019, approximately 12.15 millions of adults in USA have some form of CVD causing 647,000 deaths per year. Further, it is predicted by world heart federation, 2019 that by 2023, 23 million deaths per year will take place due to the CVD. It is also reported that a stroke in every 40 s happens to someone in USA. The above-cited facts reveal that HD is very fatal and causes maximum number of global deaths compared to all other diseases. Hence, all countries of the world are focusing on early detection, proper treatment, and creating awareness on severity of heart diseases. Therefore, early detection of HD is extremely important. To address this problem, the scientists, engineers and doctors have focussed their attentions for devising affordable methods for diagnosis and treatment of different types of heart diseases. Keeping these aspects in mind the proposed book chapter has been planned to provide a critical overview of existing literature which deals with the diagnosis of HD. It is, in general, observed that large number of articles have appeared dealing with early detection and diagnosis of heart diseases. In this current book chapter, selected but important articles of major two types of heart diseases have been chosen for critical review. These articles have been published in standard journals during 2017 to 2020. In recent past, DLNN and CNN have proven to be powerful and promising machine learning (ML) tools and have been successfully employed in many fields because of their superior potentiality for HD detection. Considering these two aspects the present book chapter has been conceived and developed to analyse the work reported in HD detection using CNN and DLNN.

2 Objectives and Organization

The section deals with the objectives and the organization of the book chapter.

2.1 *Objectives*

- To identify and collect relevant and recently published articles on classification of HD using CNN and DLNN-based methods.
- To compile and present a detailed review of the collected articles on classification of heart diseases.
- To review the selected articles in terms of source of data, methodology employed, contributions made, and concluding remarks.
- To present and explain of CNN and DLNN-based diagnosis of HD.
- To provide and analyze the various performance measures related to HD classifications which have been reported in these articles.
- To present the concluding remarks highlighting the contribution of the chapter and outlining the scope of future research work in the area of HD detection.

2.2 *Organization*

Keeping the above objectives in mind, the organization of the book chapter proceeds as follows:

In Sect. 2, the objectives of the book chapter is outlined. It also deals with the organization of the chapter. In Sect. 3, an overview of literature on HD detection using CNN and DLNN is presented. A detail review of collected literature on HD detection using CNN and DLNN are dealt in Sect. 4. The review is presented in a tabular form. In Sect. 5, the development schemes using CNN and DLNN is for HD detection is covered. A comparative performance of various classifications and detection of heart diseases using two approaches are presented and analyzed in Sect. 6. Finally, the conclusion section discusses the contributions of the chapter and the future scope of the work in this area.

3 An Overview of Literature

Fifteen relevant articles on HD detection specifiaclly using CNN and DLNN methods and published between 2017–2020 have been collected. These articles are divided into two groups and is presented in Table 9.1. Eleven of these articles employ CNN as the key tool for diagnosis of HD. Four of the remaining articles use DLNN approach for classification of the HD. Even though many ML method have been chosen for

Table 9.1 Distribution of reviewed papers based on machine learning methods used

Machine learning method	Reference number of papers
CNN	[1, 3–10, 14, 15]
DL	[2, 11–13]

Table 9.2 Distribution of reviewed papers based on types of heart diseases

Types of HD	Reference number of papers
Arrhythmia	[4, 6–9]
CAD/CHD	[1–3, 10–12, 14]
Not Specified (Common HD)	[5, 13]

this purposes, those have not been included in this chapter as the focus of the chapter is on CNN and DLNN-based methods. Table 9.2 presents the distribution of review papers based on types of HDs. Five articles pertain to arrhythmia type HD, where as seven articles deal with detection of coronary artery disease (CAD) or coronary heart disease (CHD). The remaining two articles have reported on the classification of HD but specifically have not mentioned the types of HD.

4 Critical Review of Literature

In this section, a comparative review of fifteen articles published between 2017–2020 and dealing with DLNN and CNN-based diagnosis schemes is presented.

Table 9.3 contains the details of this review of articles on heart diseases, namely, on Arrhythmia and CAD or CHD. The review table comprises of six columns. The heading of columns of review table are journal and publisher name, year, vol. no, pages, title of the paper and names of authors, source of data used, the problem addressed and the methods used, contribution of the paper, conclusion, future scope, deficiency or weakness of the article. The last three columns contain the core of the each of the papers. The fourth column addresses the problem investigated and the method used in the article. The methods employed for training and validation are also presented in this column. Further, the techniques related to features extraction and features selection or features reduction as applicable for each paper, are mentioned. In the contribution column the significant results of the proposed methods are highlighted. In some cases, the results of the comparative performance study are also presented. Finally, in the conclusion section, three important items are included. These are overall conclusion, deficiency, and scope for further extension. In some papers, all the three items are not presented in the conclusion section. It is mostly observed that the CAD detection is made by using features of ECG signal extracted from CNN and then carrying out classification task in the last few layers of CNN. In case of DLNN-based methods the features are extracted using some transform domain technique [8] and then DLNN-based approach is used for classification task.

Table 9.3 Details of literature review on heart disease

Journal and Publisher name, year, Volume, Number and pages	Title of the paper and author details	Datsets used and sources	Problem addressed and methods used	Contribution of the paper	Conclusion, future scope, deficiencies or weaknesses identified
1. Elsevier Knowledge-based systems 2017, 132, pp.62–71	Automated detection of coronary artery disease using different durations of ECG segments with convolutional neural network Authors:- U. Rajendra Acharya et.al	PhysioNet databases, namely, fantasia (for normal) and St.-Petersburg Institute of cardiology Technics (for CAD) – ECG signals (20 males, 20 females) – 7 CAD (1 male, 6 female)	– Detection of CAD using ECG signal of different durations. The CNN is used for the diagnosis of CAD. CNN consists of four convolution layers, four max-pooling layers and three fully connected layers – Ten-fold cross-validation technique is used for training and testing purpose	– The CNN provides an accuracy of 94.95%, sensitivity of 93.72% and specificity of 95.18% for 2 s ECG signal data – But in case of 5 s ECG data, an accuracy of 95.11%, sensitivity of 91.13% and specificity of 95.88% were obtained	– The proposed CAD detection method is simple to use and affordable – Further work can be done to improve the CNN structure which may be suitable for larger database – Extension of this work can be made for early diagnosis of CAD

(continued)

Table 9.3 (continued)

Journal and Publisher name, year, Volume, Number and pages	Title of the paper and author details	Datsets used and sources	Problem addressed and methods used	Contribution of the paper	Conclusion, future scope, deficiencies or weaknesses identified
2. IEEE IEEE Transactions on Biomedical Engineering 2017, 65, pp. 956–968	A regularized deep learning approach for clinical risk prediction of acute coronary syndrome using electronic health records Authors:- Zhengxing Huang et.al	Chinese PLA general hospital – Samples from 3247 patients – Each with 200 features was used as dataset	– The paper investigates on the risk prediction of ACS using regularized SDAE model	– The AUC and accuracy of the proposed approach are found to be 0.868 and 0.73, respectively – The proposed method has the potential to identify the risk factors of patients with different risk levels	– The paper has developed a risk prediction model of patients having ACS using DL – Work can be extended for prediction of risk without using the expert opinion – The prediction task can also be carried out using other DL approaches

(continued)

Table 9.3 (continued)

Journal and Publisher name, year, Volume, Number and pages	Title of the paper and author details	Datsets used and sources	Problem addressed and methods used	Contribution of the paper	Conclusion, future scope, deficiencies or weaknesses identified
3. Elsevier Information Sciences 2017, 415, pp. 190–198	Application of deep convolutional neural network for automated detection of myocardial infarction using ECG signals Authors:- U. Rajendra Acharya et.al	ECG signals were obtained from the ECG database (Physikalisch-Technische-Bundesanstalt diagnostic ECG database) – Out of 200 subjects, 148 MI and 52 healthy. Number of male (39 normal, 110 MI) and number of female (13 normal, 38 MI) – ECG beats with and without noise have been used in the study	– A novel approach for automatic detection of MI using ECG signals is presented – A CNN model is used for this purpose – A total of 10,546 normal ECG beats and 40,182 MI ECG beats were use in this study	– For Noisy and noise free cases, – The accuracies are 93.53% and 95.22% – The sensitivities are 92.83% and 93.71% – The specificities are 94.19% and 95.49%, respectively	– The overall performance of the proposed approach is quite good – The proposed model can be employed for automatic detection of MI – The doctors can be assisted by the outcome of this proposed approach

(continued)

Table 9.3 (continued)

Journal and Publisher name, year, Volume, Number and pages	Title of the paper and author details	Datsets used and sources	Problem addressed and methods used	Contribution of the paper	Conclusion, future scope, deficiencies or weaknesses identified
4. Elsevier Computers in biology and medicine 2017, 89, pp.389–396	A deep convolutional neural network model to classify heartbeats Authors:- U. Rajendra. Acharya et.al	Opensource PhysioBank MIT-BIH arrhythmia database – Number of subjects is 47 – Sampling rate of ECG signal is 360 Hz – Each ECG beat 260 samples long. A total of 109,449 ECG beats were extracted	– Two sets of data were used – The paper has developed a nine layered CNN-based classification model for heartbeats – Five different categories of heartbeats have been identified Both noisy and noise free ECGs are used for simulation study	– The proposed method has achieved an accuracy of 89.07% and 89.3% using noisy and noise free ECG data, respectively	– The proposed method can be used for clinical settings to help the cardiologists for diagnosis purpose – Online implementation of the proposed scheme can reduce the waiting time of patients and work load of the cardiologists – Work can be extended to develop a CNN-based model to predict only three classes such as normal, abnormal and severe or critical

(continued)

Table 9.3 (continued)

Journal and Publisher name, year, Volume, Number and pages	Title of the paper and author details	Datsets used and sources	Problem addressed and methods used	Contribution of the paper	Conclusion, future scope, deficiencies or weaknesses identified
5. IEEE IEEE Transactions on Biomedical Engineering 2018, 65, pp. 1924–1934	Multi-views fusion CNN for left ventricular volumes estimation on cardiac MR Images Authors:-Gongning Luo et.al	– DSBCCD dataset – 500 training subjects, 200 validation subjects and 440 test subjects were used – The validation data were used for selecting optimal model – The test datasets were used to evaluate the performance	– The paper has proposed a new data processing method on CMR – A Multi-views fusion CNN has been proposed for estimation of LV volumes	– Proposed method outperforms other LV volumes estimation methods – The various performance metrics achieved are EDV: $R^2 =$ 0.974, RMSE = 9.6 ml; ESV: $R^2 =$ 0.976, RMSE = 7.1 ml; EF: $R^2 =$ 0.828, RMSE = 4.71%	– The simulation results reveal that the proposed CNN-based method is useful for prediction of LV volumes – This method can be applied for cardiac disease screening – The proposed method can be extended for analysis of other medical images

(continued)

Table 9.3 (continued)

Journal and Publisher name, year, Volume, Number and pages	Title of the paper and author details	Datsets used and sources	Problem addressed and methods used	Contribution of the paper	Conclusion, future scope, deficiencies or weaknesses identified
6. Elsevier Computers in biology and medicine 2018, 102, pp. 278–287	Automated diagnosis of arrhythmia using combination of CNN and LSTM techniques with variable length heartbeats Authors:- Shu Lih Oh et.al	PhysioNet public database – 48 ECG recordings were obtained – Total number of segments is 16499 – Number of segments less than 1000 samples is 13535 and number of segments more than 1000 samples is 2963	– Paper has proposed an automated diagnosis method using CNN, LSTM techniques. The paper employs variable length heart beats – The diagnosis consists of normal sinus rhythm, LBBB, RBBB, APB, and PVC – Ten-fold cross validation strategy has been used	The proposed approach provides an accuracy of 98.10%, sensitivity of 97.50% and specificity of 98.70%	– The CNN is selected for picking up spatial features and LSTM is used because of learning of temporal features – The method does not require noise filtering, feature extraction, and selection – It is assumed that each ECG segment has one type of arrhythmia

(continued)

Table 9.3 (continued)

Journal and Publisher name, year, Volume, Number and pages	Title of the paper and author details	Datsets used and sources	Problem addressed and methods used	Contribution of the paper	Conclusion, future scope, deficiencies or weaknesses identified
7. IEEE IEEE Access 2018, 6, pp. 27,465–27,472	Automated ECG classification using dual heartbeat coupling based on convolutional neural network Authors:- Xiaolong Zhai and Chung Tin	MIT-BIH arrhythmia database	– The paper has suggested automatic classification of ECG signal using CNN. The method employs dual heartbeat coupling – The proposed approach detects SVEB or S beats and VEB	The proposed CNN approach provides sensitivity and positive predictive rate for S beats which is 12.2% and 11.9% more than the best performing algorithms. The Acc, sen, spec, and ppr of VEB beat for 24 testing records are 98.6, 93.8, 99.2, and 92.4, respectively	– The reported approach provides a reliable and automatic tool for detection of arrhythmia heartbeat without feature extraction – It can be implemented to develop a portable device for monitoring of cardiac arrhythmia

(continued)

Table 9.3 (continued)

Journal and Publisher name, year, Volume, Number and pages	Title of the paper and author details	Datsets used and sources	Problem addressed and methods used	Contribution of the paper	Conclusion, future scope, deficiencies or weaknesses identified
8. IEEE IEEE Access 2019, 7, pp. 92,871–92,880	ECG Arrhythmia classification using STFT-based Spectrogram and Convolutional neural network Authors:- Jingshan Huang et.al	– MIT-BIH arrhythmia database – Sampling rate 360 Hz – A segment of 10 s of ECG signals has been selected – The signals have been divided into 2520 samples	– The paper employs a CNN for classification of ECG arrhythmia. It uses spectrogram which is obtained from STFT	– The proposed model provides an average accuracy of 99%. A learning rate 0.001 and a batch size of 2500 provide highest accuracy and lowest loss – The 1D-CNN model was also used for the same dataset and an average accuracy of 90.93% was achieved	– The use of spectrogram as input to the CNN model has substantially improved the accuracy

(continued)

Table 9.3 (continued)

Journal and Publisher name, year, Volume, Number and pages	Title of the paper and author details	Datsets used and sources	Problem addressed and methods used	Contribution of the paper	Conclusion, future scope, deficiencies or weaknesses identified
9. IEEE IEEE Access 2019, 7, pp. 67,123–67,129	Morphological arrhythmia automated diagnosis method using gray-level co-occurrence matrix enhanced convolutional neural network Authors:- Weifang Sun et.al	– MIT-BIH arrhythmia database was used – Sampling rate = 360 – Data belonging to six types of cardiac arrhythmias were chosen – 680 records of ECG signals were used	– The paper has presented an improved CNN for automated diagnosis of morphological arrhythmia – It employs GLCM for statistical feature extraction	– The proposed method can efficiently extract the required feature vector for efficiently identifying arrhythmia – The experimental results show high diagnostic performance	– The proposed method can be used in clinical situation. The suggested method can also be used for other biomedical signals

(continued)

Table 9.3 (continued)

Journal and Publisher name, year, Volume, Number and pages	Title of the paper and author details	Datsets used and sources	Problem addressed and methods used	Contribution of the paper	Conclusion, future scope, deficiencies or weaknesses identified
10. Elsevier Medical Image Analysis 2019, 51, pp. 46–60	Coronary artery centreline extraction in cardiac CT angiography using a CNN-based orientation classifier Authors:- Jelmer M. Wolterink et.al	– CAT08 dataset – 32 CCTA images, Siemens medical solutions, Forchheim, Germany – UMCU dataset – 50 CCTA scans, University medical center Utrecht, Utrecht, The Netherlands – orCaScore dataset – 36 CCTA scans, Toshiba medical systems, Otawara, Japan	– The paper develops a CNN classifier for coronary artery centreline extraction from CCTA scans	– The CNN approach was able to provide seed-based iterative tracker with information about the direction of coronary centreline as well as the radius of the coronary lumen at a given point – Extraction of centreline took an average of 0.4 s and complete coronary tree extraction took around 20 s	– The proposed method can be trained with limited training dataset. It also allows fast automatic extraction of coronary artery trees from CCTA images – As an extension of the current work the set of centreline can further be processed to identify bifurcations

(continued)

Table 9.3 (continued)

Journal and Publisher name, year, Volume, Number and pages	Title of the paper and author details	Datsets used and sources	Problem addressed and methods used	Contribution of the paper	Conclusion, future scope, deficiencies or weaknesses identified
11. Elsevier Biomedical signal processing and control 2019, 52, pp. 77–83	Automatic staging model of heart failure based on deep learning Authors:- Dengao Li et. al	– CPCs of Shanxi academy of medical sciences – 573 patients – The dataset consists of ECG signals, genders, age, hypertension, history of diabetes, primary percutaneous coronary intervention	– The paper has developed DL-based HF detection – It has employed a CNN RNN model – In the pre-processing stage, the data is segmented and augmented – CNN is used for feature extraction and RNN is used for classification	– The proposed model achieves an accuracy of 97.6%, sensitivity of 96.3%, and specificity of 97.4% for two seconds of ECG segments – The corresponding values for 5 s ECG signal are 96.2%, 96.9% and 95.7%, respectively	– The proposed model has achieved a robust and generalization performance on real data set – It can be employed for additional health care purpose

(continued)

Table 9.3 (continued)

Journal and Publisher name, year, Volume, Number and pages	Title of the paper and author details	Datsets used and sources	Problem addressed and methods used	Contribution of the paper	Conclusion, future scope, deficiencies or weaknesses identified
12. Elsevier Information Fusion 2020, 63, pp. 208–222	A smart healthcare monitoring system for heart disease prediction based on ensemble deep learning and feature fusion Authors:- Farman Ali et.al	The physiological data were collected using wearable sensors (Medical and activity sensor) – These data are used for training purpose – For testing purpose, Cleveland and Hungarian data from UCI repository are used	– The paper has proposed a HD prediction system using ensemble DL – Feature fusion method is used to combine the extracted features from sensor data and electronic medical records – Information gain technique is used to eliminate irrelevant features and select the important ones. This decreases the computational effort and improves the performance	– The proposed system provides an accuracy of 98.5% which is better than the accuracies obtained by SVM, LR, MLP, RF, DT, and NB classifiers	– Compared to six standard methods the proposed ensemble DL method provides highest accuracy of classification – Some novel feature reduction method can be used to handle larger volumes of health care records – To further improve the performance, noisy data needs to be cleaned before use and irrelevant features need to be removed

(continued)

Table 9.3 (continued)

Journal and Publisher name, year, Volume, Number and pages	Title of the paper and author details	Datsets used and sources	Problem addressed and methods used	Contribution of the paper	Conclusion, future scope, deficiencies or weaknesses identified
13. Springer Health and Technology 2020, 10, pp. 207–216	Heart disease classification using hybridized Ruzzo-Tompa memetic-based deep neocognitron neural network Authors:- J. Vijayashree and H. Parveen Sultana	HD dataset from UCI repository – 303 patients and 75 attributes	– The paper employs hybridized Ruzzo-Tompa memetic approach is used for feature selection – DTNN is used for HD classification – The results have been compared with BAT-BP, GA-CNN, and ACONN methods	The proposed method provides a mean square error of 0.0103, precision of 99.835, recall of 99.875, and F-measure of 99.85% which is higher than the corresponding results of other three methods	– The proposed hybrid approach is shown to be a promising HD classification technique – In future, the proposed method can be applied for larger datasets and other optimization techniques can be used for selection of features

(continued)

Table 9.3 (continued)

Journal and Publisher name, year, Volume, Number and pages	Title of the paper and author details	Datsets used and sources	Problem addressed and methods used	Contribution of the paper	Conclusion, future scope, deficiencies or weaknesses identified
14. Elsevier Expert systems with applications 2020, 159, pp.113408	An efficient convolutional neural network for coronary heart disease prediction Authors:- Aniruddha Dutta et.al	NHANES data from 1999–2000 to 2015–2016 – 37,079 total data – 1300 CHD – 35,779 Non-CHD	– A novel CHD prediction model has been developed using CNN – A LASSO-based feature assessment is employed – In addition, majority voting-based identification of important features have been made – A simulated annealing process is used to boost the classifier accuracy	– The paper has achieved a balanced accuracy of 79.5% which is better than SVM and RF classifiers – The proposed classifier also provides higher specificity, test accuracy, high value of recall, and AUC	– The paper has suggested a novel approach for classification of CHD using unbalanced data – Other clinical datasets which are unbalanced in nature can also be used in this model to obtain improved accuracy

(continued)

Table 9.3 (continued)

Journal and Publisher name, year, Volume, Number and pages	Title of the paper and author details	Datsets used and sources	Problem addressed and methods used	Contribution of the paper	Conclusion, future scope, deficiencies or weaknesses identified
15. IEEE IEEE Access 2020, 8 pp. 130,551–130,560	ECG signal reconstruction via Doppler sensor by hybrid deep learning model with CNN and LSTM Authors:- Kohei Yamamoto et.al	Data was collected using Doppler sensor with a sampling frequency of 1000 Hz – Number of epochs to train the model = 40 – Batch size to train the model is 180 – Number of subjects = 9	– The paper develops a novel method for reconstruction of ECG signal using hybrid deep learning model of CNN and LSTM – The CNN is used for extraction of spatial and temporal features	– The experimental results show that the ECG signal is reconstructed with a correlation coefficient of 0.86 – It is demonstrated that the ECG signal can be reconstructed from the heart beat signal via a Doppler sensor	– The accuracy of reconstruction of ECG signal can further be improved by developing appropriate ML-based models

In few papers [6, 15] hybrid models are used in which the CNN is employed for features extraction and another ML method is used for classification or prediction purpose. It is, in general, observed that the CNN is mostly used both for features extraction and classification task and thus eliminates the problem of appropriate choice of features of input data. To facilitate reading and understanding, nomenclatures are used for standard technical terms. By going through all fifteen articles a list of nomenclatures has been prepared and presented in Table 9.4. It is grouped into three columns. The first column of nomenclatures is related to HD whereas the second group lists the nomenclatures commonly used for ML techniques. The nomenclatures of other technical terms are presented in the third group. The relevant test data, signals such as ECG or images of different subjects should be from standard sources. This is because the performance of various methods needs to be compared to identify the best method. The sources of data related to various heart diseases are collected from different papers are obtained and are presented in Table 9.5. The main sources of data used by various authors are: Physionet database, MIT-BIH arrhythmia database and UCI repository. It is observed that most of the papers employ either ECG signal, heart sound signal, or cardiac MR images. Various articles have used different features extraction and features selection or features reduction methods. A compilation of these methods used by different articles is presented in Table 9.6. The common methods for features extraction and features selection are convolution layers of CNN, GLCM, feature fusion, HRM, and majority voting algorithm.

5 CNN and DLNN-Based Methods for HD Detection

The reviews of papers made in this chapter are very recent and employs the CNN and DLNN methods for detection or classification of heart diseases. In this section, the basic principle of training and operation of CNN and DLNN are presented.

5.1 Development of CNN-Based Classification Model

Figure 9.1 shows the block diagram of a CNN-based classification scheme. In case of HD detection, the input to the models is either an ECG signal or images-related HD. In rare cases, features of HD patients are used as input. The CNN structure primarily comprises of convolution operation followed by pooling operation. These two stages are repeated numbers of times until desired features are achieved to provide best possible accuracy of classification. The objective of convolution operation is extraction of features. The convolution operation is performed between the input datasets and 1 or 2-Dimensional filter coefficients. The pooling operation is carried out for dimensionality reduction. In case of maximum pooling, the maximum value in the window of the segmented features is chosen. But in case of average pooling, the windowed values are replaced by the average value. After the desired features are

Table 9.4 Nomenclature used in reported articles

Heart-Related		ML Techniques		Others	
Electrocardiography	ECG	Machine Learning	ML	Area under curve	AUC
Coronary Artery Disease	CAD	Convolutional neural network	CNN	Massachusetts Institute of Technology-Beth Israel hospital	MIT-BIH
Acute coronary syndrome	ACS	Stacked de-noising auto encoder	SDAE	Correlation coefficient	R
Myocardial Infarction	MI	Deep learning	DL	Root mean square error	RMSE
Left ventricle	LV	Long short-term memory	LSTM	Short-time fourier transform	STFT
End-diastole volume	EDV	One dimensional convolutional neural network	1D-CNN	Gray-level co-occurrence matrix	GLCM
End-systole volume	ESV	Recurrent neural network	RNN	University of California Irvine	UCI
Ejection fraction	EF	Support vector machine	SVM	Least absolute shrinkage and selection operator	LASSO
Cardiac magnetic resonance	CMR	Logistic regression	LR	National health and nutritional examination survey	NHANES
Left bundle branch block	LBBB	Multi layer perceptron	MLP	Data science bowl cardiac challenge data	DSBCCD
Right bundle branch block	RBBB	Random forest	RF	Positive Predictive Rate	PPR
Arterial premature beats	APB	Decision tree	DT	World health organization	WHO
Premature ventricular contraction	PVC	Naive bayes	NB	Mean square error	MSE
Supraventricular ectopic beats	SVEB or S	Deep trained neocognitron neural network	DTNN		
Ventricular ectopic beats	VEB	Hybridized Ruzzo-Tompa memetic algorithm	HRM		

(continued)

Table 9.4 (continued)

Heart-Related		ML Techniques		Others	
Electrocardiography	ECG	Machine Learning	ML	Area under curve	AUC
Coronary artery centreline extraction in cardiac CT angiography	CCTA	Bat-based back propagation algorithm	BAT-BP		
Coronary artery tracking challenge	CAT08	Genetic algorithm optimization of a convolutional neural network	GA-CNN		
Heart failure	HF	Ant colony optimization neural network	ACONN		
Heart Disease	HD	Deep learning neural network	DLNN		
Coronary heart disease	CHD				
Chest pain center	CPC				

Table 9.5 Sources of data related to heart diseases

References	Sources
[1]	PhysioNet database, namely, Fantasia (for normal) and St.-Petersburg Institute of Cardiology Technics 12-lead arrhythmia (for CAD)
[2]	Chinese PLA general hospital with a discharge diagnosis of ACS
[3]	ECG database (Physikalisch-Technische Bundesanstalt diagnostic database)
[4]	Opensource PhysioBank MIT-BIH arrhythmia database
[5]	DSBCCD database
[6]	Physionet public database, MIT-BIH arrhythmia database
[7–9]	MIT-BIH arrhythmia database
[10]	CAT08 dataset, CMCU dataset, orCaScore dataset
[11]	CPC of Shanxi academy of medical sciences
[12, 13]	The Physiological data were collected using wearable sensors (Medical and activity sensor), UCI Repository
[14]	NHANES dataset
[15]	Data was collected using doppler sensor with a sampling frequency of 1000 Hz

Table 9.6 Features extraction and features selection or features reduction methods used in heart disease diagnosis in collected literature

References	Features extraction and features selection	Feature reduction
[1, 4, 6, 11]	Convolution and pooling process of CNN	–
[9]	GLCM	–
[12]	Feature fusion	Information gain
[13]	HRM	–
[14]	Majority voting algorithm	–
[15]	Spatial and temporal features	–

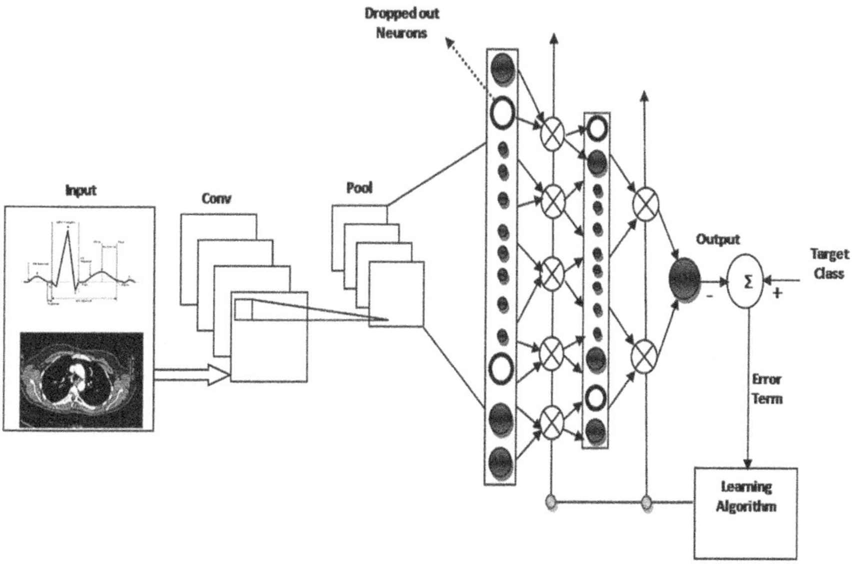

Fig. 9.1 Block diagram of CNN-based classification or prediction or detection of HD

extracted, the classification or prediction operation is performed. For this purpose, the 2-Dimensional feature sets are converted to one dimension. Subsequently, few layers of CNN similar to conventional ANN are devoted for prediction or classification. In these layers drop out of neurons is introduced to avoid overfitting problem. The output of the final layer is compared with the target output and the generated error term is used to update the connected weights between the last few layers. The training scheme is continued until the MSE attains the lowest possible value. After the completion of the training scheme, the developed CNN model is used for detection of HD. The learning algorithm used for the updating the weights in the last few classification layers are the standard back propagation algorithm.

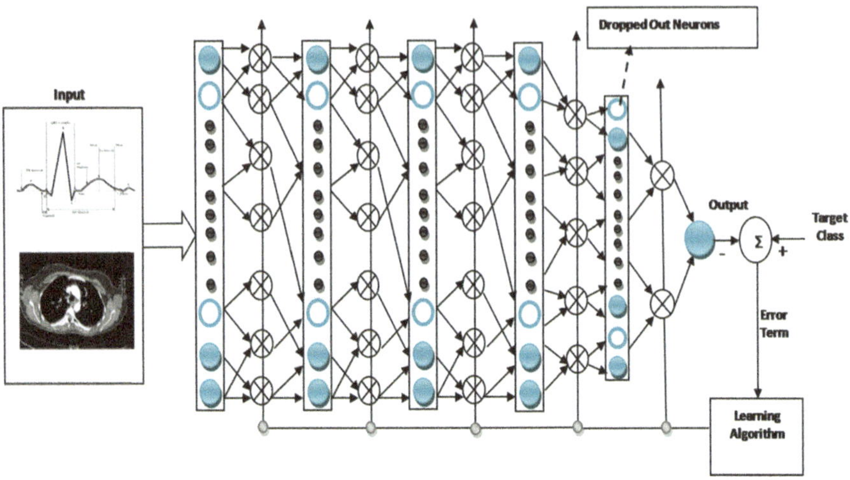

Fig. 9.2 Block diagram of DLNN-based classification or prediction or detection of HD

5.2 *Development of DLNN-Based Classification Model*

The DLNN is also an important neural network model used for forecasting, classification, and other applications. Many papers on the diagnosis of HD using DLNN have appeared in the literature and most recently published articles are [2, 11—13] used in this chapter. Simplified block diagrams of DLNN for classification or prediction task are shown in Fig. 9.2. For HD detection, the input to the DLNN is either an ECG signal or the relevant images of a patient. In this case, the numbers of layers are more than the conventional artificial neural network. To overcome the overfitting problem, random dropout of neurons is introduced in each layer. The output of the DLNN is compared with the target output and the error term is used to update the coefficients between different layers. The standard back propagation algorithm is also used in this case to update the connecting weights. In case of DLNN unlike CNN, the adaptive weights appear from the first layer to the last layer.

6 Analysis of Simulated-Based Results

Different articles have used different performance metrics to assess and compare the results obtained from simulation-based experiments. These performance metrics have been compiled and presented in Table 9.7. The associated formula of each of the performance metric is also listed in the same Table. Using real life standard data of HD patients the CNN and DLNN-based methods have been simulated for prediction and classification. The various performance metrics reported in the collected articles are presented in Table 9.8. Most of the articles have provided results in terms of accuracy

Table 9.7 Performance metrics used in heart disease

References	Performance metrics	Formulae
[1–4, 6, 8, 11, 12, 14]	Accuracy, test accuracy, average accuracy	$(T_p + T_n) / (T_p + F_p + F_n + T_n)$
[1, 3, 6, 7, 11]	Sensitivity	$T_p/(T_p + F_n)$
[1, 3, 6, 11, 14]	Specificity	$T_n/(F_p + T_n)$
[2, 14]	AUC	$\int_m^n f(y)dy$
[5, 15]	Correlation coefficient (R)	$\frac{k(\sum yz)-(\sum y)(\sum z)}{\sqrt{\left[k\sum y^2-(\sum y)^2\right]}\sqrt{\left[k\sum z^2-(\sum z)^2\right]}}$
[5]	RMSE	$\sqrt{\frac{1}{M}\sum_{i=1}^{M}(y_i - \hat{y})}$
[7]	PPR	$T_p/(T_p + F_p)$
[13]	MSE	$\frac{1}{m}\sum_{i=1}^{m}\left(y_i - \widehat{y_i}\right)^2$
[13]	Precision	$T_p/(T_p + F_p)$
[13, 14]	Recall	$T_p/(T_p + F_n)$
[13]	F-measure	$2T_p / (2T_p + F_p + F_n)$

Table 9.8 Results of various performance metrics reported in various articles

References	Results
[1]	Accuracy—94.95% / 95.11% (for 2 secs / 5 secs ECG) Sensitivity—93.72% / 91.13% (for 2 secs/ 5 secs ECG) Specificity—95.18% / 95.88% (for 2 secs/ 5 secs ECG)
[2]	Accuracy—0.73, AUC = 0.868
[3]	Accuracy—93.53% / 95.22% (for noisy and noise free) Sensitivity—93.71% / 95.49% (for noisy and noise free) Specificity—92.83% / 94.19%(for noisy and noise free)
[4]	Accuracy—89.07%, 89.3% (for noisy and noise free)
[5]	Correlation Coefficient (R)- 0.974, 0.976, 0.828 RMSE-9.6 ml, 7.1 ml, 4.71%
[6]	Accuracy—98.10%, Sensitivity- 97.50%, Specificity- 98.70%
[7]	Accuracy—98.6%, Sensitivity-93.8%, Specificity- 99.2%, PPR- 92.4%
[8]	Average Accuracy—99% / 90.93% (for STFT-CNN / 1D-CNN)
[11]	Accuracy—97.6% / 96.2% (for 2 secs / 5 secs ECG) Sensitivity—96.3% / 96.9% (for 2 secs / 5 secs ECG), Specificity—97.4% / 95.7% (for 2 secs / 5 secs ECG)
[12]	Accuracy—98.5%
[13]	MSE—0.0103, Precision—99.83%, Recall—99.87%, F-Measure—99.85%
[14]	Accuracy—79.5%
[15]	Correlation Coefficient—0.86

of classification, sensitivity, specificity, AUC, RMSE, and PPR. The analyses of the results demonstrate that mostly the accuracy of classification varies between 89 to 99%. Similarly, the ranges of sensitivity and specificity obtained by various approaches vary between 91% to 97.50% and 92.83% to 99.2%, respectively.

7 Conclusion

This chapter presents a critical overview of very recent published articles on classification of heart diseases using CNN and DLNN-based methods. A comprehensive literature review has been presented. The sources of HD data used in these articles as well as the techniques used for extraction and selection or reduction of features are also listed for the convenience of the readers. The various performance measures along with their definitions used in different articles are also presented. The details of methodology of CNN as well as DLNN used for classification purpose are also dealt. Finally, the results in terms of various performance metrics obtained in the simulation study are listed in a Tabular form for purpose of comparative analysis.

-The consolidated form of presentation of the materials relating to the CNN and DLNN-based diagnosis of HD will be of immense help to the researchers in this field. Even though many articles related to detection of HD using the CNN and DLNN approaches have already been reported, few articles have been chosen and a comprehensive review of those articles is presented in a systematic manner. The interested readers are also advised to go through the papers listed in the reference section for getting more details relating to training and validation scheme used in different papers.[1]

References

1. Acharya, U.R., Fujita, H., Lih, O.S., Adam, M., Tan, J.H., Chua, C.K.: Automated detection of coronary artery disease using different durations of ECG segments with convolutional neural network. Knowl.-Based Syst. **132**, 62–71 (2017)
2. Huang, Z., Dong, W., Duan, H., Liu, J.: A regularized deep learning approach for clinical risk prediction of acute coronary syndrome using electronic health records. IEEE Trans. Biomed. Eng. **65**(5), 956–968 (2017)
3. Acharya, U.R., Fujita, H., Oh, S.L., Hagiwara, Y., Tan, J.H., Adam, M.: Application of deep convolutional neural network for automated detection of myocardial infarction using ECG signals. Inf. Sci. **415**, 190–198 (2017)
4. Acharya, U.R., Oh, S.L., Hagiwara, Y., Tan, J.H., Adam, M., Gertych, A., San Tan, R.: A deep convolutional neural network model to classify heartbeats. Comp. Biol. Med. **89**, 389–396 (2017)

[1]Sample references. In case of doubt, kindly consult Springer to obtain detailed guidelines for accurate reference entries for particular subject fields.

5. Luo, G., Dong, S., Wang, K., Zuo, W., Cao, S. And Zhang, H.: Multi-views fusion CNN for left ventricular volumes estimation on cardiac MR images. IEEE Trans. Biomed. Eng. **65**(9), 1924–1934 (2017)
6. Oh, S.L., Ng, E.Y., San Tan, R., Acharya, U.R.: Automated diagnosis of arrhythmia using combination of CNN and LSTM techniques with variable length heart beats. Comput. Biol. Med. **102**, 278–287 (2018)
7. Zhai, X., Tin, C.: Automated ECG classification using dual heartbeat coupling based on convolutional neural network. IEEE Access. **6**, 27465–27472 (2018)
8. Huang, J., Chen, B., Yao, B., He, W.: ECG arrhythmia classification using STFT-based spectrogram and convolutional neural network. IEEE Access. **7**, 92871–92880 (2019)
9. Sun, W., Zeng, N., He, Y.: Morphological arrhythmia automated diagnosis method using gray-level co-occurrence matrix enhanced convolutional neural network. IEEE Access. **7**, 67123–67129 (2019)
10. Wolterink, J.M., van Hamersvelt, R.W., Viergever, M.A., Leiner, T., Išgum, I.: Coronary artery centerline extraction in cardiac CT angiography using a CNN-based orientation classifier. Med. Image Anal. **51**, 46–60 (2019)
11. Li, D., Li, X., Zhao, J., Bai, X.: Automatic staging model of heart failure based on deep learning. Biomed. Signal Process. Control **52**, 77–83 (2019)
12. Ali, F., El-, S., Islam, S.R., Kwak, D., Ali, A., Imran, M., Kwak, K.S.: A smart healthcare monitoring system for heart disease prediction based on ensemble deep learning and feature fusion. Inf. Fusion. **63**, 208–222 (2020)
13. Vijayashree, J., Sultana, H.P.: Heart disease classification using hybridized Ruzzo-Tompa memetic based deep trained Neocognitron neural network. Health Technol. **10**(1), 207–216 (2020)
14. Dutta, A., Batabyal, T., Basu, M., Acton, S.T.: An Efficient convolutional neural network for coronary heart disease prediction. Expert Syst. Appl. **159**, 113408 (2020)
15. Yamamoto, K., Hiromatsu, R., Ohtsuki, T.: ECG signal reconstruction via doppler sensor by hybrid deep learning model with CNN and LSTM. IEEE Access. **8**, 130551–130560 (2020)

Congruence of Deep Learning in Medical Image Processing: Future Prospects and Challenges

Aradhana Behura

Abstract Machine Learning and deep learning procedures, in particular deep reinforcement neural networks, have quickly become a smart approach for scrutinizing medical signal and image datasets. The perilous problem like Cancer takes place when the cellular reproduction procedure goes out of control when some parts of the human body's cells arise to spread into contiguous fleshy tissue and divide without discontinuing which may be a clue to death. This fatal cancer is a dangerous disease categorized by undesirable, uncontrolled, and uncoordinated cell division. So early cancer diagnosis can protect a patient. Here, various types of deep learning techniques are applied for optimized feature extraction, normalization or dataset preprocessing (used to eliminate null value, noises, and outlier), data segmentation, accurate classification, and the common description of flow chart is described in Figs. 1 and 7. The survey of deep learning is used for image classification, carotid ultrasound data investigation, cardi tocography, intravascular ultrasound report, lung CT report, brain tumor prediction from the MRI report, object detection, segmentation, breast cancer prediction, ECG (electrocardiogram) signal, EEG (electroencephalogram), PPG signal registration and psoriasis skin disease as well as cancer detection. Concise summaries are delivered of trainings per application zone: pulmonary, musculoskeletal neuro, digital pathology, abdominal, retinal, breast, cardiac. There are various type of deep learning techniques are present to improve accuracy of the medical dataset. Deep reinforcement learning, Recursive neural network, Multilayer perceptron, Recurrent neural network, Boltzmann machine, Convolution neural network are different types of deep learning techniques used to train the image and signal dataset. Generative adversarial network, Auto encoder and deep belief neural network are coming under unsupervised pretrained neural network. Some well known architectural models of convolution neural networks are ResNet (2015), VGGNet (2014), GoogLeNet (2014), ZFNet (2013) is introduced as the visualization concept of the De-convolutional network, AlexNet (2012) and LeNet are basically used to train image dataset, LSTM technique (long short term memory) is used to train

A. Behura (✉)
Computer Science and Engineering, Veer Surendra Sai University of Technology, Sambalpur, Odisha, India
e-mail: aradhanabehura@gmail.com

H. K. Tripathy et al. (eds.), *Technical Advancements of Machine Learning in Healthcare*, Studies in Computational Intelligence 936,
https://doi.org/10.1007/978-981-33-4698-7_10

signalized dataset and RHSBoost, genetically optimized neural network are used for multiple classification of datasets efficiently. Dimensionality reduction, feature extraction, overfitting, underfitting and normalization problems can be solved using various types of optimization algorithm.

Keywords Biomedical image and signal processing · Hyper-parameter · Attention module · Data prediction · Magnetic resonance image · Deep learning · Hypercolumn technique · Brain tumor · Breast cancer

1 Introduction

In the conventional machine learning system, user gives input information and logic to the computer then user can able to get result or output but in the case of machine learning, user gives input data and result then the system can able to generate logic/model or program but it needs feature selection algorithm but in the case of deep learning, it does not need feature selection procedure [1–5]. The life cycle of machine learning procedure is described (collection of data-data wrangling-analyse the data-train and test algorithm-deployment phase) in Fig. 4. Data imbalance is a crucial problem [6–11] now a days but it is very difficult to handle. From the Fig. 2 we conclude about it. The SMOTE, ADASYN, Adaboost, XGBoost, and SMOTE-ENN are the various types of techniques used to balance dataset (Figs. 1 and 3).

There are various types of learning algorithms are used [12–16]. They are may be supervised, semi-supervised, unsupervised, and reinforcement learning techniques and they are providing better result according to the data set quality or the size of the dataset by following the problem statement. We conclude all about from the Fig. 5.

Clustering is an important technique which helps to group similar types of data points and it may be exclusive, overlapping, or hierarchical [17–21] procedure. DBSCAN is a high density-based clustering technique used to handle noise data set then c means and k-means algorithm is also used to detect disease [22] from

Fig. 1 Procedure of disease classification in the dataset

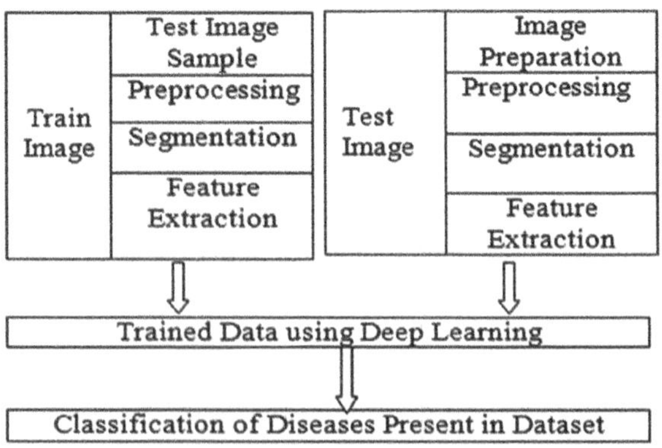

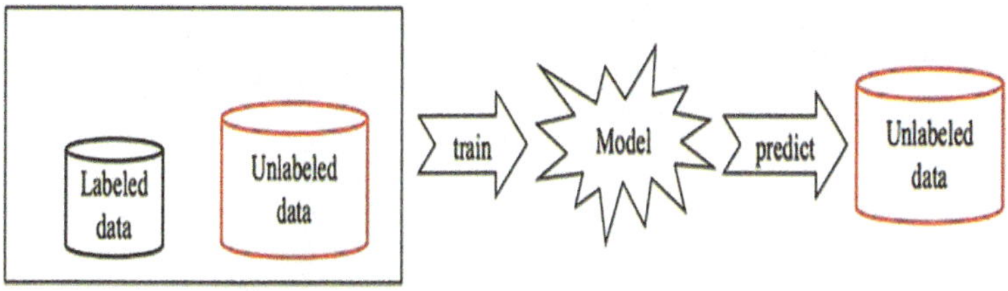

Fig. 2 Handling mechanism of data set

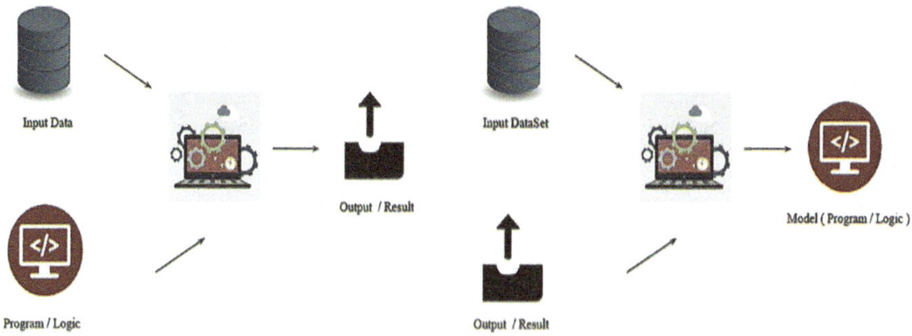

Fig. 3 Conventional machine learning versus deep learning

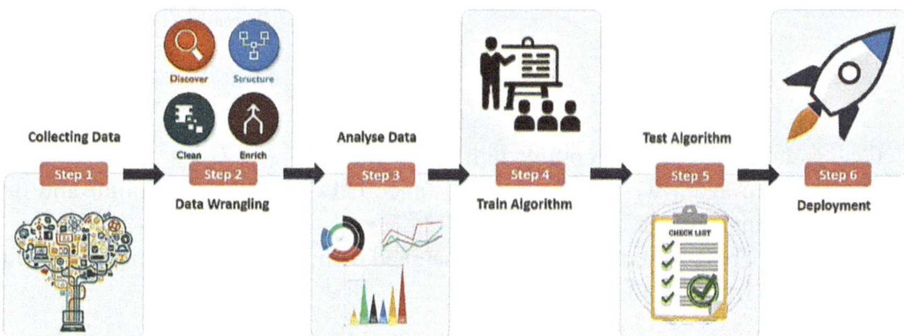

Fig. 4 Life cycle for machine learning

the MRI or CT scan [23–30] image. Now a days there are many optimization algorithms (ex. Particle swam algorithm, Genetic algorithm, ant colony algorithm, Gravitational algorithm) are used to optimize the clustering algorithm to provide better performance according to the problem statement and the data set [31–37].

K-means clustering algorithm

Let $X = \{x_1, x_2, x_3, \ldots, x_n\}$ be the set of data points and $V = \{v_1, v_2, \ldots, v_c\}$ be the set of centers.

Fig. 5 Learning algorithm

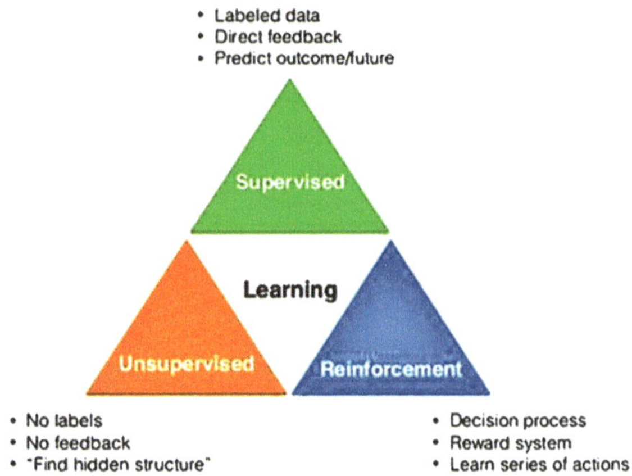

Start
Step-1: we randomly select the cluster centers (c).
Step-2: then, we calculate the distance between each data point and the cluster centers.
Step-3: now we assign the data point to the cluster center, which has minimum distance from the cluster as compare to other cluster centers.
Step-4: again we calculate the new cluster center using this formula:

$$v_i = (1/c_i)\sum_{j=1}^{c_i} x_i \tag{1}$$

("c_i" is the number of data points in ith clustre).
Step-5: once again we calculate the distance between each data point and the newly obtained cluster centers.
Step-6: If there is no data point was reassigned then we stop, otherwise we repeat the process from step 3.
End

Different type models are verified on medical signal and image processing and computer-assisted [38, 39] intervention tests catalogues including multimodal fatal brain tumor image segmentation (BRATS) 2017, 2016 and 2015, breast cancer diagnosis dataset (Wisconsin), respectively. Even with appropriate acquisition of breast cancer and brain tumor datasets, the reliable and accurate segmentation of tumors data in breast and brain are a complicated-task [40]. By following Fig. 7, we can able to solve a machine learning problem (Fig. 6).

Automatic accurate segmentation of datasets become conceivable with improvement of deep-learning procedures that carries plethora of clarifications in this chapter survey prospect. Here, our aim is to design a deep learning network named as residual

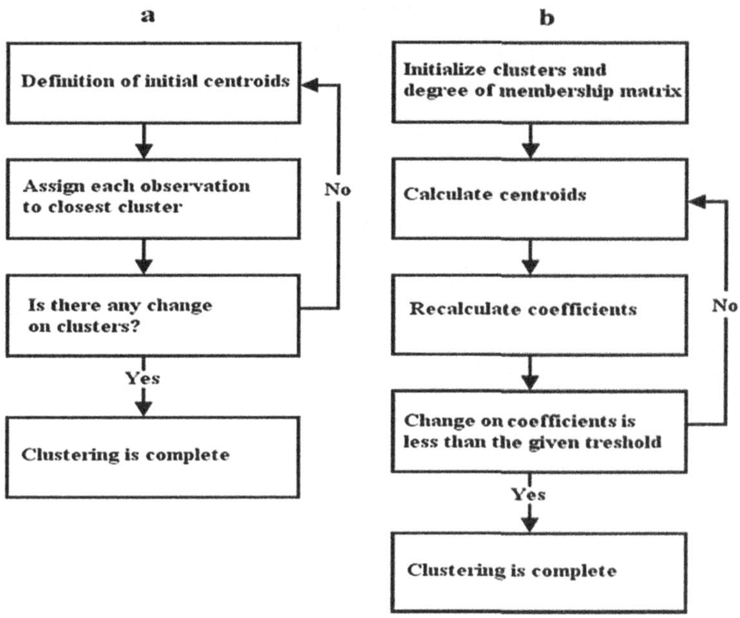

Fig. 6 Clustering Procedure

cyclic unpaired encoder-decoder network well known as RescueNet using mirroring and residual main beliefs.

1.1 Various Types of Deep Learning [20, 49] Architecture

AlexNet **(2012)**

- Trained on two GTX 580 GPUs for **five to six days** (Fig. 8).

The network they designed was used for classification with 1000 possible categories and it has five convolution layers, max-pooling layers, dropout layers, and 3 fully connected layers.

ZF Net **(2013)**

- AlexNet trained on 15 million images, while ZF Net trained on only 1.3 million images.
- Instead of using 11 × 11 sized filters in the first layer (which is what AlexNet implemented), ZF Net [21] used filters of size 7 × 7
- Trained on a GTX 580 GPU for **twelve days** (Fig. 9).

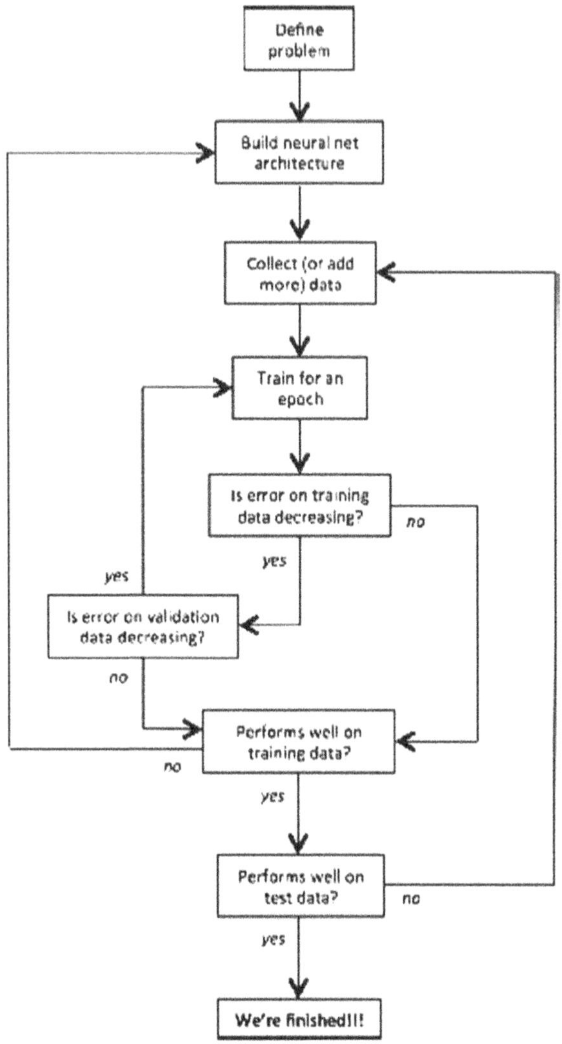

Fig. 7 Procedure of disease classification in the dataset

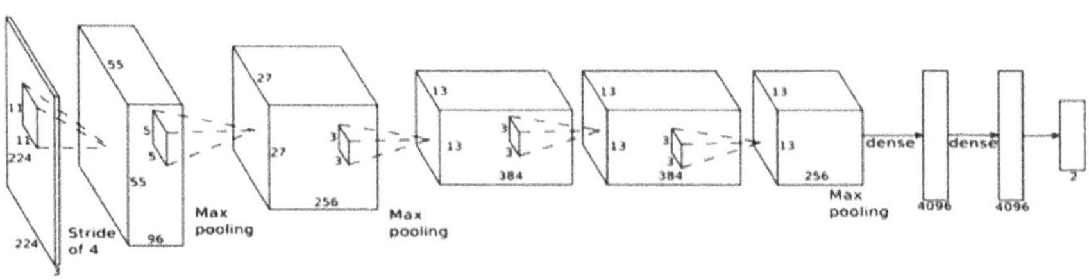

Fig. 8 AlexNet Architecture

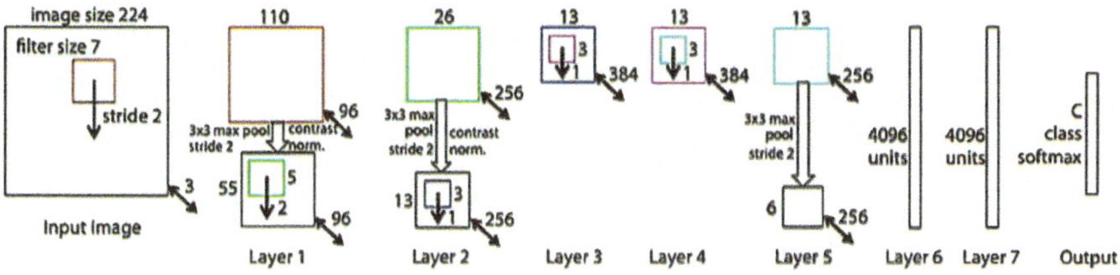

Fig. 9 ZF Net Architecture

VGG Net **(2014)**

The use of only 3 × 3 sized filters is quite different from AlexNet's 11 × 11 filters in the first layer and ZF Net's 7 × 7 filters [49] (Fig. 10).

- Trained on four Nvidia Titan Black GPUs for two to three weeks.

GoogLeNet **(2015)**

The GoogLeNet [21] has 100 layers and it helps researcher to train their model according to their problem statement and data set. This architecture is very useful to train a system but it takes a lot of time. Suppose take a case like corona virus prediction (COVID-19). GoogLeNet provides better result as compare to the other architecture. Trained on "a few high-end GPUs within a week" and it's error rate is 6.7% as compare to the other architecture.

ConvNet Configuration					
A	A-LRN	B	C	D	E
11 weight layers	11 weight layers	13 weight layers	16 weight layers	16 weight layers	19 weight layers
input (224 × 224 RGB image)					
conv3-64	conv3-64 **LRN**	conv3-64 **conv3-64**	conv3-64 conv3-64	conv3-64 conv3-64	conv3-64 conv3-64
maxpool					
conv3-128	conv3-128	conv3-128 **conv3-128**	conv3-128 conv3-128	conv3-128 conv3-128	conv3-128 conv3-128
maxpool					
conv3-256 conv3-256	conv3-256 conv3-256	conv3-256 conv3-256	conv3-256 conv3-256 **conv1-256**	conv3-256 conv3-256 **conv3-256**	conv3-256 conv3-256 conv3-256 **conv3-256**
maxpool					
conv3-512 conv3-512	conv3-512 conv3-512	conv3-512 conv3-512	conv3-512 conv3-512 **conv1-512**	conv3-512 conv3-512 **conv3-512**	conv3-512 conv3-512 conv3-512 **conv3-512**
maxpool					
conv3-512 conv3-512	conv3-512 conv3-512	conv3-512 conv3-512	conv3-512 conv3-512 **conv1-512**	conv3-512 conv3-512 **conv3-512**	conv3-512 conv3-512 conv3-512 **conv3-512**
maxpool					
FC-4096					
FC-4096					
FC-1000					
soft-max					

Fig. 10 VGG Net Architecture

type	patch size/ stride	output size	depth	#1×1	#3×3 reduce	#3×3	#5×5 reduce	#5×5	pool proj	params	ops
convolution	7×7/2	112×112×64	1							2.7K	34M
max pool	3×3/2	56×56×64	0								
convolution	3×3/1	56×56×192	2		64	192				112K	360M
max pool	3×3/2	28×28×192	0								
inception (3a)		28×28×256	2	64	96	128	16	32	32	159K	128M
inception (3b)		28×28×480	2	128	128	192	32	96	64	380K	304M
max pool	3×3/2	14×14×480	0								
inception (4a)		14×14×512	2	192	96	208	16	48	64	364K	73M
inception (4b)		14×14×512	2	160	112	224	24	64	64	437K	88M
inception (4c)		14×14×512	2	128	128	256	24	64	64	463K	100M
inception (4d)		14×14×528	2	112	144	288	32	64	64	580K	119M
inception (4e)		14×14×832	2	256	160	320	32	128	128	840K	170M
max pool	3×3/2	7×7×832	0								
inception (5a)		7×7×832	2	256	160	320	32	128	128	1072K	54M
inception (5b)		7×7×1024	2	384	192	384	48	128	128	1388K	71M
avg pool	7×7/1	1×1×1024	0								
dropout (40%)		1×1×1024	0								
linear		1×1×1000	1							1000K	1M
softmax		1×1×1000	0								

Fig. 11 GoogLeNet architecture

The architecture of layer by layer (having twenty two layers) of GoogLeNet is described in Fig. 11 and it provides better accuracy as compared to other algorithms but this process is very time consuming. This architecture holds two classifier layer which is auxiliary and associated to the Inception (4a) as well as Inception (4d) at output layers. This architecture uses unpaired adversarial training to segment the cancer datasets followed by enhance regions in a breast and brain image scan. The problem in tumor [41–44] analysis is formulating enormous labeled dataset for training of deep neural networks which is actually a time consuming as well as difficult job. To reduce this requirement of paired dataset which we used unpaired training method to train the network [45–48].

Microsoft ResNet **(2015)**

The Fig. 12 has 152 layer network and its error rate is 3.6% as compare to the other deep learning architecture.

- Trained on an 8 GPU machine for two to three weeks.
- The group tried a 1202-layer network, but got a lower test accuracy, presumably due to overfitting

1.1.1 Discriminative Feature Extraction from X-ray Images Using Deep Convolutional Neural Networks

- Digital image retrieval techniques are becoming increasingly important in the field of medical image databases (i.e., radiology, histopathology, and CT) [41, 42].

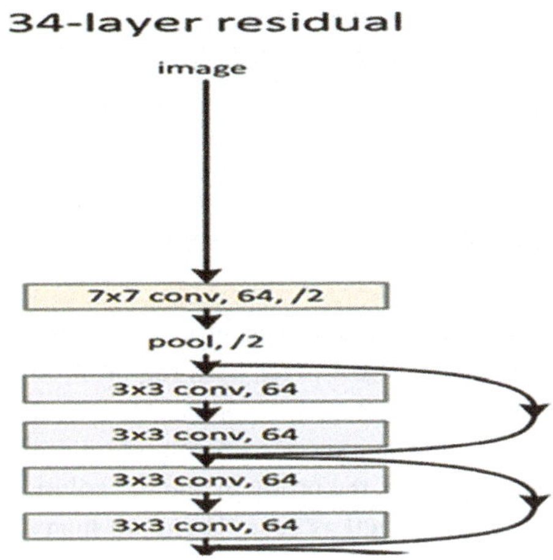

Fig. 12 Architecture of Microsoft ResNet

Problem:

- Organizing the images into various categories is an important step in the content-based medical image retrieval (CBMIR)

Experiments and Results:

From Table 1, we conclude about the performance of the dataset such as class level and comparison with different features by using Wavelet SVM, Texture SVM, HOG SVM and CNNs [20]. Support vector machine is a classifier used to classify the

Table 1 Comparision result

Class labels	With different features			
	Wavelet + SVM	Texture + SVM	HoG + SVM	CNNs
C1	96	76	100	96
C2	96	64	84	96
C3	100	56	100	100
C4	100	80	96	96
C5	96	16	100	96
C6	100	68	84	96
C7	92	28	88	96
C8	92	80	92	96
C9	0	84	100	100
C10	48	84	92	100
C11	100	20	100	100
C12	10	84	92	100
Performance	85	67	93.6	**97.6**

data set and convolution neural network is a standard deep learning technique which is used to predict the disease in the image data set and performs better than other optimized neural network which has very complex architecture.

1.2 Medical Image Segmentation Using Deep Learning

Image segmentation is the process of partitioning a digital image into multiple regions where each of the pixels in a region is similar to some characteristics or computed properties, such as color, intensity, or texture (Fig. 13).

Machine learning is an important subset of artificial intelligence which helps user to predict the problem and it's solution in an informatics way which consumes less time as well as cost. There are many clustering algorithms are used to predict the disease from the data set by taking the similarity instances among the data set. The well-known clustering algorithms are K-means, C-means, DBSCAN which is a density-based clustering algorithm used to remove noise from the data set. The well known neural network SOM (self organizing feature map) [3] is used for clustering as well as pattern recognition purposes. This neural network not only an information visualization procedure but also helps [44] to reduce dimension to observe pattern of the feature from the data set.

- Image segmentation has been widely used in various fields
  - Computer-aided diagnosis (CAD) for cancer detection [20],
  - Remote sensing image analysis,
  - Outdoor object recognition & robot vision,
  - Content-based image and marketplace decision support.

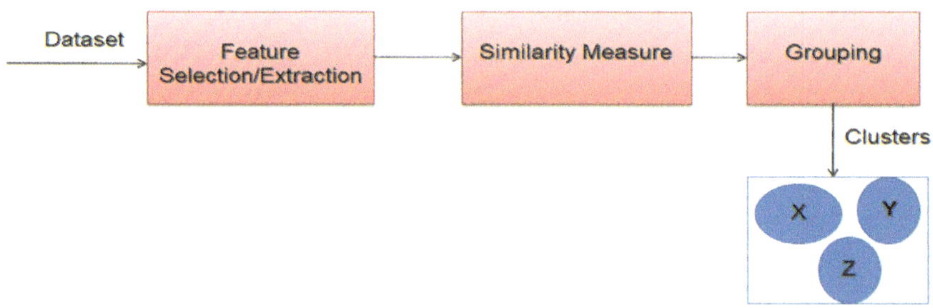

Fig. 13 Fundamental of clustering

2 Malaria Parasites Detection

Malaria is a dangerous disease now a days and the detection of malaria parasites in blood is very important. There are various types of machine learning techniques are present for actual prediction of disease. In this chapter we are using convolution neural network which is not only provide better accuracy than other machine learning algorithm but also gives better parasite detection in human blood. The convolution operation of the CNN is described in Fig. 14.

First take the blood smear image as input image then apply filtering technique on image to enhance the intensity. At last, RBC segmentation and convolution neural networks are applied for classification approach which is described in Fig. 15.

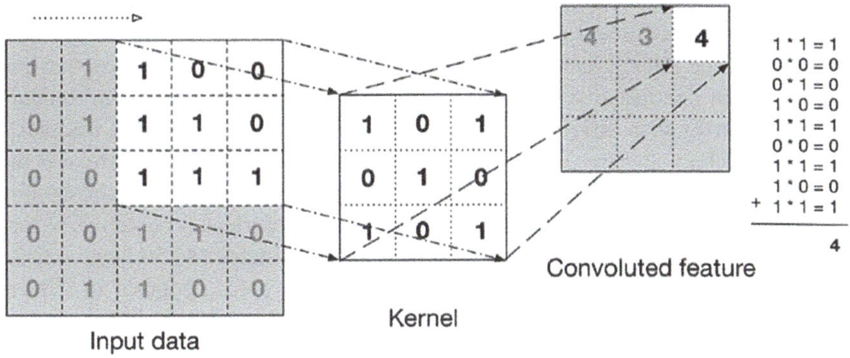

Fig. 14 CNN operation

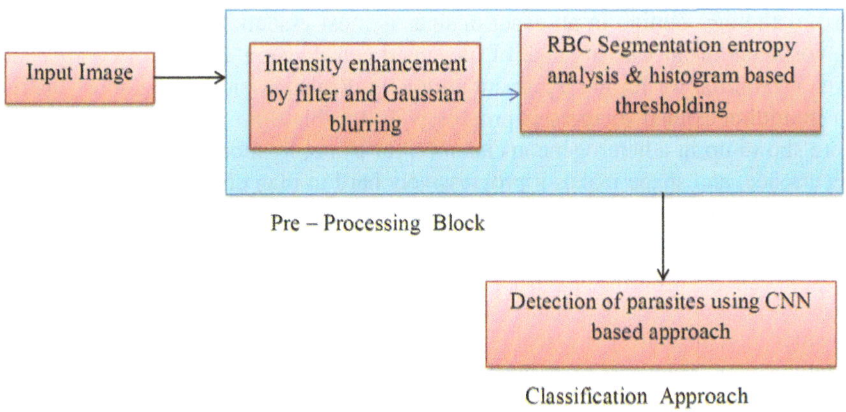

Fig. 15 Malaria parasites detection

3 Brain Tumor Detection

Cerebrum tumor recognition is a functioning territory of research in image processing. Here, a system is recommended to the section and arrange the brain tumor utilizing the MRI report. Deep Neural Networks (DNN)-based design is utilized for tumor or cell division. Here, multi-layers are utilized for the order that comprise of convolutional, ReLU, and a softmax layer. The information MRI picture is isolated into various fixes and afterward the inside pixel estimation of every fix is provided to the Deep Neural Network. It dole out marks as per focus pixels and perform division. A standout among the most loathsome sorts of unwanted cell division is known as harmful cell division or tumors [17]. Gliomas and lymphomas are the well known harmful tumor. Gliomas incorporate subsections of essential unwanted cell growth which degree from second rate to progressively infiltrative dangerous tumors. They have greatest pervasiveness with exceptionally great death rate. They are categorized into High Grade (HGG) and Low Grade Glioma (LGG). HGG is low irruption and forceful when contrasted with the LGG. Patients of HGG as a rule don't endure more noteworthy than one year after the recognition procedure. We can use radiotherapy and chemotherapy for improvement in brain tumor. Ischemia stroke is the cerebrovascular contamination and normal intention of inability and passing around the world. The influenced cerebrum area (stroke sore) experiences numerous phases of the malady sorted as sub-intense (23 h–2.5w), interminable (>2.5w), and intense (0–23 h). Segmentation [17] and ensuing quantitative sores appraisal in clinical pictures give profitable information to the assessment of mind pathologies that are crucial for treatment arranging techniques, ailment checking forecast, and movement of patient results. Moreover, careful wounds areas identify with explicit shortfalls relying upon influenced structure of the cerebrum. The useful deficiencies delivered from wallop injury are connected with harm capacity to explicit cerebrum areas. At last, pathology outline in an exact manner is most essential advance in cerebrum tumor situation in which gauge of unwanted cell division amount of components area is required for further treatment arranging. Right division of the injury district in multidimensional pictures is progressively troublesome and testing work. The sore shows up in a heterogeneous manner, for example, more variety in size, area, recurrence, and shape makes it progressively hard to plan effective division stages. It is very non-unimportant to clarify wounds and drain's in components of cerebrum tumor, for example, the necrotic canter and multiplied with chambers. The apparently increasingly precise division results can be accomplished by the manual clarification through human specialists that is additional tedious, costly, and dull undertaking. Besides, it is absolutely illogical if there should arise an occurrence of more investigations which presents extra bury spectator varieties. Increasingly effective robotized technique for tumor extraction is a noteworthy point in registering therapeutic pictures that gives independent and versatile strategies for qualitative assessment of unwanted cell growth. Brain stroke injuries have hyper-serious advent and other white issue sores in groupings. Here it is generally difficult to accomplish factually earlier data identified with injury appearance and shape. Several administered

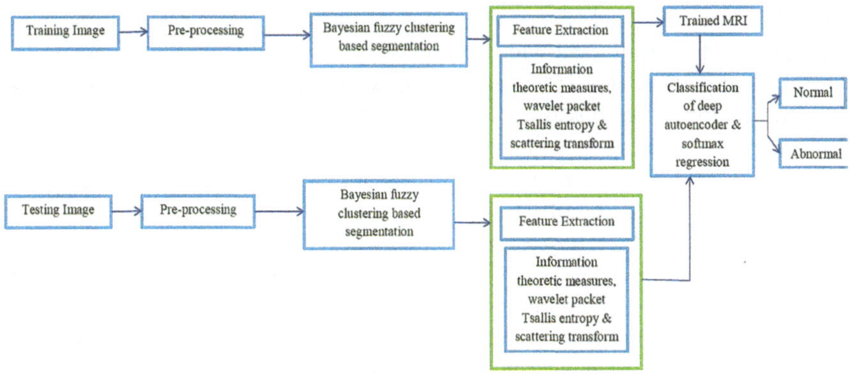

Fig. 16 Brain tumor prediction using Bayesian fuzzy clustering-based segmentation

strategies are utilized for cerebrum injuries division, for example, a popular classifier known as Random Forests classifier (RFC) and Gaussian Mixture Model (GMM) [17] (Fig. 16).

Logical and structural highlights are utilized for the identification of various sorts of cerebrum sores. Random Markov Field (MRF) is utilized for cerebrum injury division. The previously stated strategies are utilized with pointer made component removal strategy however the issues with pointer made technique are working out escalated when contrasted with profound learning strategies. At a similar time, profound learning strategies are all the more dominant when contrasted with managed techniques with the incredible capacity of model to adapt more separated highlights for assignment available. These highlights perform better just as they are pre-characterized and carefully assembled capabilities. We can utilized Convolutional Neural Networks (CNN) to investigate the therapeutic imaging risky errands to accomplish best outcomes. Right off the bat two dimensional CNN can be utilized for sectioning neural films. Three-dimensional mind division is acquired through preparing the two-dimension cut independently. In spite of the basic engineering, better outcomes are accomplished by utilizing these methods showing CNN potential. Huge assortment of parameters increasingly adaptive power and huge recollection necessities are required completely in CNN model. Patches are extricated from multi-scale figures and then joined into multi patches to evade the completely CNN systems. Real cause is disheartening the CNN use since it has moderate derivation for to adaptively as well as progressively costly. Subsequently, classifier predispositions into uncommon classes may result in cell division. A CNN prototype is intended to prepare tests through circulation of parts that are near genuine parts however over-sectioned pixels focuses toward off base grouping in primary stage. Next preparing stage is exhibited by in which fixes on separation parts are consistently extricated from info picture. Two periods of preparing arrangement may be inclined to over fitting and furthermore increasingly touchy to first classifier organize. At that point thick preparing technique is utilized for system preparing. This strategy presented in imbalance class mark that is like uniform examining. Weight cost work is utilized to beat this issue. Manual change of system affectability is given yet it turns out to be progressively hard to deal with multi-class issues by utilizing this strategy. The general article association is as per the following: (a) characterizes-related work. Nitty gritty exhibited proposed steps are referenced here. Then Deep Neural Network results are depicted in this Section. At last finish of this exploration work is outlined in various procedure. In cerebrum tumor cases, map book can be assessed at the season of division because of the variable area and state of neoplasms. Unwanted cell mass impact can be estimated by the injury development structures. The voxels gives accommodating data used to getting flatter division outcomes by the Markov Fields (MRF) [26]. MRF strategy is utilized for mind tumor cell division. Generative models well sum up shrouded information [4] with certain constraints at the preparation organize. These strategies can gain proficiency with the example of mind tumor without using a particular model. These kind of techniques for the most part consider indistinguishable and autonomous voxels circulation through setting highlights data. Because of this cause, disengaged groups of voxels might be segregated erroneously in the off base parts, now and then in anatomically and physiological impossible areas. To maintain a strategic distance from these issues, numerous scientists included neighborhood data through installing probabilistic expectations into a Random Field (RF) classifier. The Convolution Neural Network models are utilized to naturally learn chains of importance of information highlights. Convolution Neural Network can keep running over patches by utilizing the bit trap. In cell division, ongoing techniques are using Neural Network. This model is utilized with max-pooling two convolutional layers and walk with completely associated (FC) layer and softmax layer for tumor discovery in MR pictures. Multi-dimensional channels [32] are utilized for the assessment of cerebrum tumor. Three-dimensional channels can take benefits over the MR nature however adaptive burden is elevated. Double CNN is utilized to distinguish the total tumor area. At that point cells are connected to soft division outcomes before the CNN performs multi-class segregation between the tumor districts. Convolution Neural Network is prepared on separated fixes in every voxel plane and yield of last layer, softmax and Random Forest (RF) are utilized to prepare the model. Cerebrum cell division method is isolated into parallel assignments and proposed organized expectations based on CNN as a initial learning model. Marks of patches are assembled into groups and Neural Network predicts input participation on every bunch. CNN is utilized for the removal in MR pictures. It is utilized to accomplish further CNN model. We demonstrates the concise synopsis of existing techniques.

Real commitment of this critique is as per the following:

1. Modified Deep Neural Network model depends on multilayers subsequently proficiently portioning the cerebrum cell mass.
2. Info MRI picture is isolated into different patches and afterward focus pictorial element mark of each fix is determined and provided to the DNN which recovers the aftereffects of division just as grouping.
3. Accomplished outcomes are assessed with late strategies which demonstrate that DNN model performed superior to existing procedures.

4 Ovarian Cancer: Gynaecological Disorders

4.1 Feature Extraction

Feature extraction is done to reduce the dimensions in this way raw data also reduced to makes us easier for processing the data. Feature extractions simplify the amount of resources which is required for describing the large set of data accurately. By analysing the complex data one of the major problems arise from the number of variables that are involved [43]. Analysing a large number of variables basically requires a high memory and also computation power or required a classification algorithm that fits the training data and categorized the new data. Feature extraction is the methods to combine the variables to overcome these problems that describe the data with accuracy [25]. After the pre-processing phase in the character recognition system feature extraction is done. The primary task of pattern recognition is to take an input pattern and assigning it as output classes [47]. Feature extraction is divided into 2 general stages: Feature selection and classification. Feature selection is difficult in the whole process because the classifier may not be able to recognize the selected features. In constructing pattern classification feature extraction is an important step [40]. The important features are retrieve from objects to form the feature vectors in the process of feature extraction. The feature vectors are used by different classifier for recognizing the input unit to target the output unit. Which helps the classifier to classify the classes by observing the features [20]. In feature extraction, all character are represented by feature vector, for its identity. The main target of feature extraction is to retrieve a set of features, which increase the recognition rate with less amount of elements and for generating similar feature. The mostly used feature extraction methods are Deformable templates, Template matching, Graph description, Unitary image transforms Projection Histograms, Contour profiles, Zoning, Fourier descriptors, Gradient feature, Gabor features, etc.

4.1.1 Image Feature

Image feature describe the property of the image, containing several types of information regarding the image [15]. It gives some special types of information regarding the characteristics of the image. The features of an image can be classified into two groups:

- Low-level features: In this feature extraction the feature can be extracted directly from the original image [44].
- High level features: In this feature extraction the feature can be extracted from low-level features [15].

Feature extraction also divided into 2 parts. One is color analysis and other is texture analysis.

4.1.2 Color Analysis

Color is the most important features in any image feature because of its effectiveness, robustness & computational simplicity. There are 4 types of color model, namely, RGB, HIS, CMY, YIQ.

- RGB color model is used to extract the red, green, and blue component of an image
- HIS color model is used to extract the hue, intensity, and saturation component of an image
- CMY color model is used to extract the cyan, magenta, and yellow component of an image

4.1.3 Texture Analysis

It is also a type of image feature which is used for characterization of an images. The main characteristic of the texture is the repetition of the patterns over a region in an image. Texture include the term texton, which define the components of patterns of an image. Different region has different types of textons according to their, shape, size, and color. According to the degree of variation of textons, we can differentiate any two texture of an image. It can done according to the spatial statistical distribution of textons of an image. Texture cannot find similar types of images but when we combine it with a visual attribute just like color, texture can easily retrieve the or extract the images [20].

Ovary cancer is a dangerous disease now a days. There are various types of machine learning algorithms are used to detect the disease. From Fig. 17, we conclude

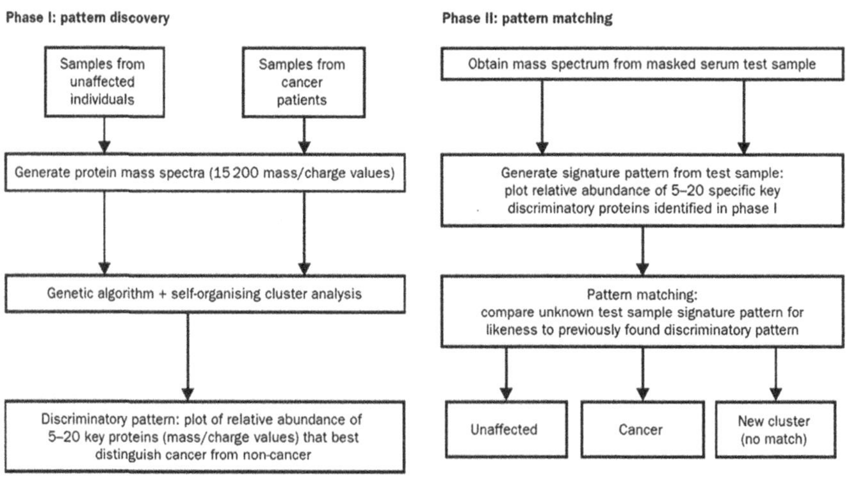

Fig. 17 Ovary cancer prediction

that two phases are used which are known as pattern discovery and pattern matching. Self organizing feature map is a neural network which helps to cluster the data set or helps in finding similar data pattern then it helps to predict unaffected or cancerous image data set and GA (genetic algorithm) is used to optimize the performance and helps to increase the accuracy of cancer prediction. Self organizing feature map (SOM) is a neural network which helps in data clustering or grouping of similar types of elements in the dataset.

5 Breast Cancer Prediction Using Deep Features

Now a days breast cancer is a very critical disease for female candidate and the proper detection of this disease can helpful for patient. By using filter which is a de-noising as well as contrast enhancement process helps physician to detect the surrounding tissues. Women's breast is consisting of micro-calcification, which is very small amount of calcium deposited in breast tissue, usually in a cluster layout; it is clearly visible as a small bright spot in the mammogram. Micro-calcification is very small in size. So that it is very difficult to detect (range of 0.05–1 mm). Image processing is a technique which is widely spread in the field of medicine, mainly for diagnose of diseases or a disruption of human body. Breast cancer is very dangerous in human body which mostly seen in female. There are mostly three types of breast cancer, i.e., Speculated Lesions, circumscribed/oval masses and micro-calcifications. The anatomical structure of breast cancer can have observed through its medical image which can be taken from high-quality imaging tools such as: X-RAY, THERMOGRAPHY, ULTRASONOGRAPH, MAMMOGRAPHY, MEDICAL RESONANCE IMAGE (MRI) (Fig. 18).

Medical images clutch significant property and are very important part of medical information. Such a part of the image is called as region of interest (roi). The ROI is helpful in providing similar diagnosis through the specialist. A little bit of distortion in ROI part in the image may additionally lead to unwanted handling for patient. For securing scientific imagery through watermarking ROI ought to be preserved and the watermarks can be carried out at the last part of the picture called as region of non interest (roni). To remove noise from the data set, we are using various types of noise removal filters (such as Gaussian filter or median filter) which is used to remove unwanted features from the data set and helps to increase the accuracy rate.

Feature extraction is an another problem of the dataset but if we will use deep learning then there is no need to require optimization algorithm. From Fig. 19, we conclude that first take image data set to detect mass from the breast image then extract the relevant feature of the training data set. After completion of data training, we use classifier such as support vector, random forest, adaboost, or xgboost algorithm to classify the data set by taking the help of activation function. Image compression is very important technique and essential to solve the real time problem. There are various types of compression algorithm such as DCT (discrete cosine transform), DWT (discrete wavelet transform), IWT (inverse wavelet transform) are used to

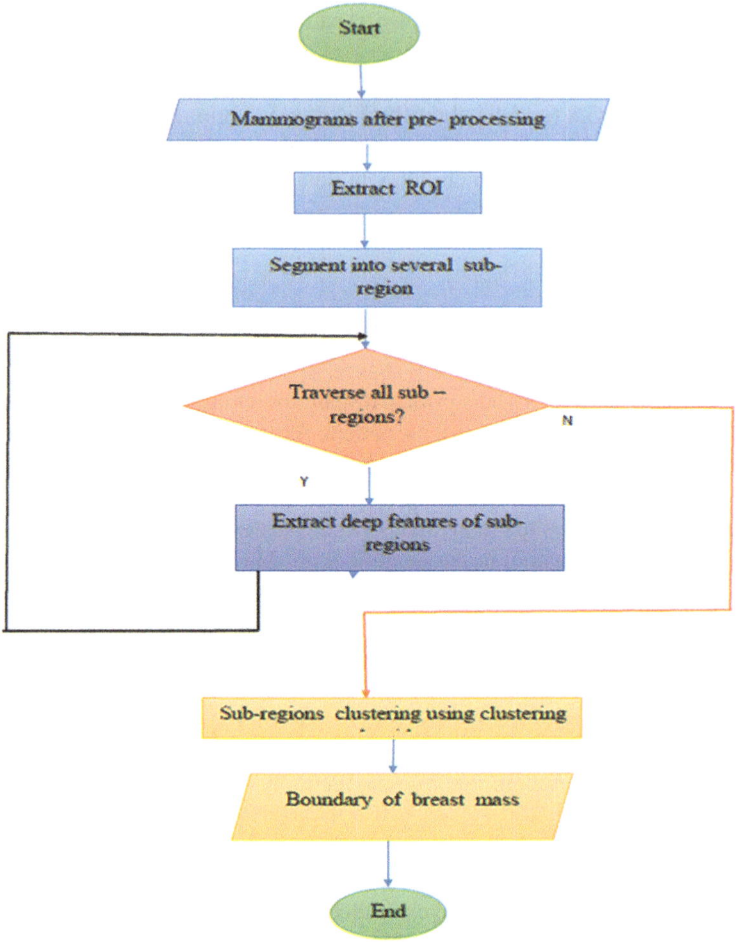

Fig. 18 Breast cancer prediction using deep learning

minimize the redundant bits in the image which helps to provide better accuracy, specificity, prevalence. Data imbalance is another problem, to handle imbalance rate, we can use data augmentation or adaptive rule. In data augmentation, we add extra relevant data in the data set so that accuracy of the training will increase. First pre-process the data set then extract the region of interest and segment into several sub-region. Extract the feature from the data set and apply clustering algorithm to picture out similar types of points from the data set.

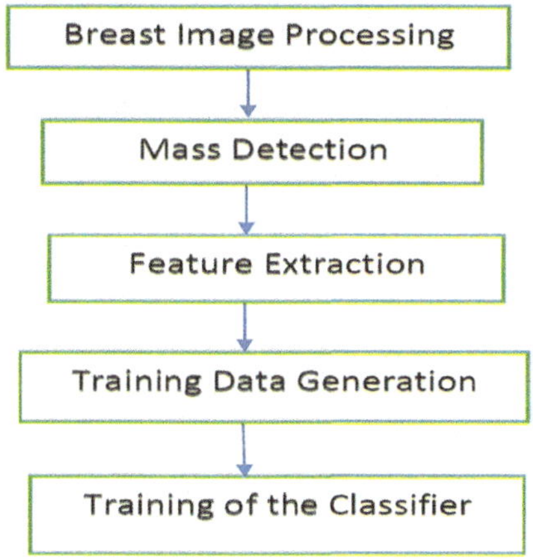

Fig. 19 Breast mass detection

6 Retinal Image Analysis

A. **Overview**

Medical Imaging is the process of producing visible images of inner structures of the body for scientific and medicinal study and treatment as well as visible view of the function of interior tissues. These medical images play an important role for treatment of various pathological disorders. Medical imaging is developing rapidly due to developments in image processing techniques including image recognition, analysis, enhancement, segmentation, etc. It increases the percentage and amount of detected tissues detected through imaging. Retinal image analysis plays a crucial role in retinal pathology for an ophthalmologist for detection and diagnosis. This provides a high rate of information, such as: retinopathy of prematurity (RoP), diabetic retinopathy, glaucoma, hypertension, and age-related macular degeneration or in prognosis of diseases related to brain and heart stocks. These are related with abnormality variation in retina vascular structure. Therefore, changes in retina's articular and vascular morphology have a principal diagnostic value. Retinal vessels segmentation consists of wide-ranging varieties of algorithms and methods which have been proposed and its implementation for the sake of automatized identification, localization, and extraction of retinal vasculature structures. A number of methods are studied in the literature using different methodologies. In literature reviews, the authors classified the retinal segmentation techniques into two broad categories. These are rule-based methods and machine learning-based methods. Rule-based methods generally deals with specific rules regarding the framework of algorithm such as kernel based, vessel tracking, adaptive local thresholding, etc. Machine Learning method uses a manually segmented image (ground truth) to form a labeled dataset which is further used as training dataset. In training images pixels are identified by either they belong to the vessels or not. The machine learning-based methods use supervised learning approach (requires training images) and unsupervised approaches (does not require

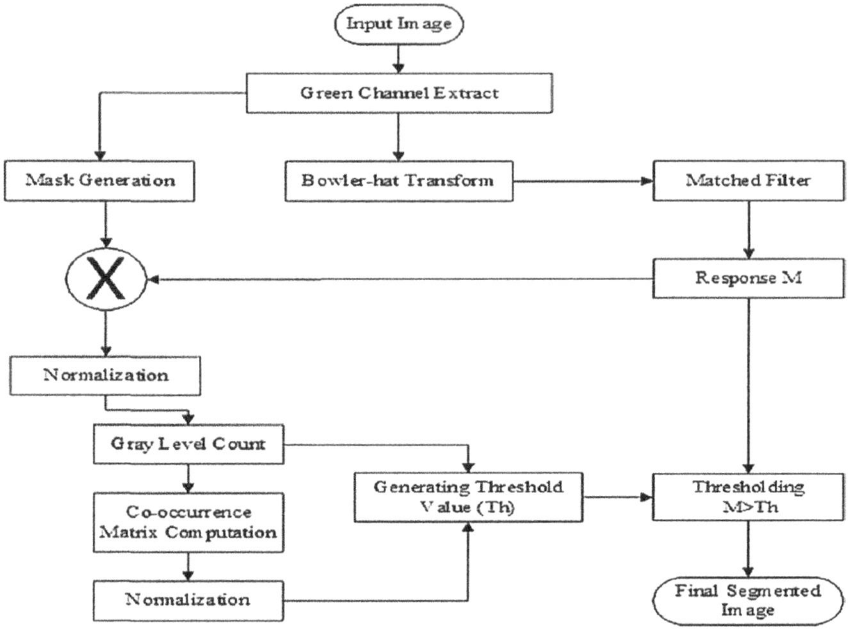

Fig. 20 Retinal vessel segmentation

training images). However, noise occurs in the process of exaggeration of the retinal images due to the lower intensity difference between the background and the vessel surface. Further, it is challenging to preserve the minute vessels, while segmenting. Usually, the contrast enhancement techniques enrich the information content as well as the noise present in its background. Therefore, selection of a suitable enhancement technique for retinal vessel segmentation plays a vital role (Fig. 20).

To address this problem, we propose here a bowler-hat transform-based enhancement technique with joint relative entropy (JRE) thresholding. The proposed method is an unsupervised approach for enhancing the contrast of retinal vessels relative to its background in the retinal image. In this paper, the Bowler-hat transform is implemented for contrast enhancement in the process of retinal vessel enhancement. In the next stage, an optimized matched filter is employed on the enhanced image for delineating the vessel structure from the background. The optimized matched filter uses a two-dimensional Gaussian-shaped kernel for improvising the segmentation performance in the retinal images. The matched filter kernel is designed with three input points. The feasibility of the points is dependent on the orientation, thickness of vessel structures, and the pixel intensity profile. Finally, JRE-based thresholding is implemented on the resulting response of the matched filter for the segmentation of retinal vessels above the background. The proposed technique is experimented with multiple retinal images obtained from the DRIVE dataset. The database provides testing images along with the manually segmented ground truths. The performance of the proposed method is compared with the different methods in terms of the quantitative evaluation parameters, such as: sensitivity, specificity and accuracy.

B. **Material Database**

Different vessel segmentation methods are evaluated using two commonly used databases: DRIVE (Digital Retinal Images for Vessel Extraction) and STARE (Structured Analysis of the Retina) [24]. The images of DRIVE database were taken from camera with specifications of Canon CR-5 non-mydriasis 3-CCD and a 45 degrees field of view (FOV). Each captured image has 768 × 584 pixels with eight bits per color channel in JPEG formatted. The 40 images are divided in two groups, namely, test set and training set each of them contains 20 images. Each set contains 20 manually segmented images which are used as ground truth image. The training set has color images, the FOV masking's for the image, and sets of monochromatic (black and white) ground truth images resulted due to manual segmentation. The test set containing color fundus images, the FOV masking's for the images, and two set of colorless ground truth images resulted due to manual segmentation by 2 different experts. The ground truth images taken for the 1st observer were used to measure the efficacy of algorithms. Normally in this thesis work we have taken DRIVE database into consideration for the implementation and performance of the proposed method.

7 Classification of Coronavirus and Other Viruses Using ML-Based Approach

Currently, viruses are the major concern for the human society throughout the globe. Viruses are the sub-microscopic infectious agents having the capability of replication itself inside the living cells of human body. Various dangerous viruses greatly affect the human body by infecting the major parts such as lungs, kidney, heart, etc. Coronavirus [45] one of them. It is very difficult for the survival of human society due to the effects of these dangerous viruses. So, it is very much essential much for the identification as well as classification of these dangerous viruses at the initial stage in order to take preventive measures at the earliest, otherwise the life risk probability will be gradually increased. Alfa, beta, delta, gamma, SARS–CoV-2vare different types of viruses. It is a challenging task to classify the virus accurately due to change of structure of viruses. This is also a serious issue to predict the future impact of viruses on the human society as well as to predict the future structure of viruses. Currently, many research works have carried out by several researchers, doctors, scientists throughout the globe for the classification of Coronavirus in order to develop suitable vaccines to increase the survival rate of human society. Different techniques such as machine learning (ML)-based techniques, deep learning-based techniques, etc., are used for such classification. ML plays an important role in the today's era for the researchers, doctors, and scientists to carry out their research work. It is considered as one of the most important application of artificial intelligence. Systems can be learnt and improved from experience in automatic manner without any explicit programming by using ML. The main focus of ML is to develop computer programs that can access data as well as use it for learning purpose. It is an important concern for the scientists, doctors, and researchers to carry out research work for the classification of viruses in the current scenario. Different ML-based techniques can be used for the classification of Coronavirus as well as other viruses. Here, several ML-based techniques such as AdaBoost, Logistic Regression, KNN, Neural Network, Decision Tree, Random Forest are implemented using Orange Tool for the classification SARS-CoV-2 and other viruses. Apart from the mentioned techniques other techniques such SVM, SGD, Naïve Bayes, etc., can be used for such purpose. Initiatives can be taken for the development of improved techniques for better classification results.

8 Conclusion

Deep learning is gathering momentum as the machine learning tool of choice for computer vision. It feeds on large amounts of hardware and data. Though immensely successful, its biological evidence remains a question mark, and this leads to the possibility of new avenues of machine learning which are unfolding as we speak, ever since after the success of nature. Other possible avenues for future work by using deep learning medical applications are context-aware deep learning techniques; fusion of statistical techniques with deep learning architectures, training procedures, and classification procedures; use of multidimensional data by deep learning, etc. Performance assessment parameters are occupied as specificity, DICE, accuracy, Sensitivity, and prevalence measure. Fitness function and minority information is calculated by distance score (D-Score) and F-Score. Dataset classification improves the performance of a data classifier. The investigational domino effect are verified on various medical dataset and the outcome leave behind the present methods for cancerious data segmentation. The arrangement of a specific domain-specific data segmentation approaches and overall-perseverance adversarial learning loomed to leverage massive benefits for medical datasets presentations and can increase the capability of automated systems to support radiologists.

References

1. Srinivas, M., Roy, D., Krishna Mohan, C.: Discriminative feature extraction of X-ray images using deep neural networks. In: Proceedings of the 41st IEEE International Conference on Acoustics, Speech and Signal Processing (ICASSP 2016), Shanghai, China, Mar 2016
2. LeCun, Y., Bengio, Y., Hinton, G.: Deep learning. Nature **521**(7553), 436–444 (2015)
3. Srinivas, M., Krishna Mohan,C.: Efficient clustering approach using incremental and hierarchical clustering methods.In: Proceedings of the IEEE International Joint Conference on Neural Networks (IJCNN), Barcelona, July 2010

4. Brezeale, D., Cook, D.: Automatic video classification: a survey of the literature. IEEE Trans. Syst. Man Cybern. Part C: Appl. Rev. **38**(3), 416–430 (2008)
5. Smeulder, A.W.M., Worring, M., Santini, S., Gupta, A., Jain, R.: Content based image retrieval at the end of the early years. IEEE Trans. PatternAnal. Mach. Intell.**22**(12), 1349–1380 (2000)
6. Srinivas, M., Krishna Mohan, C.: Classification of medical images using edge based features and sparse representation. In: Proceedings of the 41st IEEE International Conference on Acoustics, Speech and Signal Processing (ICASSP 2016), Shanghai, China, Mar 2016
7. Srinivas, M., Krishna Mohan,C.: Medical image indexing and retrieval using multi-feature extraction method.In: Proceedings of the IEEE International Conference on Computational Intelligence and Information Technology (CIIT) (Elsevier), Mumbai, Oct 2013.
8. Donoho, D.: Compressed sensing. IEEE Trans. Inf. Theory **52**, 1289–1306 (2006)
9. Guha, T., Ward, R.: A sparse reconstruction based algorithm for image and video classification. In: Proceedings of the IEEE Conference on Acoustics, Speech and Signal Processing (ICASSP), pp. 3601–3604 (2012)
10. Xiang, M., Schonfeld, D., Khokhar, A.A.: Video event classification and image segmentation based on non causal multidimensional hidden Markov models. IEEE Trans. Image Process. **18**(6), 1304–1313 (2009)
11. Pourghassem, H., Ghassemian, H.: Content based medical image classification using a new hierarchical merging scheme. Comput. Med. Imaging Graph. **32**(8), 651–661 (2008)
12. Cai, W., Feng, D., Fulton, R.: Content-based retrieval of dynamic PET functional images. IEEE Trans. Inf. Technol. Biomed. **4**(2), 152–158 (2000)
13. Krawczyk, B., Schaefer, G.: Ensemble fusion methods for medical data classification. In: Proceedings of the IEEE International Symposium on Neural Network Applications in Electrical Engineering (NEUREL), pp. 143–146, 20–22 Sept 2012
14. Peng, F., Li, L., Xu, W., Liu, W., Zhang, J., Shao, G.: The identification of breast mass based on multi agent interactive information fusion method. In: Proceedings of the IEEE International Conference on Bioinformatics and Biomedical Engineering, 11–13 June 2009
15. Mitchell, T.: Machine Learning
16. Abu-Mostafa, Y.S., Magdon-Ismail, M., Lin, H.-T.: Learning From Data. AMLBook
17. Kandi, H., Mishra, D., Gorthi, S.R.K.S.: Exploring the learning capabilities of convolutional neural networks for robust image watermarking. Comput. Secur. **65**, 247–268 (2017). https://doi.org/10.1016/j.cose.2016.11.016
18. Dvorák, P., Menze, B.: Structured prediction with convolutional neural networks for multimodal brain tumor segmentation. In: MICCAI Multimodal Brain Tumor Segmentation Challenge (BraTS), pp. 13–24 (2015)
19. Simonyan, K., Zisserman, A.: Very deep convolutional networks for large-scale image recognition (2014). arXiv:1409.1556v6
20. Hafiz, A.M., Bhat, G.M.: A survey of deep learning techniques for medical diagnosis. Adv. Intell. Syst. Comput. 161–170 (2019).https://doi.org/10.1007/978-981-13-7166-0_16
21. Siva Raja, P.M., Rani, A.V.: Brain tumor classification using a hybrid deep autoencoder with Bayesian fuzzy clustering-based segmentation approach. Biocybern. Biomed. Eng. (2020). https://doi.org/10.1016/j.bbe.2020.01.006
22. Jiao, Z., Gao, X., Wang, Y., Li, J.: A deep feature based framework for breast masses classification. Neurocomputing **197**, 221–231 (2016). https://doi.org/10.1016/j.neucom.2016.02.060
23. Hastie, T., Tibshirani, R., Friedman, J.: The Elements of Statistical Learning. Data Mining, Inference, and Prediction
24. Bishop, C.: Pattern Recognition and Machine Learning
25. Duda, R.O., Hart, P.E., Stork, D.G.: Pattern Classification. Wiley
26. Bengio, Y.: Practical recommendations for gradient-based training of deep architectures (2012). In: Sutskever, I. (ed.) Training Recurrent Neural Networks. Ph.D. thesis (2013)
27. Le, Q.V., Jaitly, N., Hinton, G.E.: A Simple Way to Initialize Recurrent Networks of Rectified Linear Units (2015)
28. Sutskever, I., et al.: On the importance of initialization and momentum in deep learning (2013)

29. Koshimizu, H., Kojima, R., Kario, K., Okuno, Y.: Prediction of blood pressure variability using deep neural networks. Int. J. Med. Inform. 104067 (2020).https://doi.org/10.1016/j.ijmedinf.2019.104067
30. Saba, T., Sameh Mohamed, A., El-Affendi, M., Amin, J., Sharif, M.: Brain tumor detection using fusion of hand crafted and deep learning features. Cogn. Syst. Res. (2019). https://doi.org/10.1016/j.cogsys.2019.09.007
31. Li, F.-F., Karpathy, A.: CS231n: Convolutional Neural Networks for Visual Recognition (Course Notes)
32. Srivastava, N., et al.: Dropout: A Simple Way to Prevent Neural Networks from Overfitting. Ibid (2014)
33. Zeiler, M.D., Fergus, R.: Stochastic Pooling for Regularization of Deep Convolutional Neural Networks (2013)
34. Wertheim, J.A., Petrowsky, H., Saab, S., Kupiec-Weglinski, J.W., Busuttil, R.W.: Major challenges limiting liver transplantation in the United States. Am. J. Transplant. **11**, 1773–1784 (2011)
35. Weismuller, T.J., Fikatas, P., Schmidt, J., et al.: Multicentric evaluation of model for end-stage liver disease-based allocation and survival after liver transplantation in Germany dlimitations of the "sickest first"-concept. Transpl. Int. **24**, 91–99 (2011)
36. Dutkowski, P., Linecker, M., DeOliveira, M.L., Mullhaupt, B., Clavien, P.A.: Challenges to liver transplantation and strategies to improve outcomes. J. Gastroenterol. **148**, 307–323 (2015)
37. Han, G., Liu, F., Tian, Y., Wang, H., Wang, J., Wang, Y.: Detection of glucose concentration in a turbid medium using a stacked auto-encoder deep neural network. Infrared Phys. Technol. **105**, 103198 (2020). https://doi.org/10.1016/j.infrared.2020.103198
38. Khan, H., Shah, P.M., Shah, M.A., ul Islam, S., Rodrigues, J.J.P.C.: Cascading handcrafted features and convolutional neural network for IoT-enabled brain tumor segmentation. Comput. Commun. (2020).https://doi.org/10.1016/j.comcom.2020.01.013
39. Das, H., Naik, B., Behera, H.S.: Medical disease analysis using Neuro-Fuzzy with Feature Extraction Model for classification. Inform. Med. Unlocked **18**, 100288 (2020). https://doi.org/10.1016/j.imu.2019.100288
40. Havaei, M., Davy, A., Warde-Farley, D., Biard, A., Courville, A., Bengio, Y., Pal, C., Jodoin, P.-M., Larochelle, H. (2017). Brain tumor segmentation with deep neural networks. Med. Image Anal. **35**, 18–31.https://doi.org/10.1016/j.media.2016.05.004
41. Toğaçar, M., Ergen, B., Cömert, Z.: BrainMRNet: brain tumor detection using magnetic resonance images with a novel convolutional neural network model. Med. Hypotheses 109531 (2019).https://doi.org/10.1016/j.mehy.2019.109531
42. Vijh, S., Sharma, S., Gaurav, P.: Brain tumor segmentation using OTSU embedded adaptive particle swarm optimization method and convolutional neural network. In: Lecture Notes on Data Engineering and Communications Technologies, pp. 171–194 (2019). https://doi.org/10.1007/978-3-030-25797-2_8
43. Amin, J., Sharif, M., Gul, N., Raza, M., Anjum, M.A., Nisar, M.W., Bukhari, S.A.C.: Brain tumor detection by using stacked autoencoders in deep learning. J. Med. Syst. **44**(2) (2019). https://doi.org/10.1007/s10916-019-1483-2
44. Nema, S., Dudhane, A., Murala, S., Naidu, S.: RescueNet: an unpaired GAN for brain tumor segmentation. Biomed. Signal Process. Control **55**, 101641 (2020). https://doi.org/10.1016/j.bspc.2019.101641
45. Litjens, G., Kooi, T., Bejnordi, B.E., Setio, A.A.A., Ciompi, F., Ghafoorian, M., Sánchez, C.I.: A survey on deep learning in medical image analysis. Med. Image Anal. **42**, 60–88 (2017). https://doi.org/10.1016/j.media.2017.07.005
46. Abdelaziz Ismael, S.A., Mohammed, A., Hefny, H.: An enhanced deep learning approach for brain cancer MRI images classification using residual networks. Artif. Intell. Med. 101779 (2019).https://doi.org/10.1016/j.artmed.2019.101779
47. Ghassemi, N., Shoeibi, A., Rouhani, M.: Deep neural network with generative adversarial networks pre-training for brain tumor classification based on MR images. Biomed. Signal Process. Control **57**, 101678 (2020). https://doi.org/10.1016/j.bspc.2019.101678

48. Amin, J., Sharif, M., Gul, N., Yasmin, M., Shad, S.A.: Brain tumor classification based on DWT fusion of MRI sequences using convolutional neural network. Pattern Recognit. Lett. (2019). https://doi.org/10.1016/j.patrec.2019.11.016
49. https://medium.com/analytics-vidhya/

Deep Learning Model for Efficient Mammogram Analysis

Debolina Mahapatra, Ratula Ray, and Satya Ranjan Dash

Abstract Breast cancer is one of the main causes of death due to cancer in women all over the world. There is an urgent need for effective identification of the onset of breast cancer so that it can be treated in its early stages, and thus, save many lives. Breast cancer can be detected at a treatable stage with the aid of screening mammography. However, these tests often suffer from false-positive and false-negative cases due to their limited sensitivity and specificity. CAD systems have been used for a long time, to produce digitized mammograms and to perform an automated analysis for the detection of suspected regions. This has helped to provide a second opinion to radiologists, thereby increasing the diagnosis rate. Although CAD systems were equipped with hand-crafted features and machine learning algorithms, they failed to solve the problem of false-positive cases, and also spent more time on image interpretation. Deep Learning uses a complex architecture comprising of neural networks, and is becoming a favored method for medical image analysis. Deep Neural Networks can process an enormous amounts of data, perform automatic feature extraction, and give better results than the existing state-of-the-art methods. In this work, we have proposed a model which uses deep learning for an efficient analysis of mammograms. We have addressed the issue of unnecessary biopsies being conducted due to improper mammogram analysis. Our model focuses on three main areas—micro-calcification detection, analysis of lesions, and tissue texture analysis.

Keywords Breast cancer · Neural networks · Deep learning · Feature extraction

---

D. Mahapatra
Department of Computer Science and Engineering, Silicon Institute of Technology, Bhubaneswar, India
e-mail: mahapatra.debolina201@gmail.com

R. Ray
School of Biotechnology, KIIT University, Bhubaneswar, India
e-mail: ratularay@gmail.com

S. R. Dash (✉)
School of Computer Applications, KIIT University, Bhubaneswar, India
e-mail: sdashfca@kiit.ac.in

H. K. Tripathy et al. (eds.), *Technical Advancements of Machine Learning in Healthcare*, Studies in Computational Intelligence 936,
https://doi.org/10.1007/978-981-33-4698-7_11

1 Introduction

Rapid advancements in technology have created an impact on every aspect of our society. According to a report by McKinsey Global Institute, Artificial Intelligence (AI) is estimated to create a total value of around 13 trillion US dollars annually by the year 2030 [1]. AI has the ability to affect developing economies, jobs, and various industries and sectors like software, retail, transportation, healthcare, manufacturing, and materials. Artificial Intelligence, along with its related technologies like Data Analytics, Machine Learning, and Deep Learning has the potential to transform several aspects of healthcare [2]. It has played a major role in the reduction in the overall costs thereby making healthcare facilities affordable and accessible to everyone. Almost every country has faced concerns regarding its healthcare costs, and by tapping into technology, it is possible to revolutionize the healthcare sector altogether.

Due to the large availability of biomedical data, there have been tremendous opportunities and challenges to healthcare research [3]. Biomedical data is complex, noisy, sparse, time-dependent, and heterogeneous and also has high dimensionality. Another key challenge is the exploration of associations among the different pieces of information in these datasets. Some other types of data in healthcare research are the data collected from sensors, texts, images, and electronic health records. AI is already transforming disease diagnosis and prognosis techniques.

Machine Learning is a programming paradigm that learns using the data and infers the rules by determining the distinctiveness of specific patterns in the data. ML algorithms are being used in clinical research to identify irregularities in medical images. Machine Learning has the ability to process huge datasets and obtain insights from this data that can help physicians. It can also aid to achieve better outcomes, reduce the expenses, thus, leading to patient satisfaction. Traditional machine learning algorithms required using hand-crafted features. Neural networks came into existence during the 1960s, and are still widely popular.

Deep learning methods [4] enable the automatic discovery of representations needed for prediction from data. Deep Learning provides a feature engineering component, and is capable of handling data that is very complex and has high dimensionality, thus giving superior performance in comparison to other existing techniques for prediction. There have been several recent advancements in medicine. Google's London-based AI subsidiary DeepMind has developed a model [5] for early detection of breast cancer using less information than human doctors and relying on the identification of cancerous tumors on mammograms. This AI-based model has successfully reduced the number of false negatives by 9.4% and false positives by 5.7% for women in the US. Researchers have trained deep learning algorithms for the intelligent diagnosis of skin cancer, using nearly 130,000 medical images related to skin diseases [6]. In diabetic patients worldwide, diabetic retinopathy is considered to be the cause of blindness. A deep learning algorithm having high sensitivity and specificity was developed. This algorithm has proved to be capable of detecting diabetic retinopathy using images of the retinal fundus [7]. Overall, one can say that deep learning has powered modern healthcare systems and it paves the way for advanced healthcare research and development.

The number of people affected by cancer every year is staggering, and the problem of cancer is not only increasing in incidents, but it is also a major cause of deaths every year. In order to save more lives, the early detection of cancer is necessary. The investigation of medical images obtained using Computer Aided Diagnosis (CAD) systems is an important step toward cancer detection. To overcome the drawbacks of common machine learning algorithms and to simplify the extraction of features, methods such as deep learning are being used. Convolutional Neural Networks (CNNs) can transform raw images into a high-level representation, thereby increasing the performance of cancer detection systems.

1.1 Terminologies

We describe some of the common medical terminologies related to cancer below.

- Cancer: It is a phenomenon which results in an uncontrolled growth of cells (that are not normal) in any part of the body. The disease of cancer has the ability to spread further to other areas in the body, due to its rapid multiplication capability, and the term for this event is referred to as 'metastasis'.
- Tumor: When an abnormal tissue growth leads to the formation of a lump, or swelling in a body part, it is called a tumor. It can either be benign (non-cancerous) or malignant (cancerous).
- Neoplasm: It is also a type of an abnormal growth of tissue, which may or may not form a swelling.
- Metastasis: In terms of cancer biology, metastasis refers to the spread of cancer from the primary site (where it first arose) to the distant organs. Metastasis is a lethal event in the progression of cancer and can eventually lead to fatality.

Cancers can be classified into four types according to their tissue of origin.

- Carcinoma—This type of cancer occurs in the epithelial tissue. Such tissues form the internal and external lining of the body. A common type of carcinoma, called adenocarcinomas, usually develop in organs having glands, such as the prostate, lungs, esophagus, pancreas, liver, and breasts.
- Sarcoma—These cancers appear in bones, muscles, and connective tissues. It is not very common, and comprises less than 10% of all cancers.
- Leukemia—It is the cancer of the blood cells that originates in the bone marrow.
- Lymphoma—In this type of cancer, the immune system of the human body gets affected. It occurs in lymphocytes.

In the following sections, we provide a brief discussion on breast cancer, and the methods to perform screening.

1.2 Breast Cancer

Breast cancer affects women all over the world. It is diagnosed in 2.1 million women per year worldwide, and also accounts for about 15% of all cancer deaths in women. It leads to around 40,000 deaths per year in the US, making it one of the common causes of deaths due to cancer. Early diagnosis of breast cancer is necessary to increase the possibilities of survival by providing prompt access to medical treatment services.

Breast cancers are classified by their location and by their histological subtype (tissue or cellular). Primary breast cancers are infiltrating ductal cancers which constitute about 80% of all cases, followed by lobular and nipple cancers. In order to prevent breast cancer in women having high risks, there are very limited strategies. However, there exist ways to prevent these cancers by maintaining a proper diet, by staying physically fit, and maintaining an appropriate body weight.

Some of the breast cancer risk factors are as follows:

Age: Women in the age group of 45–55 are usually considered to be at a risk, as breast cancer is more common in this age group.

Family history: If a woman happens to have a close relative (first degree) with breast cancer, it increases her risk.

Genes: Certain genes such as BRCA1 and BRCA2, if present, increase the risk of breast cancer significantly.

Lifestyle: Obesity, decrease in physical activity, smoking, high alcohol intake, usage of oral contraceptives are some of the lifestyle issues that may possibly lead to breast cancer.

1.2.1 Types of Breast Cancers

The various ways of categorizing breast cancers are mentioned below.

a. Invasive vs. In-situ: True cancers are called ‘invasive’ or infiltrating because they have invaded the blood vessels and lymph vessels, and they have the ability to spread. Invasive breast cancer, namely, invasive lobular carcinoma (ILC) and invasive ductal carcinoma (IDC) can grow into the surrounding breast tissue. They can be anywhere from stages I to IV. Pre-cancers are localized and do not have the ability to spread, which is why they are referred to as ‘in-situ’. As opposed to invasive cancers, in-situ cancers are also called intra-ductal or DCIS (Ductal Carcinoma In Situ). This is also called stage zero.
b. Histological sub-types: Histologic subtype refers to the cell of origin of the cancer. The two main histologic sub-types of breast cancer are ductal and lobular. About 80–85% of breast cancers originate from the ducts, and about 10–15% come from the lobules of the breast. Lobular cancers follow a single file pattern, and maybe bigger than anticipated. In ductal cancers, the cells join together forming a clump.

c. Molecular sub-types: This classification is based on the receptors that the cancer cells express, such as ER (estrogen receptor), PR (progesterone receptor), and her2 (tyrosine kinase).
d. Grade: It is used to determine what these cancer cells look like under the microscope according to their degrees of differentiation.
e. Stage: It is used to tell the behavior of the cancer. Stage of a cancer is based on the size of the tumor, the status of lymph nodes, and distant metastases which further helps to understand the spread of the cancer.

1.3 Screening

The early detection of breast cancer is very important so as to prevent deaths from this deadly disease. Screening tests are necessary for the purpose of finding the cancer before symptoms appear. It is possible to treat a breast cancer successfully when it is found early, and is small and still confined to the breast. Screening tests should be safe, inexpensive, and having low risks. There are different methods to perform screening for breast cancer. The simplest of all is self or clinical-breast examination. Such an inspection yields certain key information, such as symmetry, changes in the skin color or texture, dimpling or puckering, presence of lump, and sudden nipple retraction or inversion or discharge.

Most often, imaging techniques are also used for screening of breast cancer. Some of the popular methods are mammography, ultrasound, and breast MRI [8]. By far, the most common breast imaging technique is mammography. Mammography is an examination of the breast using X-rays. It has really revolutionized the treatment of breast cancers as it enables to detect cancers very early. Historically, analog or screen film was used for mammography, but now it is digital. Digital mammography gives better resolution images on the computer.

Another imaging technique is ultrasound, which is very helpful in examining dense breasts and also, in distinguishing breast masses (cystic or solid). Ultrasound is mostly used to look at an area that was not clear on a mammogram. Breast MRI is usually recommended for women who are suspected to be at a greater risk for breast cancer. It is also a very sensitive test, associated with high false-positive rates. Breast MRI is also helpful in cases of suspected chest wall involvement, or undiagnosed primary lesions.

1.3.1 Mammography

Performing a mammography does not reduce the risk of breast cancer. Rather, it aids in the detection of breast cancer at an early and treatable stage, thereby reducing mortality. Before detecting by palpitation, mammography allows the detection of breast cancers, tumors (maybe benign or malignant), and cysts. When a mammogram raises a significant suspicion of tumor or cancer, the tissue belonging to the detected area is removed for a biopsy, and is examined closely.

Mammograms are of two types: screening and diagnostic. In women who do not display any symptoms or signs, a 'screening mammography' is used to detect changes in the morphological features of the breast. This test involves the use of a low intensity X-ray in order to obtain the imaging of each breast. Using this screening methodology, it is possible to detect a tumor before any symptoms occur.

In case any unusual breast changes are observed on a screening mammogram, a 'diagnostic mammogram' can be used. This technique is used to detect abnormalities such as a palpable lump, breast pain, sores that seem erosive, thickening of breast skin or a sudden change in the shape of breasts. A diagnostic mammogram can be considered as a basic medical tool and serves as a good method to examine changes in the breasts. However, women who are older than 30 years are usually advised to undergo diagnostic mammography. At times, this imaging method is also used to examine those women who have history of breast cancer.

Mammography is the most intensely scrutinized as well as a debated medical procedure. It has a better combination of specificity and sensitivity, compared to other breast imaging techniques. However, there are certain limitations, which when overcome, can make mammography a much better method.

1.3.2 Limitations of Mammograms

Mammography is considered to be the most preferred screening test for breast cancer. However, mammography does not perform equally well for all women. The proportion of true-positive results can be given by sensitivity values, and the proportion of true-negative results can be given by specificity values. The sensitivity of screening mammography ranges from 83 to 95%. This implies that around 17% of breast cancer cases might not be detected by mammography. The specificity of mammograms lies between 90 and 98%.

The occurrence of false-positive and false-negative results is high. A false-positive mammogram does not seem normal, even though no cancer is present in the breast. In such cases, additional tests are required. The chances of occurrence of a false-positive mammogram are about one out of ten. A mammogram which is false-negative, may appear normal, though it might have the underlying cancer cells. Screening mammograms may miss one out of six tumors. This happens when the breast tissues are dense. Moreover, as mammography is essentially an X-ray test, it exposes the human body to radiation. During pregnancy, radiation exposure may lead to birth defects.

Mammograms are black and white images. Breast cancers and micro-calcifications appear as whiter areas on mammogram images. Calcifications appear as fine little white spots, and they can be the first signs of cancer. There are different categories of mammographic density. Breasts are made up of fibrous tissues which appear white on a mammogram, and the fatty tissues look black. It would be difficult to detect a white cancer hiding in a white background, in case of dense breast tissues, due to the lack of contrast between them. This leads to false-negative cases. Since mammography has a widespread use, its optimization can be done to make it an effective screening technique for breast cancer.

1.3.3 Evolving Techniques for Breast Imaging

Latest breast imaging techniques are now being developed. Breast Tomosynthesis (3D mammography) is one such technique which is already being used, and it takes pictures similar to a CT scan through the breast tissue, thus giving individual slices of images and finally, a 3D digital reconstruction of the breast takes place.

Molecular breast imaging (MBI) is an imaging test in which a radioactive chemical is injected into the blood stream. With the help of a special camera, this test helps to examine the extent to which the breast cancer has spread in dense tissues. However, it exposes the body to radiation.

Contrast-enhanced spectral mammography (CESM) is a new technique which involves injection of a contrast dye having iodine to be injected into the vein before the test is conducted. Thereafter, two sets of mammograms are taken at different levels of energy. It helps the X-rays assess the abnormal areas in a standard mammography. Some other such new and developing techniques include positron emission mammography (PEM) and optical imaging tests.

During the past decade, technical advancements have led to the improvement of both the technique and the results. With newer and developed methods, the risks due to radiation have decreased considerably, and are almost negligible nowadays. The quality of images produced has also improved. Using digital mammography, breast imaging techniques have been enhanced particularly for women having age less than 50 years, with dense breast tissues, and who are peri-menopausal or pre-menopausal. Compared to the traditional screen film mammography, digital mammography systems can produce images with better contrast and lower spatial resolution. Also, this method uses a lower radiation dose for imaging.

In the following section, we shall discuss the steps involved in medical imaging. We shall understand the process of automated detection of abnormalities present in digital mammograms using CAD systems. We shall also describe the various Deep Learning architectures proposed for the analysis of mammograms.

2 Mammogram Image Analysis

Mammography has been in use for the past three decades. It is the best-known technique for screening of breast cancer, and is widely used. The task of interpreting medical images is performed by radiologists, and it depends on the quality of the image and its interpretation. Electronic images of the breasts obtained by digital mammography can be further enhanced and stored on computers. These images can also be highlighted by the computer-aided detection (CAD) systems for further analysis by the radiologists. These systems provide a second opinion to the radiologists in the task of detecting suspected regions in a mammogram. There is a need for the automated analysis of mammograms so as to ease the process of screening, as well as assist the radiologists by reducing manual work. Without using CAD, the sensitivity of cancer detection is around 80%, and by using CAD, this sensitivity can be increased to 90%.

Traditional Machine Learning (ML) methods have been extremely useful in the field of medical imaging. Several advancements have led to intelligent CAD systems [9] and the learning ability of the systems comes from ML methods. The CAD systems may also support the analysis of digitized mammographic images for the presence of calcifications, suspected masses, or areas having an abnormal density which may indicate the presence of breast cancer. Automated detection using CAD can help to reduce false-positive cases, thereby increasing the diagnosis rate.

The process of mammogram image analysis undergoes several processing steps [10]. First, the images are preprocessed using certain image preprocessing techniques so as to remove noise and enhance its clarity. Next, image segmentation is performed so as to divide the image into regions in accordance with its visual characteristics. The region of interest (ROI) is obtained using this process. ROI is a sample within a dataset, and it contains information related to the boundary of a suspected mass or tumor for the purpose of further analysis. After having identified the ROI(s), feature extraction, and selection are performed. In this stage, the extraction of features is done and then the distinct features are selected. These selected features enable the detection of cancerous regions and differentiate them from normal regions in the image. Analysis of screening mammogram images deals with the detection of masses, micro-calcifications, and architecture distortion.

2.1 Mammograms Analysis Using Machine Learning

Machine Learning (ML) algorithms have been in use for the purpose of analysis and classification of medical images. Several researchers have used these methods to develop models for the automated detection and classification of suspected masses in mammogram images.

Mina et al. proposed a system [11] for breast abnormality detection. In this system, the authors have performed feature extraction using a 2-dimensional wavelet decomposition analysis. For the classification of breast tissue images obtained from mammograms, the ANN learning algorithm was used. During the preprocessing stage, the low-frequency components were removed so as to highlight micro-calcifications depicted by high-frequency components. Feature extraction was performed using a series of steps. The back-propagation algorithm of ANN was used to classify and distinguish abnormal tissues from normal ones. Upon testing this proposed system on MIAS dataset, it achieved an accuracy of 91.64%.

Saini and Vijay [12] have compared the performance of Feed-forward and Cascade-forward back-propagation ANNs. To extract features from the mammogram image, Gray Level Co-occurrence Matrix (GLCM) has been used. GLCM feature extraction method is a statistical method that considers the spatial relationship between the different gray-level pixels and helps to compute second-order features. Both the ANNs used the back-propagation algorithm to classify mammogram images into benign and malignant. The feed-forward network achieves an accuracy of 87.5% whereas the accuracy of the cascade forward network was 67.8%.

An automatic system for the classification of digital mammograms obtained from the mini-MIAS image dataset was proposed in [13]. In this work, the Fuzzy C-means algorithm, an unsupervised algorithm for pattern recognition, has been used for the purpose of segmentation of mass region from the breast ROI. Feature extraction has been done using GLCM, which helps to obtain texture characteristics. Using three different classification techniques, namely, Back Propagation Neural Network (BPNN), Ada Boost, and Sparse Representation Classifier (SRC), a comparative analysis has been done. Upon analyzing performance measures, it was observed that SRC achieved the highest accuracy of 93.75%, outperforming the other classification algorithms.

In 2017, Perez et al. proposed a classification system for mammograms using texture characteristics [14]. The image dataset used was taken from the Digital Database for Screening Mammography (DDSM). Haralick's descriptors were extracted from the images using GLCM. A back-propagation neural network (BPNN) consisting of one hidden layer, was trained on the extracted features, and the classification accuracy was estimated using leave-one-out cross validation. An average accuracy of 84.72% was achieved by the proposed model.

Using Radial Basis Function Neural Networks (RBFNN), Pratiwi et al. [15] proposed a model for mammograms classification using GLCM texture-based features. According to their experimental results, RBFNN outperforms BPNN and achieves an accuracy of 93.98% in classifying abnormal and normal masses, and an accuracy of 94.29% for the classification of malignant and benign tumors. In another work, Hussain et al. employed SVM, Bayesian, and Decision Tree classifiers to distinguish benign mammograms from normal ones [16] and the performance was evaluated on five different categories of features extracted from the images.

One of the early signs of breast cancer is architecture distortion (AD), that is, the normal architecture of breast tissue gets distorted. This often goes undetected on screening mammograms leading to false negatives. A study done by Kamra et al. [17] focused on texture analysis of the ROI from the original mammogram, and found that the selection of the size of ROI must be appropriately done in order to achieve better results. In order to differentiate between ROIs having architecture distortion and non-architecture distortion ROIs, a Support Vector Machine (SVM) classifier was used to achieve an accuracy of 92.94% on DDSM dataset.

Another early sign of breast cancer is the presence of micro-calcification clusters in mammograms. Abirami et al. [18] proposed a model for detection of micro-calcifications in the mammogram images using an artificial neural network (ANN)-based classifier. Discrete Wavelet Transforms were used for feature extraction from the images. Using RBFNN, the model achieved an accuracy of 93%.

The study of automated mammogram analysis and classification systems highlights the importance of early detection of breast cancer. Segmentation of mammogram images is done to find the regions of interest (ROIs). These ROIs include masses as well as normal tissues that may appear suspicious. This, in turn, leads to the problem of false positives during the screening process. To reduce the occurrence of false positives, better and more advanced techniques such as Deep Neural Networks, are being used.

2.2 *Need for Deep Neural Networks*

Currently used CAD systems are based on analyzing a mammogram using hand-crafted features that are pre-designed, and machine learning algorithms are being used for classification on top of these features. However, CAD systems lead to higher false-positive rates and increased interpretation time. Deep Learning has become a popular learning technique for understanding natural as well as medical images.

Deep Neural Networks (DNNs) are the most complex form of machine learning that have the ability to process huge amounts of data and uncover the underlying features, and it is powered by graphics processing units (GPUs) for faster processing of such complex architectures. Deep Learning is increasingly being used for detection of cancerous tissues or lesions in radiology images, and also for extraction of clinically relevant features from the image data. Recent studies have also proven that deep learning-based diagnosis systems perform with greater accuracy in comparison to computer-aided detection (CAD) systems. Feature extraction and selection is also automatically performed by DNNs (Fig. 1), and these features have outperformed hand-crafted or heuristically crafted descriptors for recognition tasks.

With the increasing adoption of Deep-CNNs, medical image analysis has been revolutionized. Akselrod-Ballin et al. introduced a novel deep learning method [19] to detect suspected masses and calcifications in mammogram images. The proposed approach is based on an ensemble of individual Faster-RCNN models, each of which was trained for detecting a set of abnormalities as per clinical categories. With the aim of reducing false-positive cases, the model was built using a DNN that consists of a cascade having three stages, which includes a modified Faster-RCNN and a classifier CNN.

Ribli et al. [20] proposed a fully automated CAD system based upon Faster RCNN, which is a state-of-the-art object detection framework, for detection and classification of lesions on a mammogram. The evaluation of the method was done on the INbreast dataset, and it achieved an AUC of 0.95, and an AUC of 0.85 on the final validation dataset. The proposed system has a high sensitivity, with a significant reduction in false-positive cases. Lotter et al. [21] proposed a deep learning-based approach to address the problem of large amounts of annotated data, and achieved state-of-the-art performance. Their proposed model is annotation-efficient, and it not only classifies mammograms accurately, but also extends to 3-dimensional mammogram classification successfully.

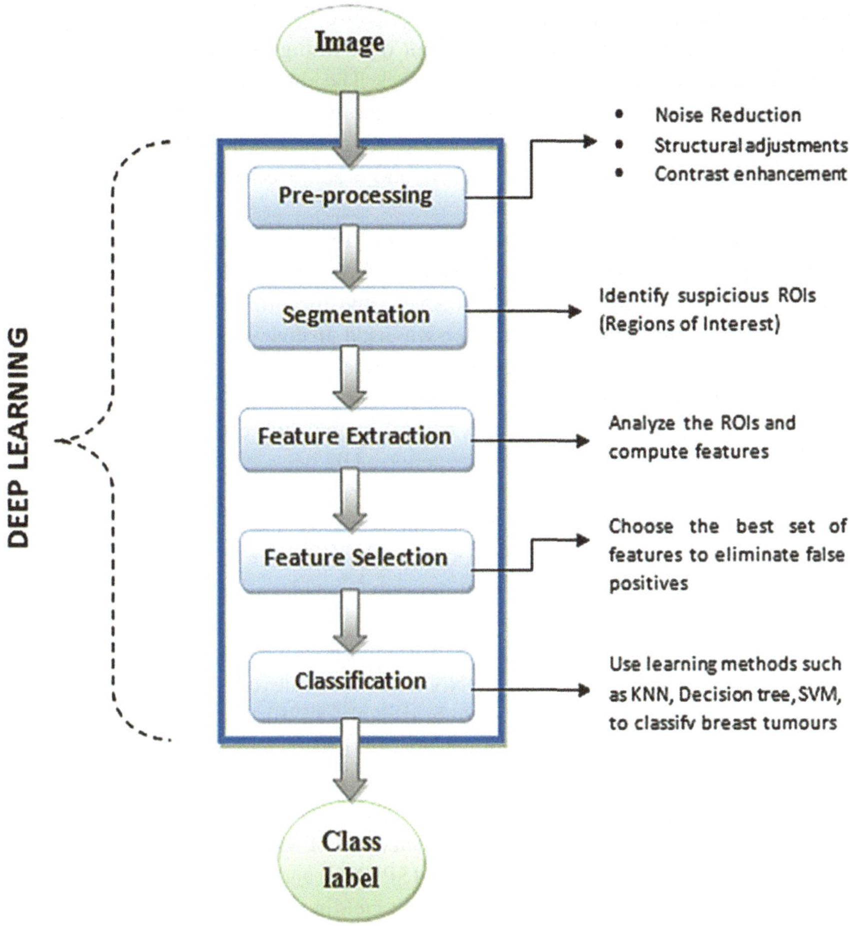

Fig. 1 A typical image processing pipeline that begins with basic image processing, followed by image segmentation and feature extraction, and thereafter, selection of best set of features. The final set of features obtained is fed to the classifier to perform the classification task

A CNN-based model was proposed by Dubrovina et al. [22] to perform tissue classification on mammograms, and to learn the discriminatory features in a automatically as an application to segmentation. The architecture of the deep neural network is composed of 3 stages of convolutional layers, ReLU activation layers, and max-pooling layers, followed by three fully connected layers. The model was tested on annotated mammograms, and it successfully classifies different categories of breast tissues while also performing image segmentation.

Jadoon et al. presented two methods [23] for a classification model based on deep learning in order to classify a large dataset of mammograms into three classes, that is, normal, malignant and benign. Convolutional neural network-discrete wavelet

(CNN-DW) and CNN-curvelet transform (CNN-CT) are the two methods used. Data augmentation is performed to prevent over-fitting. The contrast of mammogram images is enhanced on very small patches. The enhanced mammogram images are decomposed using two-dimensional discrete wavelet transform (2D-DWT) in the CNN-DW method. This method achieves an accuracy of 81.83%. In CNN-CT, discrete curvelet transform (DCT) is used, and it achieved an accuracy of 83.74%, respectively.

Lévy and Jain proposed a CNN-based model to classify breast masses [24] and achieved state-of-the-art results using the DDSM dataset. The breast masses on mammograms were pre-segmented. To overcome the limitation of the amount of training data available, data augmentation was used. In this work, three network architectures, namely, a shallow CNN (the baseline model), an AlexNet and a GoogLeNet (with certain modifications) were evaluated. Transfer learning was also applied in order to learn low-level features from natural images and effectively use them for medical image classification. The model achieved 93.4% recall and 92.4% precision.

Wang and Yang [25] addressed the issue of frequent occurrence of false positives in the detection of clustered micro-calcifications. This is because of the local image patterns which influence the response of the classifier. In their work, they have proposed a context-sensitive DNN that not only considers the local image features, but also the surrounding tissue background. After evaluating the proposed model, it was observed that this approach achieves FP (false positive) rate equal to 0.5 clusters per image, and the context-sensitive DNN classifier achieved a sensitivity of 87.4%.

Guo et al. have proposed a novel hybrid method [26] to improve the detection rate of micro-calcifications in mammograms. Initial image processing is performed to remove label and pectoral muscle, and the subjective image quality is improved to enhance the micro-calcifications (MCs). The suspicious calcification areas are obtained using contourlet transform. The detection of MC clusters is done by using Simplified Pulse-Coupled Neural Network (SPCNN) and thereafter, post-processing enables the removal of isolated points, finally yielding the MC clusters.

Another challenge in the medical domain lies with the detection of regions of interest (ROI) in mammogram images and their diagnosis.

Platania et al. proposed a framework called BC-DROID [27] for the automatic detection and diagnosis of breast cancer. In this work, Convolutional Neural Networks have been used for automated ROI detection and diagnosis. The model is initially trained on regions defined by physicians, and later trained on full mammogram images. BC-DROID framework achieves an accuracy of around 90% for ROI detection, and a classification accuracy of 93.5%.

Gardezi et al. presented the utility of Visual Geometry Group (VGG) based CNN model [28] for classification of mammograms. VGG provides significant improvement in performance of the system due to the increased depth of layers. In this work, mammogram ROIs have been obtained from the IRMA dataset, and VGG-16 CNN architecture has been used. Using convolution filters, the feature matrix was computed. Four different classifiers (simple logistic, binary decision tree, SVM, KNN) were applied on the feature matrix and the results were evaluated using tenfold cross validation.

We provide a brief summary of the above discussed machine learning and deep learning methods used for mammogram classification in Table 1.

Table 1 A comprehensive summary of learning methodologies used for mammogram analysis and classification

Learning algorithm	Purpose	Feature extraction	Results
Back-prop ANN	Breast abnormality detection by identifying presence of micro-calcifications	2D wavelet decomposition analysis	Testing with MIAS dataset, 91.64% acc
SRC	Classify suspected masses from ROIs	Fuzzy C-means for image segmentation of mass region from ROIs; GLCM to obtain texture characteristics	Using mini-MIAS dataset, 93.75% acc
SVM	To classify architecture distortion in ROIs	GLCM, fractal-based features and fourier power transform have been used	On DDSM dataset, achieved 92.94% acc
RBFNN	Detection of micro-calcifications from mammograms	Discrete wavelet transforms were used to extract features	Achieved an acc of 93%
Faster-RCNN	Detect and classify lesions	Convolutional layers extract the features, and RPN (region proposal network) detects and localizes objects/regions	Using Inbreast dataset, AUC of 0.95 on training data
CNN	Tissue classification and image segmentation	Conv-layer (3 stage) extracts features automatically	Measured using dice coefficient, nearly 70%
GoogLeNet, AlexNet and baseline CNN	Breast mass classification	Conv-layer; transfer learning for low-level features from natural images	GoogLeNet achieved highest acc of 92.9%
CNN	Automatic ROI detection and diagnosis	Object detection model (YOLO) was adapted to identify ROIs; features learned using CNNs	90% acc for ROI detection, and 93.5% classification acc
VGG-16	Classification of mammogram ROIs	Feature matrix was computed using convolutional filters	Using IRMA dataset, model obtained AUC 1.0

3 Proposed Model

A screening mammogram is the most widely used method to detect suspicious tumors or lesions, and it assists in the early detection of breast cancer, thereby saving many lives. Usually, when there is a suspicious lesion in a mammogram, a patient undergoes a needle biopsy in order to analyze whether the lesion is malignant or benign. Studies conducted have roughly estimated that out of the total number of biopsies conducted, 70% of them are benign, 20% are malignant, and the rest 10% constitute those lesions having a higher risk of breast cancer.

High Risk Lesions (HRL) can also be termed as Atypical Ductal Hyperplasia (ADH) and Lobular Carcinoma In Situ (LCIS). These lesions are considered high risk because their occurrence indicates the future risk of the patient developing breast cancer. For most cases, due to HRLs, patients are recommended to undergo a painful and time-consuming biopsy. However, this surgery does not confirm elimination of all risks, and there may possibly be some undetected cancerous cells that do not comprise the HRLs. In such cases, Deep Learning has the power to assist the radiologists in making decisions.

Over the last few years, medical image analysis techniques have become more efficient by the application of deep learning frameworks. It is now possible to learn features directly from the medical image, without any human intervention to hand-craft features. DNNs are capable of learning features and extracting the required information directly, and it is the complex architecture which has enables these learning techniques to exceed the performance of traditional machine learning methods. Another application of DNNs is in medical image segmentation, in which identifying small structures pose domain specific challenges.

We propose an approach for improving breast cancer detection using deep learning. We focus on three main tasks—micro-calcification detection, lesion analysis and breast tissue texture analysis. These enable us to evaluate the risks of developing a breast cancer, and using DNNs, we are also able prevent the risk of undetected cancers. A diagrammatic representation of the proposed methodology is shown in Fig. 2, starting with the problem statement description and the strategies for obtaining an efficient solution.

In order to separate the normal cases from the positive ones in the screening process, there is an utmost need for the automated detection, localization, and qualification of suspicious or abnormal mammograms. This helps a radiologist by not only allowing him to concentrate on serious and challenging cases, but also to avoid unnecessary biopsies of the breast.

Micro-calcifications (MCs) appear as tiny white spots on a mammogram. They are specks of calcium deposits that are usually not a result of cancer. However, when they appear as clusters, or in some specific patterns, they may indicate precancerous cells. With the aid of a DNN classifier, local features that are relevant to the MC can be obtained. To enhance the accuracy of classification, context information and features can be extracted from the surrounding tissues as well. Existing image processing techniques may also help to preprocess the mammogram for a better micro-calcification

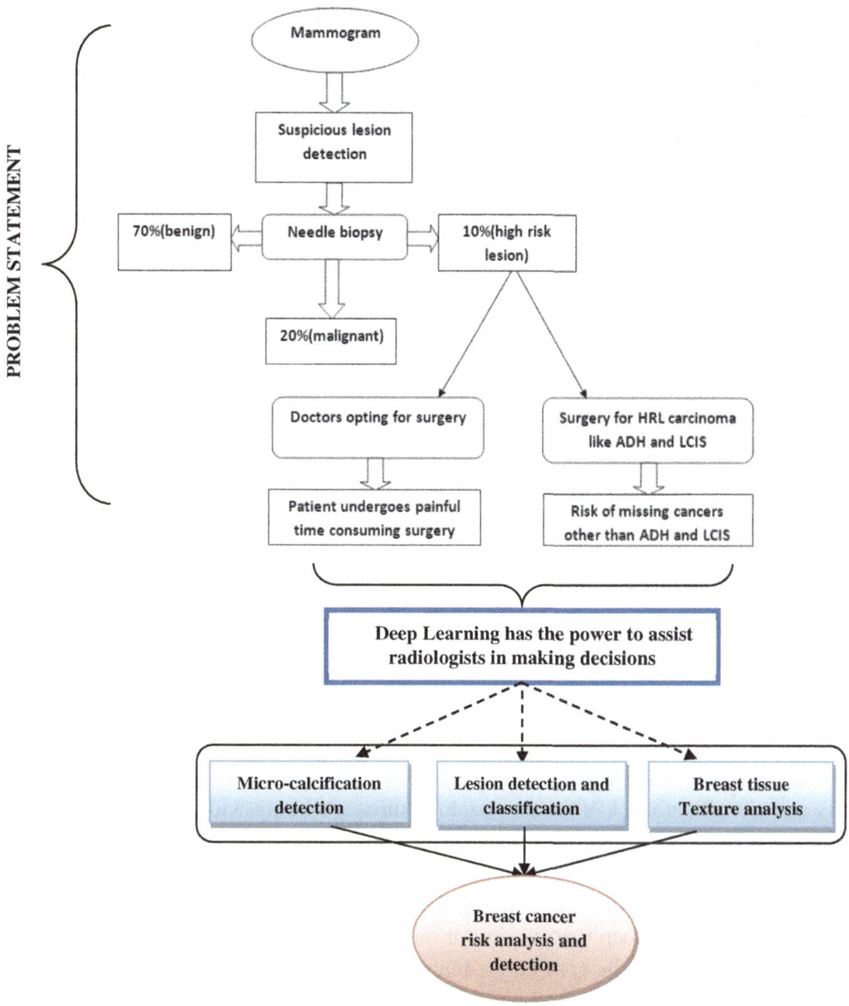

Fig. 2 A flowchart representation of the problem statement and proposed solution

detection performance. Logarithmic transforms, wavelet transforms, and contourlet transforms are some of the methods applied to obtain calcification areas, which are later processed and analyzed by deep neural networks, thus accurately classifying MC clusters.

Lesions are an abnormal change in the tissue which maybe malignant or benign. Malignant lesions are a threat and cancerous in nature, and can also be present even after a biopsy. Lesion detection can also be performed with convolutional neural networks. Complex CNN-based architectures such as VGG, which consist of very deep layers, assist in region of interest detection so as to reduce the dimension of the image. Such learning methods have the ability to detect and classify lesions present in mammograms. Convolutional layers can also be used to extract features and perform image segmentation.

Breast tissue texture analysis is essential to spot abnormalities which may possibly be cancerous. Hand-crafted texture descriptors have been in use for this purpose. CNNs serve as an efficient approach to extract high-dimensional patterns from mammograms. Texture feature maps are derived from mammograms, and upon analyzing interactions between localized patterns, rich information can be obtained that can be used to study associations with breast cancer.

4 Conclusion

Screening techniques such as mammography can help in early detection of abnormalities. However, mammography techniques face certain limitations of sensitivity and specificity, and there are also a considerable number of false-positive and false-negative cases. Since mammography is popular and easily available everywhere, a lot of recent works have been focusing on the automation of mammogram analysis. Initially, CAD systems were equipped with the ability of automated screening using traditional machine learning algorithms.

Deep Learning has revolutionized the analysis of medical images, particularly, the ability to process large datasets and performing automatic feature extraction. DNNs have been applied to different areas ranging from computer vision, natural language processing, and speech recognition, and have produced state-of-the-art results. Deep Neural Network models are increasingly becoming popular for medical image analysis and classification. CNN-based architectures are being widely used due to their ability to provide discriminative image representations, without manual intervention. Deep learning has been used for micro-calcification detection, architectural distortion detection, tissue classification, region of interest detection, and suspected mass or lesion detection. Deep learning is not only limited to performing classification of images, but it can also be applied for feature extraction and image segmentation.

In our proposed model, we aim to leverage the power of Deep Neural Networks to assist radiologists in decision making from mammogram images. We addressed the problem of unnecessary biopsies being conducted, while missing out certain other types of cancers apart from high risk lesions (HRLs). We suggested the use of DNNs for HRL analysis to identify the risks before conducting a biopsy, for analysis of breast tissue texture to spot abnormalities (if any), and micro-calcification detection. Future work shall be done to develop a model combining all these three analysis methods, and their subsequent implementation using deep learning. Due to lack of availability of data and annotations present, it might cause certain limitations in applying the DNN methods on the datasets. Techniques such as image and data augmentation have been in use as a means to overcome such limitations as well.

References

1. Bughin, J., Seong, J., Manyika, J., Chui, M., Joshi, R.: Notes from the AI Frontier: Modeling the Impact of AI on the World Economy. McKinsey Global Institute (2018)
2. Davenport, T., Kalakota, R.: The potential for artificial intelligence in healthcare. Future Healthc. J. **6**(2), 94 (2019)
3. Miotto, R., Wang, F., Wang, S., Jiang, X., Dudley, J.T.: Deep learning for healthcare: review, opportunities and challenges. Brief. Bioinform. **19**(6), 1236–1246 (2018)
4. Tobore, I., Li, J., Yuhang, L., Al-Handarish, Y., Kandwal, A., Nie, Z., Wang, L.: Deep learning intervention for health care challenges: some biomedical domain considerations. JMIR mHealth and uHealth **7**(8), e11966 (2019)
5. McKinney, S.M., Sieniek, M., Godbole, V., Godwin, J., Antropova, N., Ashrafian, H., Back, T., Chesus, M., Corrado, G.C., Darzi, A., Etemadi, M.: International evaluation of an AI system for breast cancer screening. Nature **577**, 89–94 (2020)
6. Esteva, A., Kuprel, B., Novoa, R.A., Ko, J., Swetter, S.M., Blau, H.M., Thrun, S.: Dermatologist-level classification of skin cancer with deep neural networks. Nature **542**, 115–118 (2017)
7. Gulshan, V., Peng, L., Coram, M., Stumpe, M.C., Wu, D., Narayanaswamy, A., Venugopalan, S., Widner, K., Madams, T., Cuadros, J., Kim, R.: Development and validation of a deep learning algorithm for detection of diabetic retinopathy in retinal fundus photographs. JAMA **316**(22), 2402–2410 (2016)
8. Lima, Z.S., Ebadi, M.R., Amjad, G., Younesi, L.: Application of imaging technologies in breast cancer detection: a review article. Open Access Maced. J. Med. Sci. **7**(5), 838–848 (2019)
9. Gardezi, S.J.S., Elazab, A., Lei, B., Wang, T.: Breast cancer detection and diagnosis using mammographic data: systematic review. J. Med. Internet Res. **21**(7), e14464 (2019)
10. Yassin, N.I., Omran, S., El Houby, E.M., Allam, H.: Machine learning techniques for breast cancer computer aided diagnosis using different image modalities: a systematic review. Comput. Methods Programs Biomed. **156**, 25–45 (2018)
11. Mina, L.M., Isa, N.A.M.: Breast abnormality detection in mammograms using artificial neural network. In: 2015 International Conference on Computer, Communications, and Control Technology (I4CT), pp. 258–263. IEEE (2015)
12. Saini, S., Vijay, R.: Mammogram analysis using feed-forward back propagation and cascade-forward back propagation artificial neural network. In: 2015 Fifth International Conference on Communication Systems and Network Technologies, pp. 1177–1180. IEEE (2015)
13. Vaidehi, K., Subashini, T.S.: Automatic characterization of benign and malignant masses in mammography. Procedia Comput. Sci. **46**, 1762–1769 (2015)
14. Pérez, M., Benalcázar, M.E., Tusa, E., Rivas, W., Conci, A.: Mammogram classification using back-propagation neural networks and texture feature descriptors. In: 2017 IEEE Second Ecuador Technical Chapters Meeting (ETCM), pp. 1–6. IEEE (2017)
15. Pratiwi, M., Harefa, J., Nanda, S.: Mammograms classification using gray-level co-occurrence matrix and radial basis function neural network. Procedia Comput. Sci. **59**, 83–91 (2015)
16. Hussain, L., Aziz, W., Saeed, S., Rathore, S., Rafique, M.: Automated breast cancer detection using machine learning techniques by extracting different feature extracting strategies. In: 2018 17th IEEE International Conference on Trust, Security and Privacy in Computing and Communications/12th IEEE International Conference on Big Data Science and Engineering (TrustCom/BigDataSE), pp. 327–331. IEEE (2018)
17. Kamra, A., Jain, V.K., Singh, S., Mittal, S.: Characterization of architectural distortion in mammograms based on texture analysis using support vector machine classifier with clinical evaluation. J. Digit. Imaging **29**(1), 104–114 (2016)
18. Abirami, C., Harikumar, R., Chakravarthy, S.S.: Performance analysis and detection of micro calcification in digital mammograms using wavelet features. In: 2016 International Conference on Wireless Communications, Signal Processing and Networking (WiSPNET), pp. 2327–2331. IEEE (2016)

19. Akselrod-Ballin, A., Karlinsky, L., Hazan, A., Bakalo, R., Horesh, A.B., Shoshan, Y., Barkan, E.: Deep learning for automatic detection of abnormal findings in breast mammography. In: Deep Learning in Medical Image Analysis and Multimodal Learning for Clinical Decision Support, pp. 321–329. Springer (2017)
20. Ribli, D., Horváth, A., Unger, Z., Pollner, P., Csabai, I.: Detecting and classifying lesions in mammograms with deep learning. Sci. Rep. **8**(1), 1–7 (2018)
21. Lotter, W., Diab, A.R., Haslam, B., Kim, J.G., Grisot, G., Wu, E., Wu, K., Onieva, J.O., Boxerman, J.L., Wang, M., Bandler, M.: Robust breast cancer detection in mammography and digital breast tomosynthesis using annotation-efficient deep learning approach. arXiv:1912.11027 (2019)
22. Dubrovina, A., Kisilev, P., Ginsburg, B., Hashoul, S., Kimmel, R.: Computational mammography using deep neural networks. Comput. Methods Biomech. Biomed. Eng. Imaging Vis. **6**(3), 243–247 (2018)
23. Jadoon, M.M., Zhang, Q., Haq, I.U., Butt, S., Jadoon, A.: Three-class mammogram classification based on descriptive CNN features. Biomed. Res. Int. **2017**, 1–11 (2017)
24. Lévy, D., Jain, A.: Breast mass classification from mammograms using deep convolutional neural networks. arXiv:1612.00542 (2016)
25. Wang, J., Yang, Y.: A context-sensitive deep learning approach for micro-calcification detection in mammograms. Pattern Recogn. **78**, 12–22 (2018)
26. Guo, Y.N., Dong, M., Yang, Z., Gao, X., Wang, K., Luo, C., Ma, Y., Zhang, J.: A new method of detecting micro-calcification clusters in mammograms using contourlet transform and non-linking simplified PCNN. Comput. Methods Programs Biomed. **130**, 31–45 (2016)
27. Platania, R., Shams, S., Yang, S., Zhang, J., Lee, K., Park, S.J.: Automated breast cancer diagnosis using deep learning and region of interest detection (BC-DRIOD). In: Proceedings of the 8th ACM International Conference on Bioinformatics, Computational Biology, and Health Informatics, pp. 536–543 (2017)
28. Gardezi, S.J.S., Awais, M., Faye, I., Meriaudeau, F.: Mammogram classification using deep learning features. In: 2017 IEEE International Conference on Signal and Image Processing Applications (ICSIPA), pp. 485–488. IEEE (2017)

An Automated Glaucoma Detection Model to Estimate Glaucoma Abnormalities in Fundus Images Using CNN

A. Prashanthi, P. V. Rao, Santhosh Kumar, V. Sreepathi, and A. Y. Prasad

Abstract An eye situation glaucoma is analysed effectively with the damages occurred in the optic nerve of the eye and it will become for a long period. This becomes proactive in successive stages mainly pressure built up in the optic nerve inside the eye. The current Scenario state that most predominant glaucoma type is of primary open angle glaucoma (OAG) management Glaucoma cannot be identified easily until it becomes more serious in life. Most of the glaucoma type is of primary open angle glaucoma management. An attention is made on one of the eye diseases conditionally, glaucoma which hurts the optic nerve in addition after some time emerges as being severe. The condition is induced internal to the attention with the aid of way of the increase of intraocular stress, the internal tissue layer structure of a retina acts as foreground of a watch that senses light and sends photographs to the mind. This state of affairs will display up salient and might not display in some other time right away. If the disorder is detected early then it prevents field of vision distress. Primary Open Angle Glaucoma Administration is certainly one of the maximum essential as well as most difficult factors of the glaucoma discovery. The numerous findings which depend upon clinical analysis of glaucoma are intraocular pressure, visual view loss and also optical nerve cup. This incurred visual loss growth rate tremendously increases that is purely caused due to open anterior angles,

A. Prashanthi · P. V. Rao (✉)
VBIT, Hyderabad, India
e-mail: raopachara@gmail.com

A. Prashanthi
e-mail: alaminnu401@gmail.com

S. Kumar
UBDTCE, Davanagere, India
e-mail: santhoshdr@ubdtce.org

V. Sreepathi
RRCE, Bengaluru, India
e-mail: sreepathiv@gmail.com

A. Y. Prasad
ACSCE, Bengaluru, India
e-mail: ayprasad26@gmail.com

H. K. Tripathy et al. (eds.), *Technical Advancements of Machine Learning in Healthcare*,
Studies in Computational Intelligence 936,
https://doi.org/10.1007/978-981-33-4698-7_12

visual abnormal characteristics identity and intraocular pressure of the eye. Glaucoma discovery can be determined through numerous methods: perimetry, tonometry, OCT, ophthalmoscopy, tachymetry and genotype. In this work, the author developed a novel algorithmic model to detect and provide a suitable diagnosis approach for glaucoma identification in the patients using 50 colour fundus images very accurately. In this proposed method Convolutional Neural Network (CNN) was targeted for segmentation and classification of the input fundus images to detect glaucoma by measuring cup and disc values. CNN algorithm is taken, and analysed to classify glaucoma images. The final effects of reminiscence are fed to an average clear out for pre-processing and wavelet sub-band decomposition for extraction of attributes that are fed to CNN classifier. Two ways the simulations were performed, one using GUI based simulation environment and second one the metrics evaluation using statistical properties. In this proposed work approximately 100% accuracy and CDR 0.80 values have been achieved with CNN novel approach for glaucoma detection using CDR values for 50 database eye fundus images obtained from the hospitals.

Keywords Glaucoma · Cup to disc ratio · Optic disc · Optic cup · Convolution neural networks · Accuracy

1 Introduction

In medical image processing applications content performance glaucoma detection strategies play a major attention for researchers to evaluate the disorder of the eye locations that was caused due to the damage of the optic nerve structural changes to prevent the permanent vision loss of human beings. The opticians widely adapted diagnosis methods for glaucoma detection that are: manually obtained from the medical history of the patients, visual loss test and evaluation of optic disc and cup disk in general by manual ophthalmoscope by procuring the details of the optic nerve of fundus eye images. These accurate structural boundaries of the optic nerve help the opticians in diagnosis and detecting glaucoma by adapting more advanced image processing techniques and software tools which lead to estimate the optic disc. From which cup and disc area have been identified to measures the metrics used in detecting the glaucoma efficiently. It is developed by internal stress built inside the retina. The situation of an eye where we can lose the eyesight is glaucoma. Kim et al. [1] highlight two novel approaches to determine the CDR values by segmenting from the ROI to localize cup and disc areas using fully conventional networks U-Net architecture of RIGA database and region of interest for the fundus images. By evaluating the three-performance metrics Jaccard index, F-measure and accuracy. Thakur et al. [2, 19] focused on the various glaucoma detection approaches found in the literature survey to measure CDR values. The maximum important open angle glaucoma management (OAG) is actually one of the maximum critical and moreover maximum tough aspects of the glaucoma discovery. The unique findings based upon analysis of glaucoma are intraocular stress, sight view loss and additionally optical

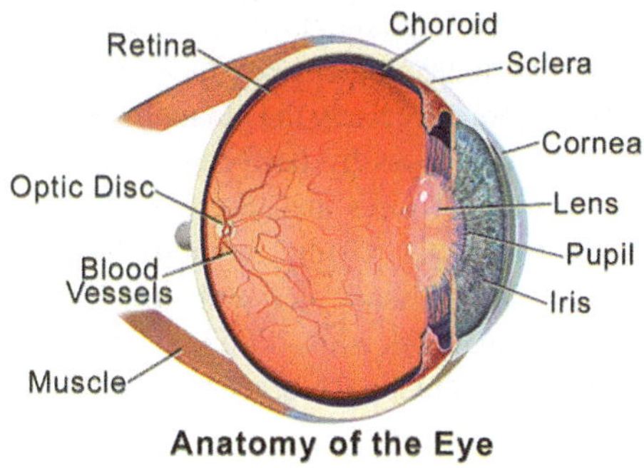

Fig. 1 Internal structure of an eye

nerve cup. Opticians can take more time in diagnosing the critical conditions to recognize the abnormality of eye circumstance. To cope with the trouble wavelets custom designed beneath bands are related to unfastened up the glaucoma strength degrees as well as the algorithms Multi-Layer Perceptron, Back Propagation and Artificial Neural Network is analysed and proposed. From the database procured from the literature papers, collected number of the images from various resources are added to database and moreover the same eye images were used in detecting glaucoma [3]. An electricity degree was separated from picture via the use of wavelet sub-bands. Figure 1 shows an internal structure of an eye.

The favoured and moreover values are calculated from the given image as well as CDR, the CDR defines cropping of optic disc to optic cup. The picture that is selected is chopped for particular region and moreover does the department to the cropped locate on. The Cup to Disc Ratio can be given as optic cup to optic disc. Images that are taken from the database are being processed for further stages using MATLAB. Bajwa et al. [4, 5] explore two-stage machine learning technique for localizing and extracting the optic disc by region-based convolution neural networks and to extract optic disc by deep convolution neural networks of fundus images by developing rule based semiautomatic ground truth generation method for automated disc localization [6–8]. For this processing the Morphological operation is used. In the proposed method CNN algorithm is used. CNN has convolution/Filtering which identifies object. CNN uses system like MLP that has been designed for reduced processing requirements. By using GUI, we check the results of CNN, Glaucoma Detected or not as well as the performance of the parameters from the selected images. The novel technique developed in this research work with the efforts made to improve the overall metrics performance of a glaucoma detection system by partitioning into the region of optic disc and optic cup independently that helps in evaluating the accuracy and CDR value from the fundus images of databases.

Further, the remaining section of this research work related to the current paper is organized into sub-sections as: Sect. 2 explores the different evaluation algorithmic relative approaches used for optical disc segmentation of the fundus images for different databases. Section 3 focuses on the different methods to provide the complete segmentation and evaluation approaches to detect glaucoma. Section 4 explains the fundamentals of an automated glaucoma detection method by considering two measurement key factors accuracy and CDR value of fundus images to identify more precisely the glaucoma in human beings; and also to prevent the growth rate of vision loss by performing diagnosis tests manually, Sect. 5 highlights the experimental results and discusses the obtained results for better performance by comparing with existing methods found in the literature survey. The last section presents a discussion on the obtained simulation results and also shown a provision to extent this work with additional factors to further implement to enrich performance measures in the glaucoma detection process in this work as a future scope.

2 Related Literature Work

Glaucoma is affected due to structural changes in the ONH, retinal rim and vasculature; so all these structural changes in a retina have been analysed by a manual observation leading to a time consuming process in diagnosing it. So, we discussed some of research works whose contributions and continuous efforts helped in easy and accurate diagnosing methods by adapting the anatomical structural changes in the retinal automatically. The diagnoses require regular monitoring, which is costly and time consuming. Both the accuracy and reliability metrics of a diagnosis process is limited by the experts with wide domain knowledge in analysing and identifying the causes for the retinal changes that leads to glaucoma. So, more focus is made towards the automatic diagnosis of glaucoma which made a lot of attention in developing novel algorithmic approaches by the researchers. R. Gayathri, P. V. Rao and Annu S., explored an innovative algorithmic method by assigning different threshold values in measuring CDR values for fundus images in a high quality glaucoma detection model and also extracting the energy features for glaucoma classification by the Naive Bayes in a MLP-BP ANN neural system. This proposed method is classified based on the wavelet energy features of fundus images and to achieve 95% accuracy [9].

Li and Kuo [10], explored two spatial–contextual SVM approaches in hyperspectral image classification schemes. The spatial information is obtained from the original space (SCSVM). Markov random fields RFs) based on the spatial information in the feature space for the IPS data set with 16 classes.

Salam et al. [11], proposed an algorithmic approach to detect and verify the possibility of glaucoma identification for 100 fundus images of local database incorporating hybrid features by combining CDR-structural and also texture and intensity non-structural features [6].

Arumuga Maria Devi et al. [12], proposed Hyperspectral image classification techniques using segmentation with Spatial and Spectral features for different image applications. Here, a framework is divided into training and testing phase, that are used to extract the features using Morphological profiles, DWT, Grey level Co-occurrence Matrix. They are used to classify the images and minimise or completely eliminate noises from the eye images. It improves the model accuracy using the image classification scheme.

Rajendra Acharya et al. and Due [6, 13], both individually proposed an automated image-based diagnosis procedures to detect glaucoma of an eye from Haralick Texture features of fundus images. This work highlights the importance of extracted texture features and from which the pixel values will be calculated based on Haralick Co-occurrence matrix values. Kharirina et al. [7], proposed three statistical features: mean smoothness and 3rd moment to detect glaucoma based on fundus image. These extracted features were being used to classify using K-NN algorithm and obtained a better accuracy of 95.24%. Chandrashekar et al. [8], explored various ways for analysing detection and classification schemes of the optic images to detect the glaucoma. In this proposed work, by extracting the wavelet energy band features from the images of the database and these features are used as in-built operators in MLP-BP algorithm to measure the metric accuracy. Arasi et al. [14], proposed an automatic diagnosis approach to detect glaucoma in the fundus images using wavelet features. Here the statistical properties like: Mean and Entropy values are obtained for a fundus image using daubechies (db3) wavelet filter and achieved an accuracy of 79% and specificity of 100% respectively. Shen et al. [15], focused on the pixel-based hyperspectral image classification using three dimensions Gobar wavelet. Hyperspectral imaging is an improved version of conventional spectroscopy which provides additional information of a fundus eye image to identify each pixel accurately with colour as well as material identification. This work provides better accuracies with metric values of 95.36 and 96.04%. Anindita Septiarini, D. Evangelin Hepsiba, A. Josephine; and Aruna S. et al., proposed an automatic glaucoma detection using cup to disc ratio in evaluating the metric CDR with an accuracy of 95% [3, 11, 16–18].

3 Related Work

At First, in biomedical imaging glaucoma detection systems, the researchers have made tremendous efforts in detecting; and helping the doctors in diagnosing an accurate Glaucoma from the fundus images of the databases is one prime requirements to prevent its growth rate and avoid permanent vision loss (blindness) In General, the segmentation techniques were developed to help in diagnosis and analysis by finding out the ROI differences observed in the optic cup and optic disc. Second, in a day to day life, the rapid growth in technology developments in medical image processing applications, will be motivating factors for the researchers to adapt the 3D fundus images rather than using 2D fundus images prominently in optical cup segmentation techniques and this will provide better performance solution in diagnosing the glaucoma from the fundus image databases in preventing early loss of vision in human beings. This becomes a challenging task for the researchers to identifying and segmenting fundus images to classify the boundary of optic disc and optic cup using 3D fundus images.

3.1 DataBase

In this proposed method, the authors have collected 50 samples of both normal and abnormal Fundus Images from R.L. Jalapa Medical College and Research Institute of Technology (RLJMCRIT), Bangalore, India. We have granted to take the permission from doctors of Ophthalmology department to collect 50 fundus images database from medical college. The images that are collected were stored in a database. And we have collected another set of 125 fundus images from a private medical college and some other fundus images from internet sources. These fundus images were taken as input images to evaluate abnormalities of the images with image processing techniques to locate the ROI, the vertical heights of optic disc and optic cup help to measure the performance of glaucoma detection. The fundus images from databases will be taken by measuring the CDR and statistical properties also help more accurately in glaucoma detection by an ophthalmist in less time and accurately, so that the overall performance of glaucoma detection system can be improved.

Glaucoma occurs in the eye situation by which the objects are not visible clearly. Glaucoma mostly occurs in children below 10 years and also people who cross 40 years. Doctors also faced problems to find abnormal situation in eye. To eliminate this problem more often and preferably CNN algorithm method for glaucoma detection is proposed and analysed with classifiers at the final stage. Figure 2 shows different phases that normally exist in glaucoma affected optic images and illustrate the possible conditions in the eye. Here, three stages of the fundus images are classified as: normal eye, abnormality and severity. These stages are classified with threshold values under different conditions, verified with localized classification schemes to detect the glaucoma abnormalities from the input eye image.

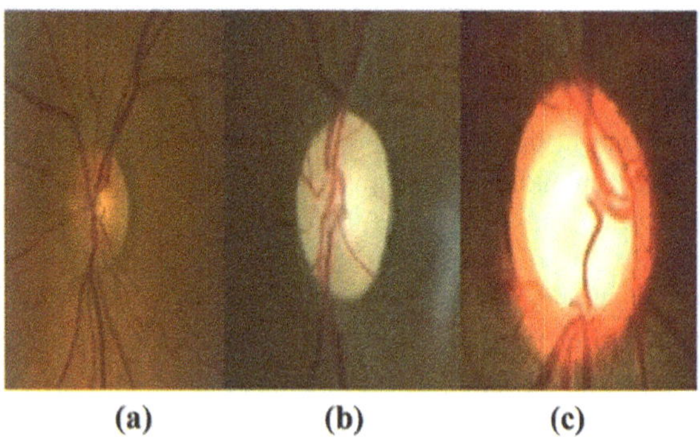

Fig. 2 **a** Normal eye. **b** Abnormality. **c** Severity

4 Proposed Method

This work highlights a novel glaucoma detection technique based on two performance metrics CDR and Accuracy in one way and statistical properties in another way are used to detect the abnormality of the glaucoma for the fundus images of the databases. The simulation results of glaucoma detection for each input fundus are verified for two conditions: normal or glaucoma image. Recent survey explored the different techniques highlighted by the researchers by incorporating the operators in glaucoma detection system, like: threshold value, ROI area, morphological operators and statistical metrics [19]. Gwenolé Q elaborates the technique in which the significant role of pixels with better quality heatmap generation and optimization solution in the fundus images plays to predict the image level classification by training using a ConvNet with backpropagation [2].

The fundamental steps of a proposed glaucoma detection method are shown in Fig. 3. This glaucoma detection model consists of different blocks. They are: 1. Image database, 2. Image pre-processing, 3. Segmentation 4. Cup to Disc Ratio and 5. CNN Classifier. Khunger et al. [18], explained the different factors that result into optic nerve damaged that leads to complete vision loss permanently in human beings. Here, the investigating procedure for live fundus images captured from high resolution cameras in diagnosing in real time applications.

4.1 Image Database

In this work, all the collected fundus images are stored in a database. Some of the normal images and image areas that possesses glaucoma are taken from the database, that are analysed to help in diagnosing the disease to prevent the patients from either progression or causing permanent loss of vision. The identified images are placed in the database as further reference. These image identities are kept in database and shown in tabular forms in various possible conditions used for detecting glaucoma problem.

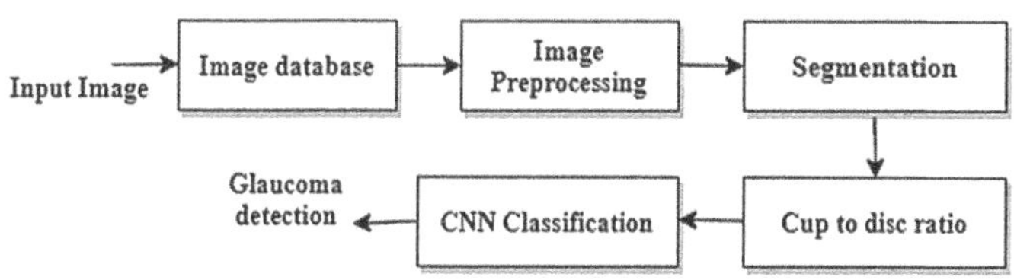

Fig. 3 Proposed block diagram of glaucoma detection

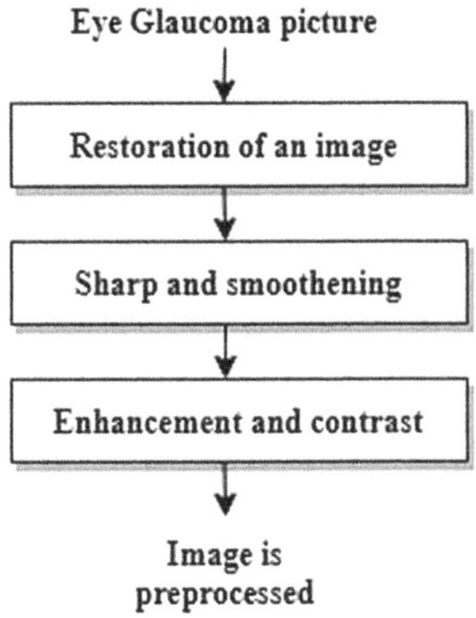

Fig. 4 Steps in pre-processing of a glaucoma image

4.2 *Image Pre-processing*

The RGB image database is structured based on the features that were extracted with the information available like fundus images and labelling of images. While extracting features from the fundus coloured images (as an input data), fundus images are considered as input raw image data to the simulation experiments. It is performed in two steps; Locating the Region of Interest (ROI) of an eye image and enhancing the features of an image. In coloured fundus images, optic disc represents mostly the brightest region of light intensity and is labelled as ROI of the fundus image. The ROI of an image is cropped and then organized into standard pixel dimensionality of 256 × 256. The other region extracted from the raw image is to indicate the optic cup region. Thus region of optic cup and disc has been measured from the fundus images. The image taken from the database is of low contrast which consists of speckle noise. Pre-processing is done for the removal of noise. The steps involved in pre-processing are: (i) Restoration of Image/Picture, (ii) Sharp and Smoothing and (iii) Enhancement.

Figure 4 explains the following steps adapted commonly involved in image Pre-processing.

Here, normally the performance evaluation of the novel proposed glaucoma detection system is measured in terms of metrics like; CDR and Accuracy, as well as statistical properties.

4.3 *Cup to Disc Ratio (CDR) and Accuracy*

Optic disc and cup segmentation is an integral part of Glaucoma detection to measure the abnormalities of fundus images more accurately and precisely. An optic disc is

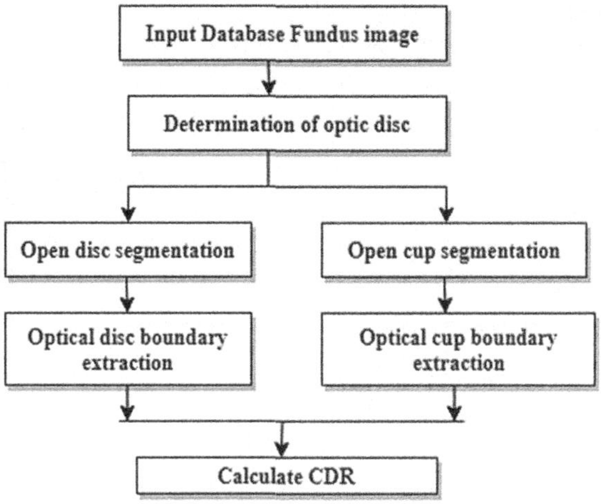

Fig. 5 Flow chart of CDR evaluation process

one of the main parts of retinal image. The optic disc (OD) is of elliptical/oval shape and further it is divided into two separate zones like: Central Zone (Cup Zone), Peripheral Zone (Neuroretinal Rim).

If there are any changes in colour, shape or depth of optic disc, probably it is the glaucoma status in the fundus images. The optic cup (OC) segmentation is used to detect cup boundaries. Figure 5 shows the measurement method for optic disc and optic cup vertical heights of an eye image in glaucoma detection.

The optic cup and disc is calculated basically to obtain CDR. Cup to Disc Ratio defines the Vertical Cup diameter to Vertical Disc Diameter, and it accommodates cropping of optic disc.

$$\text{CDR} = \frac{\text{Size of Optic Cup}}{\text{Size of Optic Disc}} = \frac{VCD}{VDD} \tag{1}$$

$$\text{Accuracy} = \frac{TP + TN}{TP + TN + FP + FN} \tag{2}$$

True Positive (TP) = Number of detected glaucoma images by an expert and the current technique,

True Negative (TN) = Number of images detected as normal images by an expert in the current technique.

False Positive (FP) = Number of images detected as normal by an expert and as glaucoma by the current technique.

False Negative (FN) = Number of images detected as glaucoma by an expert and as normal by the current technique.

Here, the parameter of optical cup to optical disc ratio is determined to find CDR using Eq. (1) and the accuracy is determined by Eq. (2). If threshold level is more than CDR value, then we can say that the image (eye) is of glaucoma, if not, it is in normal condition. In this method we obtain CDR of 0.8 [3, 18].

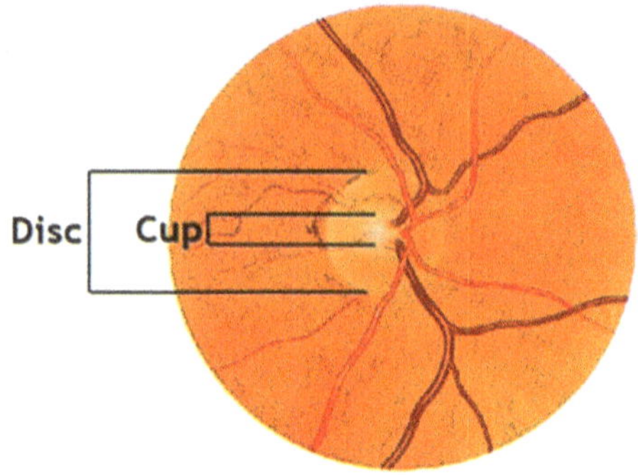

Fig. 6 Optic cup and optic disc

Table 1 Abnormality of fundus image/CDR values to detect Glaucoma

CDR values	Reason
CDR $\leq$ 0.45	1. No glaucoma detected 2. No diabetic retinopathy 3. No diabetic maculopathy
0.45 $\leq$ CDR < 0.6	1. Glaucoma detected 2. Medium risk 3. Diabetic retinopathy
CDR > 0.6	1. Glaucoma detected 2. Very high risk 3. Diabetic maculopathy

The flowchart explains the steps in CDR evaluation processing as shown in Fig. 6. The linguistic values with proper conditions (No glaucoma detected, No diabetic retinopathy, No Diabetic maculopathy or a small spot in the retina) are assigned to measure the CDR values to detect glaucoma as shown in Table 1 and it checks the abnormality condition of 50 fundus images of database.

The abnormality condition of fundus images by assigning cut off CDR values with the various possible ways for different databases are being simulated and those simulated reports are being tabulated for the conditions that are being used in the evaluation process as shown in Table 1.

The author made an attempt by assigning typical values of CDR to decide the testing conditions the different stages of glaucoma located in the fundus images these could normally help the doctors in easy diagnosing the abnormalities in the patients so that it can help from early damage of the vision loss. The author made an attempt by assigning typical values of CDR to decide the testing conditions the different stages of glaucoma located in the fundus images these could normally help the doctors in easy diagnosing the abnormalities in the patients so that it can help from early damage of the vision loss.

4.4 Image Segmentation

Images will be divided into several fragments called Segmentation. Further, it is easier to divide an image into smaller segment areas and perform processing operation to achieve maximum accuracy. The picture is managed to break up the image into smaller area regions similarly to do the processing strategies more precisely. The pictures break up right into the shape of sections for finding the cup location in addition to disc area.

4.5 CNN Classification

A Convolutional Neural Network (CNN) consists of several parts of elementary units, each unit has many weighted inputs and one output. The convolution is done with weights of input signals and transfers the output with some form of nonlinearity. These elementary units are arranged in the form of rectangular lines and their locations to layer correspond to the pixels in an input image. Figure 7 shows the internal structural details of Convolutional Neural Networks with layer types: Convolutional layers, Pooling layer and Fully Connected layer.

Convolutional layer calculates the output of neurons that are connected to main areas in input. Each unit calculates the convolution product of the weights of neurons and a small portion of region. Pooling layer performs the down sampling operation that results in calculating the volume, height and width. The primary characteristics like: Parameter sharing, Local connectivity and Pooling of hidden units of CNN are organized by the spatial arrangement [20].

A convolutional Neural Network (CNN) is used in identifying object and also in filtering process. A classifier is a nonlinear model that is used to identify the ailment. In this method, diverse algorithms are utilized for results such as Support Vector Machine (SVM), K-means Clustering (KNN), and Bayesian classifier for

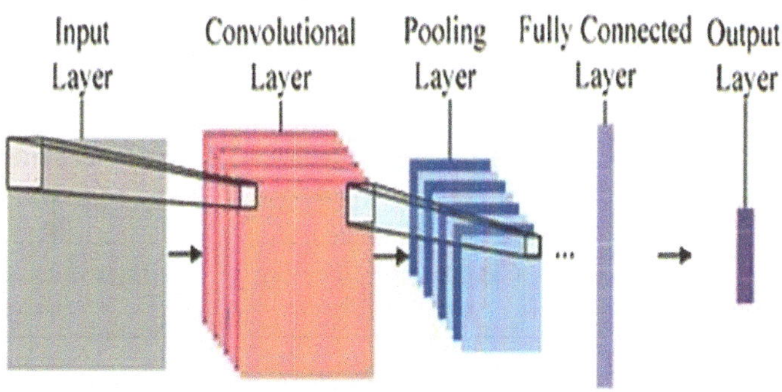

Fig. 7 Convolutional neural network

classification. CNN basically uses very fewer pre-processing techniques. CNN is used in handwritten digit recognition, emotion detection [8]. The proposed automatic glaucoma detection of fundus images using convolution neural network is shown in Fig. 8. In this work 50 images of private database are collected from medical reports and second set of images from internet database and images have been adapted in the simulation experiments using MATLAB R.14 tool. Image Pre-Processing is used to eliminate the unwanted noise from the input image to enhance the quality of image through filtering and noise elimination. The ROI is extracted from the fundus image with the help of colour channel separation in MATLAB software. The steps are shown in Fig. 9.

Region of Interest (ROI) is a portion of an image that is used to convert into a binary mask image. Extracting the ROI by

- Converting RGBImage to Grey Scale image
- From Grey scale image, eliminate unwanted noise using filters (Gaussian)
- Avoid degradation of blurred images performance while locating the sharp edges

Feature Extraction reduces resource utilization by reducing the number of resources that are used to explain with a huge dataset that merges the variables into features. It is used to reduce the data that must be processed. Feature extraction is used to enhance the speed and effectiveness of supervised learning. In this proposed work the algorithmic approach that is being adapted is shown in the flow chart. At first, the given input image is being cropped to fix the predefined region to fit into GUI block, all the pixel positions of localized region are being transformed

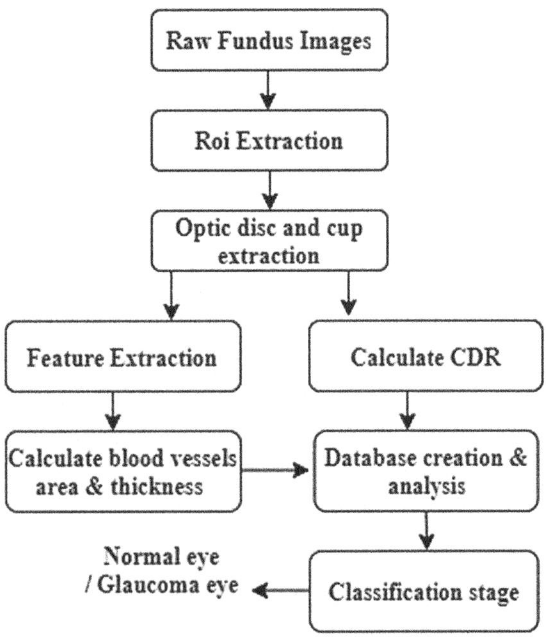

Fig. 8 Glaucoma detection model using CNN

Fig. 9 Pre-processing steps for fundus images

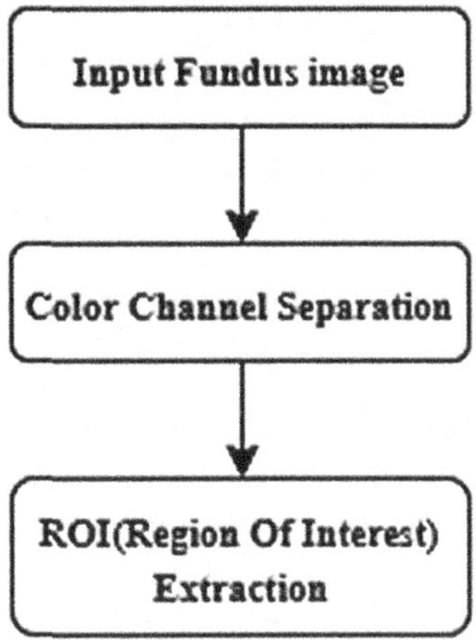

into binary valued, CNN check is performed to detect the glaucoma for the fundus images shown in Fig. 10. Table 2 shows the algorithmic steps adapted during the CNN based glaucoma detection method.

Fig. 10 Flow chart of proposed algorithm for CNN

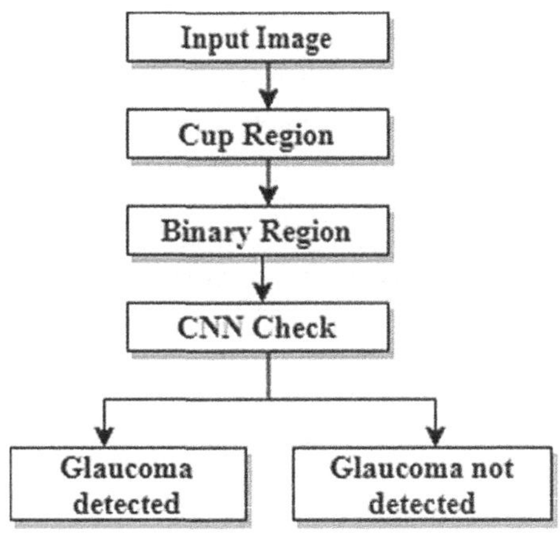

Table 2 Steps in proposed algorithm

Step 1: Take the image from input database
Step 2: Find cup region area for the selected image
Step 3: Find binary region area from selected image
Step 4: Obtain results from CNN
Step 5: Find the performance parameters of all images
Step 6: Evaluate the results for glaucoma cases
Step 7: Find performance parameters of binary image

4.6 Flow Chart

In this proposed glaucoma detector approach, the experiments were performed to obtain the simulation results MATLABtool 16a based on using CNN classifier. Here, the experimental set up was executed, analysed and tested for CDR value for the images stored in two databases. In this work, we collected few fundus images from different hospitals for testing.

The RGB image is pre-processed and converted to grey scale image with different threshold values. The converted grey scale image is represented by binary values. The binary values of this image region are given to CNNs. The evaluated CDR value of the input image will justify the condition of the glaucoma in the selected image and its severity conditions to identify and prevent the loss of vision. The performance parameters have been evaluated for the fundus images to decide any one of three possible conditions of the glaucoma status. In this proposed work, The CNN classifier achieves an accuracy of approximately 100% and 0.8 CDR.

5 Experiment Simulation Results

Nowadays the diagnosis of patients eye image reports on regular visits which indicate the aggressive nature of the glaucoma disease that helps the doctors to diagnose in stopping the progression of the disease and makes it easy to prevent from permanent vision loss. In every appointment, the patients fundus images stored in a database play key information which can help the ophthalmologist to diagnose with previous investigation reports during next visit. In this work, three linguistic approaches as low, moderate and high were adapted to evaluate the risk level of glaucoma. The execution results are obtained using MATLABR2016a. The results of CNN are obtained using GUI as shown in Fig. 12 and the results of glaucoma detection are shown in Fig. 13. The fundus images are analysed and implemented using MATLAB R16a tool and the system is trained with two sample data sets (medical report-based data and internet source) for the model to understand and familiarize the glaucoma detection. The results of an existing method and the results of proposed method are shown in Figs. 11, 12, 13 and 14.

5.1 Simulation Results of This Work

The simulated results of various probability conditions using GUI were obtained using CNN algorithmic model. In this model, the eye images will be taken from 50 fundus images database and tested the results for two conditions (Normal and abnormal) [6, 7]. The circles are applied to the original image and that image is converted to grey scale, from this it is able to calculate the statistical values and

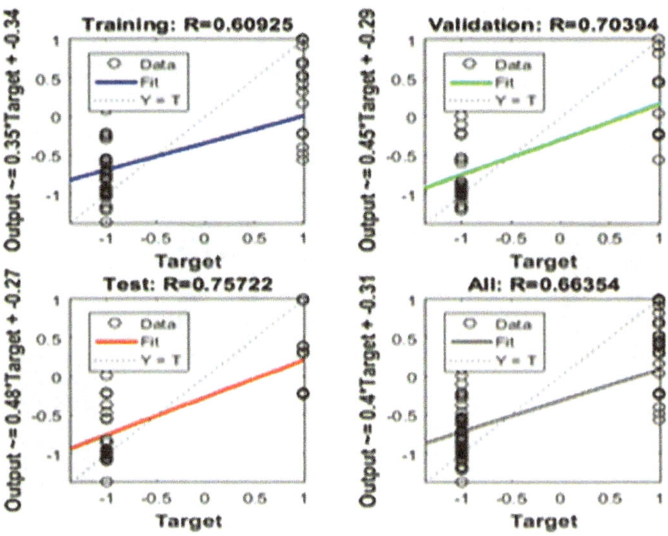

Fig. 11 Training, validation, test/all plots of ANN

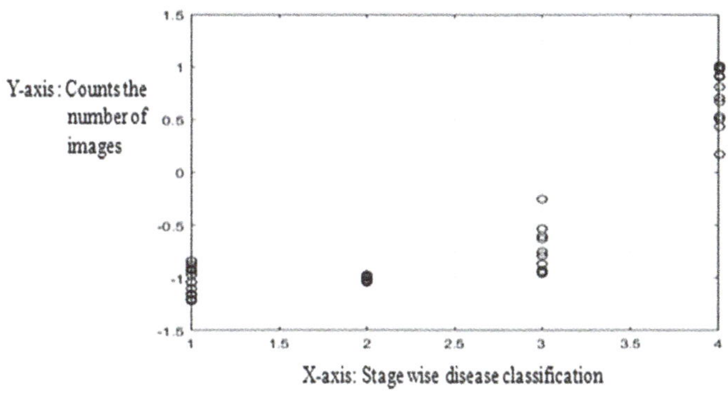

Fig. 12 ANN classification output

CDR values from CNN. From this CNN check the results obtained for the metrics, CDR and accuracy. Image parameters can be taken for all 50 fundus images. By identifying the region of interest (ROI) of the images and evaluating the CUP and DISC area which is identified by applying CNN technique algorithm recursively or by using threshold method. The classification schemes were being analysed using N Bayes and MLP-BP to evaluate the metric accuracy.

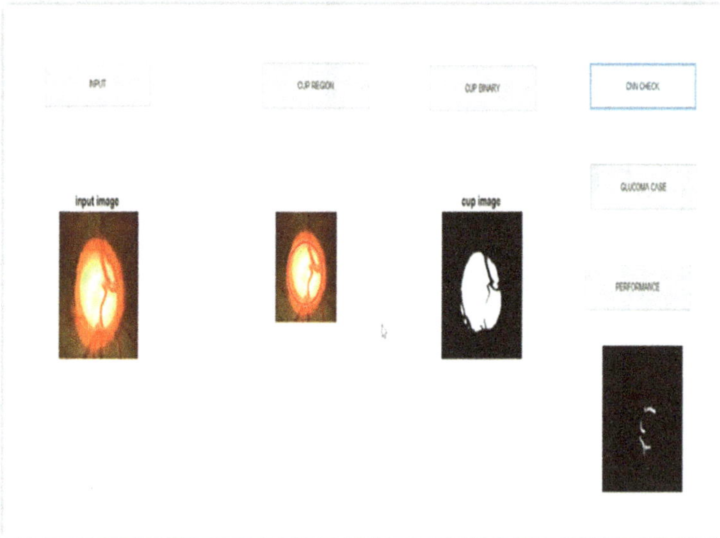

Fig. 13 GUI interfaced simulation results for CNN

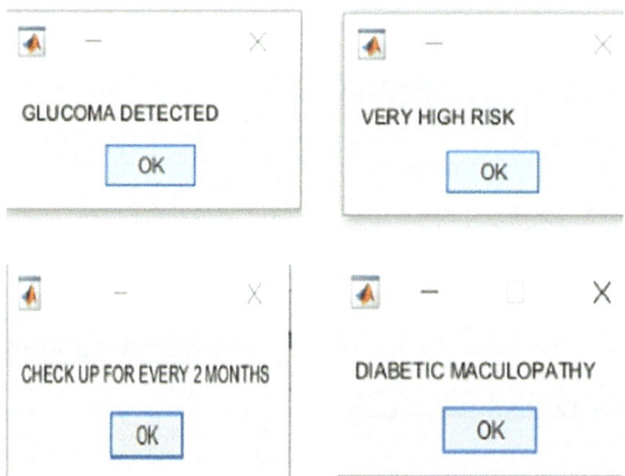

Fig. 14 Results of glaucoma detection process

The experiment setup was setup with GUI which makes the approach to measure the metrics easier and able to add the features in evaluating the CDR value and Accuracy metrics. In this technique, the fundus image from the database has been brought into GUI interface with already assigned required dimensionality to all the images before pre-processing.

5.2 Result of the Proposed Method Using CNN

Required image size and then the cropped image is transformed to gray scale image and classification schemes are used to measure the accuracy and CDR value to differentiate the different stages of the abnormalities.

The above glaucoma case results are obtained based on GUI. In these results, glaucoma detection indicates the loss of vision in the eye situation which is of very high risk and it may lead to blindness. If the small spots or dark strings appear in the retina where the vision develops highly and the objects will appear blur which indicates diabetic maculopathy. Diabetic Maculopathy is a situation that can result from retinopathy and is damage to macula. Macula is a part of an eye that provides central vision. Diabetic maculopathy can be treated by doing laser treatment. The abnormality condition of an eye can be reduced by taking treatment for every two months. Table 3 shows the possible parameter analysis report and compared with the literature survey methods.

In Table 3, the number (No) in column indicates the number of images used in this experiment and the alphabets used in the row highlight various statistical properties that were used in testing the conditions of glaucoma of eye images used from database sets. Here are the abbreviations used for the metric in this simulation experiment to identify the evaluation process for abnormality of glaucoma.

The letters in first row will indicate: the following statistical properties number of images—NO, Contrast—C, Energy—EN, Homogeneity—H, Mean—M, Standard Deviation—SD, Entropy—ET, Variance—V, Smoothness—SN, and Skew-ness—SK. All these are the statistics from GLCM—(Grey Level Co-Occurrence Matrix). GLCM is widely used to measure the joint probability occurrence of specific pixel-pairs. In this work, the proposed method was tested by taking 50–100 fundus images

Table 3 Performance parameters in GUI

NO	C	EN	H	M	SD	ET	V	SN	SK
1	0.124	9503	9959	212	1439	1479	202	9995	6.6532
2	119	9449	9940	221	1469	1530	207	9995	6.5052
3	103	9395	9949	257	1583	1725	241	9996	5.9919
4	91	9348	9954	288	1673	1884	270	9996	5.6337
5	58	9711	9971	116	1072	914	112	9990	9.1134
6	26	9829	9987	72	848	619	69	9985	11.620
7	134	9235	9933	326	1777	2074	301	9997	5.2609
8	124	9436	9938	226	1486	1557	210	9995	6.4276
9	152	9257	0.9924	305	1720	1969	282	9996	5.4606
10	142	9238	9929	320	1760	2043	298	9997	5.3182

Abbreviations: Number of Images—NI, Specificity—SP, Sensitivity—S, Accuracy—A
**All the values in this table are scaled up $*10^{-4}$

Table 4 Measurement of accuracy and CDR

Author	Parameters				
	NI	CDR	SP (%)	S (%)	A (%)
Salam A. A.	100	0.9	87	100	–
P. V. Rao	300	0.7			90
Aruna S.	120	0.6			95
Jangwoo Kim	750	0.88			99
Gayathri R.	300	0.6			89.6
The current work	50, 100	0.8			100

that were collected from different hospitals. In this proposed method two kinds of structural features are used. The two Structural features are CDR and Accuracy.

The performance measures for CDR and Accuracy that is obtained by our proposed method are compared with the other methods to evaluate our proposed work as shown in Table 4. In our proposed work, we achieved the accuracy of approximately 100% and 0.8 CDR. In this work we achieved a better accuracy as compared to above tabulated values.

6 Conclusion and Future Scope

In this proposed work, the main focus is targeted on the study of the simulations results at Glaucoma detection in fundus images of databases using segmentation and filtering using CNN in evaluating the ROI, Optic cup, Optic disc, Accuracy and CDR. The final output is analysed with the structural features like: CDR (Cup to Disc Ratio) and accuracy to identify the progressive rate of glaucoma in the fundus images of the patients. Here structural features CDR and accuracy were being estimated from the extracted ROI of two-dimensional retinal images, and verifying the abnormality of glaucoma images. With the vertical heights of optic cup and optic disc, ROIs were obtained by segmentation; the segmented portions accordingly are applied for CNN and whose results were compared with that of normal retina images. In this work, the author made an attempt with two structural metrics: Accuracy and CDR to detect the abnormality of an eye about its progression of glaucoma which leads to permanent damage of an optic nerve. CNN classifies the image from database to get an accuracy of approximately 100% and 0.8 CDR. As a second part of experiment with simulation results, the statistical parameters were analysed with simulation experiment in order to measure these metric and tabulated and compared for better performance evaluation. This additional information can enrich the accuracy, CDR value and precision in glaucoma detection. This shown work provides the better parameters performance and these design concepts can be promoted to incorporate into the computer-based diagnosis process for ophthalmologist.

6.1 Future Scope

The author shown in depth to adopt three more additional parameters would be taken into consideration into future work to enhance the Glaucoma detection of an eye with various possible databases. In the future, the actual organization might be including RNN to perceive the retinal snapshots as healthful and balanced plus dangerous that consequently may want to assist inside the detection of Glaucoma. The device is additionally made use of such artificial intelligence to categorize the exquisite irregularities of your plenty better eye.

Acknowledgements The authors of this research work deeply express their thanks for providing support of the computational lab-facilities by MIST, DST, R&D-ECE, VBIT, and support by the management of VBIT, JNTUH, Hyderabad, India, during implementation of this work.

References

1. Kim, J., Tran, L., Chew, E.Y., Antani, S.: Optic disc and cup segmentation for glaucoma characterization using deep learning. In: 32nd IEEE International Symposium on Computer Based Medical Systems, pp. 489–494 (2019). https://doi.org/10.1109/CBMS.2019.00100
2. Quellec, G., Charrière, K., Boudi, Y., Cochener, B., Lamard, M.: Deep image mining for diabetic retinopathy screening. In: Medical Image Analysis, vol. 39, pp. 178–193. Elsevier, 1 July 2017. https://doi.org/10.1016/j.media.2017.04.012
3. Patil, N.C., Rao, P.V.: Review on methods designed for automated detection of glaucoma using fundus images. Int. J. Adv. Electr. Comput. Eng. (IJAECE) **4**(1), 29–32 (2017). ISSN(Online): 2349-9338, ISSN(P): 2349-932X
4. Rao, P.V., Gayathri, R., Sunitha, R.: A novel approach for design and analysis of diabetic retinopathy glaucoma detection using cup to disk ration and ANN. In: 2nd International Conference on Nanomaterials and Technologies (CNT 2014). © 2015 Pub-Elsevier Ltd. ISSN: 2211-8128, Procedia Materials Science 10, vol. 4, pp. 446–454 (2015)
5. Bajwa, M.N., Malik, M.I., Siddique, S.A.: Two stage framework for optic disc localization and glaucoma classification in retinal fundus images using deep learning. BMC Med. Inform. Decis. Mak. **19**(136), 1–16 (2019). https://doi.org/10.1186/s12911-019-0842-8
6. Rajendra Acharya, U., Due S., Du X., Kuang, C.: Automated diagnosis of glaucoma using texture and higher spectra features. IEEE Trans. Inf. Technol. Biomed. **15**(3), 449–455 (2011). Print ISSN: 1089-7771
7. Septiarini, A., Khairina, D.M., Kom, M., Awang, H.K.: Automatic glaucoma detection method applying a statistical approach to fundus images. Health Inform. Res. Korean Soc. Med. Inform. **24**(1), 53–60 (2018). https://doi.org/10.4258/hir.2018.24.1.53. PISSN: 2093–3681
8. Chandrashekar, C., Chandrika, J., Ramesh, B.: Comparative study on the detection and classification of glaucoma images. Int. J. Eng. Econ. Manag. **3**(4), 28–32 (2015). ISSN: 2319-7927
9. Gayathri, R., Rao, P.V.: Automated detection of glaucoma system based on wavelet energy features, cup to disc ratio and artificial neural networks. J. Adv. Res. Dyn. Control Syst. **10**(02), 1032–1042 (2018)
10. Li, C.-H., Kuo, B.-C.: A spatial contextual Support vector machine for remotely sensed image classification, IEEE Trans. Geo-sci. Remote Sens. **50**(3), 784–799 (2012). https://doi.org/10.1109/TGRS.2011.2162246. ISSN: 0196-2892

11. Salam, A.A., Khalil, T., Akram, M.U., Jameel, A., Basit, I.: Automated detection of glaucoma using structural and non-structural features. SpringerPlus **5**(1), 1519, 1–21 (2016). https://doi.org/10.1186/s40064-016-3175-4
12. Arumuga Maria Devi, T., Rekha, N.: Hyperspectral image classification using spatial and spectral features. Int. J. Sci. Eng. Res. **4**(7), 1843 (2013). ISSN: 2229-5518
13. Dua, S., Rajendra Acharya, U., Pradeep, C., Vinitha Sree, S.: Wavelet-based energy features for glaucomatous image classification. IEEE Trans. Inf. Technol. Biomed. **16**(1), 80–87 (2012). https://doi.org/10.1109/.2011.2176540. ISSN: 1089-7771
14. Hepsiba, E., Arasi, J.P.: An enhanced automated diagnosis method for glaucoma detection using wavelet. IOSR J. Electron. Commun. Eng. (IOSR-JECE) **9**(3), Ver. VI, 20–22 (2014) e-ISSN: 2278-2834
15. Shen, L.: Three-dimensional gabor wavelets for pixel based hyperspectral imagery classification. IEEE Trans. Geosci. Remote Sens. **49**(12) (2011). ISSN: 0196-2892
16. Gayathri, R., Rao, P.V.: Glaucoma detection using cup to disc ratio and artificial neural networks. Int. J. Eng. Technol. **1**(5), 135–140 (2018)
17. Hanchinal, L.B., Vijapur, N.A., Shrinivasa Rao Kunte, R.: Survey of different techniques for glaucoma detection and approach for glaucoma detection using reconfigurable processor. Int. J. Emerg. Technol. Comput. Sci. Electron. (IJETCSE) **14**(2), 79–83 (2015). ISSN: 0976-1353
18. Khunger, M., Choudhury, T., Sata, S., Ting, K.C.: Automated detection of glaucoma using image processing techniques. In: Emerging Technologies in Data Mining and Information Security. Advances in Intelligent Systems and Computing Book Series (AISC), vol. 814, pp. 323–335. Springer, 02 Sept 2018. https://doi.org/10.1007/978-981-13-1501-5_28
19. Thakur, N., Juneja, M.: Various techniques used for optic disc and optic cup segmentation for glaucoma diagnosis. Int. J. Adv. Res. Comput. Sci. Softw. Eng. **4**(12), 933–936 (2014). ISSN: 2277-128X
20. Mianji, F.A., Zhang, Y.: SVM-based unmixing-to-classification conversion for hyperspectral abundance quantification. IEEE Trans. Geosci. Remote Sens. **49**(11), 4318–4327 (2011). https://doi.org/10.1109/.2011.2166766

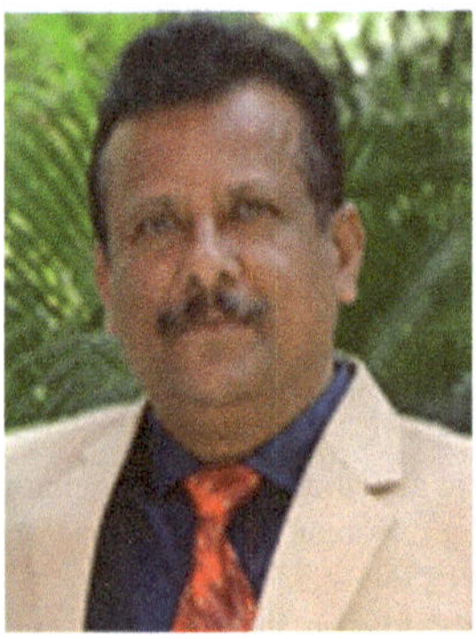

Dr. P. Venkateswara Rao, working as Professor and R&D Coordinator, Dept. of ECE, Vignana Bharathi Inst. Of Technology, Hyderabad. He pursued B.Sc.-Electronics (1986), SV University, AP, B.E.-Electronics Engineering (1991), Marathwada University, Aurangabad-Maharastra, M.E.-Digital Electronics (1999), Karnatak University, and Ph.D. in Low Power VLSI Signal Processing, (2011), DRMGR University, India. His research areas of interest are Low.

Power VLSI, Signal and Biomedical Image Processing, and Nano-Sensors. 3 Research scholars awarded Ph.D. from VTU, and SixResearch scholars from Jain University, Karnataka under his supervision and 3more Research scholars perusing Ph.Ds. He Published total 82 International Journals & Conference papers, executive and life member of professional bodies FIETE, MISTE, ITES and IMAPs. And also Reviewer and Editor for Journals.

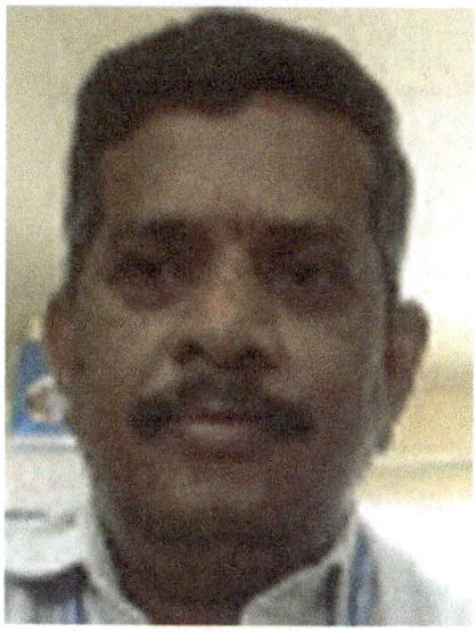

V. Sreepathi, working as Associate Professor, Dept. ECE, Rajarajeswari College of Engineering, Bengaluru, India. He pursued his AMIE-ECE, 1995, IEI, India, ME-Power Electronics in 2000, BangaloreUniversity and he is currently pursuing Ph.D.-Image Processing area, VelTech University, Chennai. He has got 22 years of experience in academic teaching and member of Professional bodies ISTE, IEI (India).

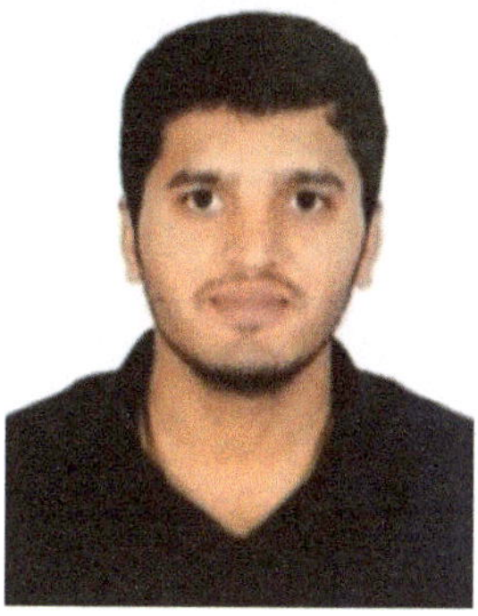

Dr. A. Y. Prasad is working as Assistant Professor, Dept. CSE, A C S College of Engineering, Bengaluru, India. He pursued Ph.D. degree in Computer science Engineering, 2020, M.Tech in CSE-2011, B.E. in CSE-2009, all degrees awarded from Visvesvaraya Technological University, Belagavi. Karnataka, India. His research areas of interest are in the field of wireless sensor networks, data mining, AI and Block chain Technology.

Sparse Approximation Techniques for Efficient Medical Image Representations

Sujoy Datta and Monideepa Roy

Abstract Doctors and researchers in the medical field rely heavily on the availability of accurate images of internal organs of patients for their diagnoses, since they cannot always have a direct view. So the higher the quality of the images, the better will be the accuracy rates of the diagnoses of the doctors. At present there are several techniques like X-rays, CT scans, and MRIs which are available to help a doctor. However as the number of patients increase, one runs into increasingly larger volumes of data and one of the key challenges here is finding an effective scheme for the economic storage for such huge volumes of data, to be used when processing is needed to be done in the future. It has been seen when that type of data is represented in sparse form then it can be encapsulated into a smaller format, but it does not affect the image quality of the recovered image. In this chapter we present a survey and comparison of the various sparse learning algorithms that can be applied for the efficient and lightweight restructuring of medical images.

Keywords Sparse learning · Image compression · Medical image analysis · Computer-aided analysis · Deep learning

1 Introduction

In the earlier days it was difficult for doctors to diagnose a patient or identify ailments of internal organs since they had no way of directly being able to view the inside of the patients. Gradually with the evolution of science, various technologies were developed in the area of medical imagery for enabling the doctors to view within a patient's body. The initial form of medical images was X-rays which were capable of rendering projected 2D images of bones, similar things, etc., inside the body of

S. Datta · M. Roy (✉)
School of Computer Engineering, KIIT Deemed University, Bhubaneswar, Odisha, India
e-mail: monideepafcs@kiit.ac.in

S. Datta
e-mail: sdattafcs@kiit.ac.in

H. K. Tripathy et al. (eds.), *Technical Advancements of Machine Learning in Healthcare*, Studies in Computational Intelligence 936,
https://doi.org/10.1007/978-981-33-4698-7_13

the patient. Although they helped the doctors to a large extent, they did not give a three dimensional image, and a lot of training was needed to study the X-rays to accurately interpret these images and was a complex task. Gradually with the advent of time there were more advanced technologies like MRI (Magnetic Resonance Imaging), CT (Computer Tomography) scans, etc., were developed, which were able to create slices of cross-sectional images of a patient's body. When these slices were assembled together, they gave a fairly accurate view of the overall picture of the internal organs. Also these images were more powerful in the context of revealing anatomical structures, like tumors or arterial blockages, which could not have been possible with X-ray images.

Such medical images are widely used in most clinics, because the diagnosis of the disease and checking its stage of progression first requires an accurate interpretation of the available medical images of patients. But if this is done manually, it is a fairly time consuming process, because it may involve in some cases a large amount of medical images. Therefore, automatic analysis of such medical images can lead to significantly higher diagnostic performance in terms of computational time and space complexity. There are at present several existing techniques like X-rays, CT scans and MRIs which can aid a doctor in making accurate and precise diagnoses. But usually most of the images need to be stored so that further processing or references to it can be made, which generally take up huge amounts of storage space. Therefore it is very crucial to find an efficient way to store the informational content of an image in an economic way, as well as successful lightweight conversions and subsequent reconstruction of the images, without losing out on the quality or precision of the image.

Research in the field of natural image processing has seen a significant progress because of the application of various efficient algorithms in data representation and knowledge extraction. Adaptive sparse coding is one such successful technique which has led to significant development in the way we represent and visualise images, especially medical images. Sparse coding consists of decomposing signals into a few linearly combined elements from a basic dictionary of some basic stimuli to construct images. Sparse image representation is a specific technique for reducing data. So, instead of presenting the information content of the images by the pixels intensity, they are changed with the objective to reduce the numbers of data points to reproduce the identical information. Since this gives rise to images which are significantly lightweight in nature this becomes an useful criteria we are concerned with storage and transmission of a very huge amount of images for various medical purposes. It is crucial to reduce the cardinality of medical data for remote diagnosis and treatments. It has also received a lot of impetus because it has the potential to lead to earlier disease detection, when used along with neural networks and deep learning methodologies can be used for the automatic analysis of such images [1, 2].

The rest of this chapter is organised as follows: Sect. 2 explains the concept of sparse matrices and their advantages ad storage structures, Sect. 3 describes the importance of medical images for a better healthcare system, Sect. 4 gives an introduction of the most commonly used sparse representation techniques, Sect. 5 describe how sparse matrices can help in machine learning, and Sect. 6 discusses the advantages of sparse approximations in medical images, followed by the conclusion in Sect. 7.

2 Defining Sparse Matrices

Matrices are of two main types: *dense* and *sparse*. Sparse matrices are characterised by having a large number of zero values whereas dense matrices have more non-zero values. If the matrices contain mostly zero values then they are called sparse and are distinct from dense matrices which contain values of which most are non zero. A majority of the data or signals that are used in the real world are found to be sparse at least in some transform domain. So signals of images, seismic data and sound are capable of being compressed and stored in terms of their projection by the application of an appropriate model basis. When the selection of a suitable model basis is done, most of the projection coefficients are found to become very small or even zero and can therefore be neglected.

Sparse image representation can therefore be a significant factor in improving and achieving this target. Instead of using the pixels intensity to represent the image informational content, the image is altered with the objective of lessening the number of data points needed to reproduce the equivalent information. Also if deep learning methodologies are used on those images it can facilitate preliminary and automatic analysis of the images without expert intervention [3].

In numerical analysis and scientific computing, we define a sparse matrix or a sparse array as a matrix a majority of its elements are zero. However, the matrix is said to be dense in comparison, when most of the elements contained in it are non-zero. In computer programming, we can define a matrix as a 2-D array. An array containing m columns and n rows represents an m X n matrix. In case there is a situation where a matrix contains a larger number of ZERO values as compared to NON-ZERO values, then that matrix is called a sparse matrix.

If a 2-D array is used to represent a sparse matrix, then a lot of space is wasted in representing that matrix. For example, suppose we have a matrix of size 100×100 which contains only 10 non-zero elements. So in this matrix, only 10 spaces will be occupied by non-zero values while the rest of the spaces of the matrix will be filled with zeros. So essentially, a total of $100 \times 100 \times 2 = 20{,}000$ bytes of space will be needed for storing this integer matrix.

Additionally, when we access theses 10 non-zero elements, around 10,000 scans need to be made. So to simplify this, we take the help of sparse matrix representations.

The representations for Sparse Matrices are done in various ways out of which the two most common are:

- Array representation
- Linked list representation.

0	0	0	0	8	0
0	9	0	0	0	0
2	0	0	4	0	0
0	0	0	0	0	6
0	0	7	0	0	0

Row	Col	Value
5	6	6
0	4	8
1	1	9
2	0	2
2	3	4
3	5	6
4	2	7

Fig. 1 An array representation of a sparse matrix

In the first case an array (Fig. 1) is used to represent a sparse matrix where there are three rows which are as follows:

- Row: the index of the row where the non-zero elements are located
- Column: the index of the column, which contains the location of the non-zero elements
- Value: the value of the non-zero element whose location is at the index—(row, column).

In the second case, a linked list (Fig. 2) is used where each node contains the four following fields:

- Row: the index of the row where the non-zero elements are located
- Column: the index of the column, which contains the location of the non-zero element
- Value: the value of the non-zero element whose location is at the index—(row, column)
- Next node: contains the address of the next node.

3 Importance of Medical Images for a Better Healthcare System

The use of medical imaging has enhanced greatly, the living standards of numerous people worldwide, as well as saving the lives of many others. In the last thirty years, medical imaging has revolutionised the ways in which medical professionals have used them to interpret, diagnose and treat complex ailments and life threatening diseases. So in recent times medical imaging consistently ranks as one of the most

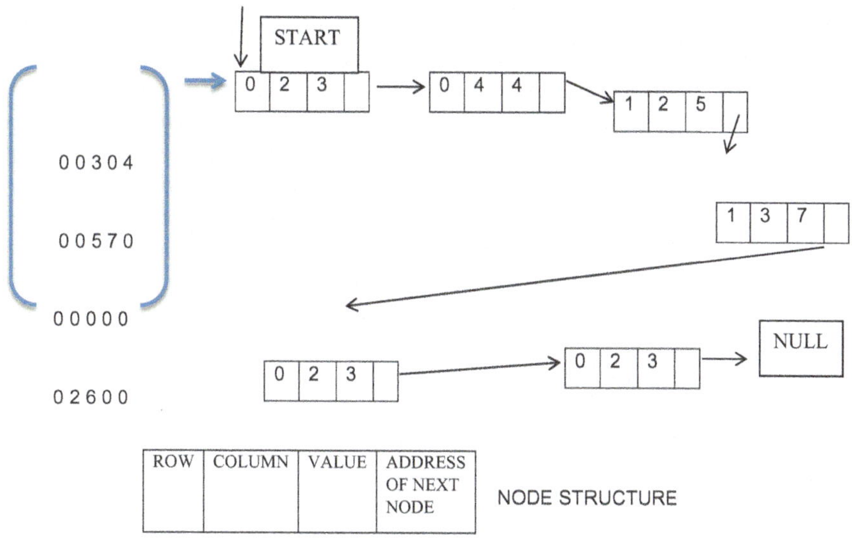

Fig. 2 A linked list representation of a sparse matrix

crucial and important area in the list of the top medical developments for this reason. While diagnosing an illness, doctors usually advice the patients to undergo diagnostic scans such as X-rays, CT scans or an MRI.

Although the basis on which a doctor diagnoses is his medical knowledge, it is vital to confirm his diagnoses with the support of adequate medical imaging. It also assists the doctors in deciding the future course of treatment and care for a patient. It also gives the information about internal problems that a doctor may not be able to detect on external examination. It is also indispensable in tracking an ongoing illness, and to monitor the effectiveness of the treatment and make adjustments if an when required. Medical images give more detailed information about a patient thus enabling them to get more comprehensive care.

The diagnoses that were previously done by invasive exploratory procedures can now be done by tests using non-invasive medical imaging techniques. They have several advantages. Firstly, medical imaging has allowed doctors early detection and a better chance at success by beginning the fight against the disease early. This has directly led to an increase in the life expectancy for individuals. Secondly, contrary to invasive exploratory procedures, the health risks involved in most medical imaging is minuscule. Thirdly, the expenditures involved in invasive medical procedures can be quite high as compared to non-invasive procedures, and allows the patients to return to their normal lives faster. The technology of medical and diagnostic imaging is improving everyday, with the quality of images becoming sharper and clearer. It also leads to more rapid and precise diagnosis, more modified treatment, fewer problems before and after surgery and an augmented understanding of the effect of the treatment on the diseases. Medical imaging also further helps in preventive care.

A mammography can help in the detection of early signs of breast cancer and it has been observed that an increase in the use of mammograms has led to a decrease of almost 30% in the number of deaths due to breast cancer, since 1990.

The kinds of medical imaging that are most frequently used consist of X-rays, CT(computed tomography) scan, MRI(magnetic resonance imaging), ultrasound. CT scans make use of multiple X-rays for the production of cross-sectional layers and are used for viewing images inside the body, like bones, organs, tissues, etc. MRI makes use of magnetic fields and radio waves for displaying images of bones, ligaments and cartilage, etc. Ultrasound (US) uses high-frequency sound waves to produce moving images onto a screen of the inside of the body, including organs, soft tissues, bones and babies in the womb.

MRI is a very useful technique for examining the soft tissues inside the body which have high water content (e.g. muscles, cartilages, nerves) that may not be as nicely visible with other techniques. It is a painless procedure and without the use of radiation. An MRI can be used for examining most parts of the body like: internal organs, brain and spine, blood vessels, bones, heart, etc.

Ultrasound imaging is an extremely important technology for expectant mothers. US technology has made vast advances in the past ten years and the sonogram images now produce a much higher resolution to create finely detailed images. Obstetricians can now get highly improved images of the health and progress of a baby inside the womb, and if there are problems with the pregnancy, then they can be found at an early stage. Ultrasound is also used extensively in other parts of the body which include the soft tissues in the neck, abdomen, pelvis, etc. It can also help in biopsies of soft tissues.

Medical imaging is also used to aid surgeons in conducting surgical procedures. CT scans can provide 3D images of various cross sections of the body, which is of great help when a surgeon is preparing to operate on such areas. They are also used for guiding the doctors through complex and delicate internal operation

4 A Review of the Existing Sparse Representation Techniques

A signal space works in the finite-dimensional, complex inner-product space $C^{d.}$ The signal space contains elements which are usually called signals. For an input signal (also called a target signal), an approximation problem creates the nearest signal which will satisfy some additional constraint. In classical problems, the approximant is often drawn from a subspace or a convex subset. In contrast, sparse approximation problems involve highly nonlinear constraints that are related to the cost of the approximation.

A dictionary for the signal space is a finite collection D of unit-norm elementary signals. The elementary signals in D are usually referred to as atoms.

The existing sparse representation methods can be categorised into four groups, i.e. the greedy strategy approximation, constrained optimisation strategy, proximity algorithm-based optimisation strategy and homotopy algorithm-based sparse representation, with respect to the analytical solution and optimisation viewpoints [7].

Greedy algorithms were used as early as in the 1950s. The basis of this method is to find out the position based on the relationship between the atom and probe sample, and subsequently use the least square to calculate the value of amplitude. The greedy algorithms are capable of always producing the global optimal solution or an approximate overall solution.

To solve the sparse representation problem using the *greedy strategy approximation*, the target is to primarily find a solution to the sparse representation method with l_0-norm minimisation. Since this is an NP-hard problem, using the greedy strategy will provide an approximate solution to take care of the difficulty. This method finds the best optimal solution for each iteration, to obtain the holistic solution. The greedy strategy does not directly solve the optimisation problem and it only tries to find an approximate solution. The greedy strategy approximation chooses the k most appropriate samples, called the *k*-sparsity, to approximate the measurement vector. The algorithms which use this strategy are Matching Pursuit algorithm, Orthogonal Matching Pursuit algorithm and several variations of matching pursuit algorithms.

The constrained optimisation strategy is used to find the solution of sparse representations with the l_1- norm regularisation. The presentation of the methods which deal with the non-differentiable unconstrained problem is done by reformulating them as smooth differentiable constrained optimisation problems.

The *constrained optimisation strategy* transforms a non-differentiable optimisation problem into a differentiable optimisation problem by replacing the l_1—norm minimisation term, (convex but non-smooth), with a differentiable optimisation term, (convex and smooth). So the l_1—norm minimisation term is substituted by the constrained optimisation strategy by an equal constraint condition on the original unconstraint problem. If we reformulate the original unconstraint problem into a differentiable problem with constraints, it becomes a simple problem because l_1—norm minimisation is global non-differentiable. The methods under this category are: Gradient presentation Sparse Representation, Interior point method based Sparse Representation Strategy, Alternating Direct Method (ADM) based Sparse Representation Strategy.

The basic idea behind proximity algorithms is to utilise the proximal operator such that it iteratively solves the sub-problems, which makes it more computationally efficient than the original problem. It is usually used for the solution of non-smooth constrained, convex optimisation problems.

Proximal algorithms are used for solving non-smooth, constrained, large-scale, or distributed versions of the optimisation problem. Here the primary job is to reconstruct the original problem into the specific model of the corresponding proximal operator which are the soft thresholding operator, the hard thresholding operator and the resolvent operator. It then uses the proximity algorithms to address the original sparse optimisation problem. The methods of this type are: Soft Thresholding or Shrinkage operator, Iterative Shrinkage Thresholding Algorithm (ISTA), Fast Iterative Shrinkage Thresholding Algorithm (FISTA), Sparse Reconstruction by Separable Approximation (SpaRSA), Augmented Lagrange Multiplier based Optimisation Strategy, and Other Proximity Algorithm based Optimisation methods.

The concept of homotopy is derived from topology and this method is usually used for addressing a nonlinear system of equations problem. This method was initially developed for solving the least squares problem with the l_1 penalty. The basic logic here was solving the original optimisation problems by the trace of a continuous parameterised path of solutions with variable parameters.

The *homotopy algorithms* use iterations for tracing the final desired solution by beginning from the starting point to the optimal point while the homotopy parameter is successively adjusted. The homotopy algorithm in homotopy algorithm based sparse representation, is utilised for solving the l_1—norm minimisation problem with k-sparse property. The methods under this category are: Lasso Homotopy, Basis Pursuit Denoising (BPDN) Homotopy, Iterative Reweighting l_1—norm Minimisation via Homotopy, and other Homotopy Algorithms for Sparse Representations.

Some methods which are most commonly used are as follows.

One type of a greedy iterative algorithm is the Matching Pursuit (MP) which approximately solves the type of problems listed above. It gradually finds the locations of the non-zeros one by one at a time. The basic objective here is finding stepwise, the column (atom) that best correlates with the current residual initialised to and subsequently updates this residual by taking the new atom and its coefficient into its calculation. It may be possible that the Matching pursuit may be picking the same atom a multiple number of times.

The Orthogonal Matching Pursuit is very similar to the Matching Pursuit, but it has one major difference: at each step of the algorithm, the Least Squares is used to update all the non-zero coefficients. As a result of this change, the residual is orthogonal to the already chosen atoms, thereby ensuring that the same atom is not picked up more than once.

Stage-wise Greedy Methods: There are some variations which improve over the algorithms given above, and these algorithms use the greedy strategy along with two added critical features:

(i) it has the ability to add groups of non-zeros at a time (instead of the previous one non-zero per round); and
(ii) it includes in each round a pruning step where many of the atoms are discarded from the support.

The Basis Pursuit replaces the l_0 norm with an l_1 norm to solve the convex relaxed version of the problem by the replacement of t. However, with this only a new objective is defined, but it leaves the question of what algorithm to be used for getting the desired solution, open [15, 16].

5 Sparsity in Machine Learning

Physicians all over the world are overwhelmed by the huge volumes of medical data they need to classify and diagnose manually everyday, and it takes up a huge part of their working time. If there were computer algorithms in place which could be trained by some similar existing data sets to accurately classify the future data without human intervention, then it would save the physicians a huge amount of time as well as assist them in case of complex or multiple images.

> Machine Learning is an application of artificial intelligence (AI) that provides systems the ability to automatically learn and improve from experience, without being explicitly programmed.

It aims to develop computer programs which are capable of accessing data and thereby using it for learning on their own. This process starts with observation or data, which consist of examples, direct experience or instructions and searches for patterns in the given data and for making better decisions on the data provided by us in the future. So the basic objective here is to make the computers to be learning automatically, in the absence of human intervention or help and adjusting the actions accordingly. These data sets are usually made up of objects in the vector form and are called the raining examples. Other structures like graphs strings, and trees can also be used.

Machine learning algorithms are broadly classified as supervised and unsupervised.

Supervised machine learning algorithms are capable of applying whatever it has learnt previously, by the use of labelled examples on new data, for making future predictions. The learning algorithms start by analysing known training data sets, and produce an inferred function that that is capable of predicting the future values. The system is also capable of providing targets for any new input after adequate training. The learning algorithms are also capable of comparing their outputs with the accurate expected output and finding errors so that the model can be modified if necessary.

Unsupervised machine learning algorithms are generally applied if the information that is used to train is neither classified nor labeled. It studies how a system can infer a function to describe a hidden structure from unlabelled data. It does not find the correct output, but it explores the data to draw inferences from the datasets to describe the hidden structures from the unlabelled data.

Sparse matrices are widely applied in machine learning as they provide several advantages. Sparse models contain fewer features and hence are easier to train on limited data. Fewer features also mean that there is a lesser chance of over fitting. In MRI images sparse models help in faster image acquisition [8] (Table 1).

Since sparse matrices have a lot of values which are zero, special algorithms can be applied for two main reasons:

- *compress the memory footprint of the matrix object is compressed*
- *for speeding up many of the machine learning routines.*

Table 1 The various types of sparse representation algorithms

Type of sparse representation algorithms						
Greedy strategy	Matching pursuit algorithm	Orthogonal matching pursuit algorithm	Series of matching pursuit algorithms			
Constrained optimisation	Gradient projection sparse representation	Interior point method based sparse representation strategy	Alternating direct method (ADM) based sparse representation strategy			
Proximity algorithm based optimisation strategy	Soft thresholding or shrinkage operator	Iterative shrinkage thresholding algorithm (ISTA)	Fast iterative shrinkage thresholding algorithm (FISTA)	Sparse reconstruction by separable approximation (SpaRSA)	Augmented lagrange multiplier based optimisation strategy	Other proximity algorithm based optimisation methods
Homotopy algorithm based sparse representation	Lasso homotopy	Basis pursuit denoising (BPDN) homotopy	Iterative reweighting l_1—norm minimisation via homotopy	Other homotopy algorithms for sparse representations		

Since the storage of all the zero values is a misuse of resources, the application of data compression techniques is done for minimising the amount of data that is needed to be stored. But there are additional advantages also. All the native machine learning algorithms need data matrices to be in memory. Therefore the process of machine learning is disrupted when a data matrix (also known as a data frame) does not fit into the RAM. One of the advantages of the conversion a dense data matrix into a sparse one is that in a lot of cases it is possible to compress it such that it is capable of being fit into the RAM.

In addition, suppose we consider the case of multiplication of a sparse matrix with a dense matrix. In spite of the fact that the sparse matrix contains many zeros, and zero multiplied by anything is always zero, the standard approach nevertheless needs this unnecessary operation to be performed. This results in slowing the processing time. So obviously it is a much more efficient plan to perform operations only on those elements which will return non-zero values. Therefore, any algorithm which utilises some of the basic mathematical computations like multiplication can take advantage of a sparse matrix implementation.

So the application of sparse representation for machine learning is now being explored widely for enabling the process of automatic classifications and analysis of medical images. This will make the process of classification much faster and accurate and without human intervention [8–10].

6 Advantages of Sparse Representation in Medical Images

Sparse image representation refers to the process of using some particular techniques for the reduction of data. Instead of representing informational content of the image with the help of the intensity of the pixels, the image is transformed with the objective of lessening the number of data points needed to reproduce the equivalent information. The lessening of the cardinality of the medical data is very important for diagnosis and treatments done remotely. So applying sparse representation techniques in the area of medical imaging shows a lot of promise because it has the potential to lead to the advantage to detect diseases earlier by the use of neural networks and deep learning methodologies for the automatic analysis of X-rays, MRIs, CTs, US, etc., which are the most commonly used techniques for medical images analysis [4].

Sparse approximation problems are defined by two characteristics:

1. A linear combination of elementary signals is approximated to obtain an input signal. In a large number of modern applications, the elementary signals can be drawn from a large, linearly dependent collection.
2. The imposition for a preference for "sparse" linear combinations is done by penalising the non-zero coefficients. The most common penalty is the number of elementary signals that are participating in the approximation.

The problem domain must justify the linear model, the choice of elementary signals, and the sparsity criterion.

CT scans and MRI were developed to generate cross-sectional images of slices of the human body. These slices can then be assembled together to get the complete picture for diagnosis. CT and MRI function on two different types of principles. CT scanners generate images by "shooting X-rays through a patient from all angles and interpolating between the resulting projections to obtain a cross-sectional image".

MRI works by "subjecting a patient's body to varying (gradient) magnetic fields in order to force protons within the subject to process magnetically different frequencies depending on their position. These processing protons will induce a signal through a receiver coil, which can be interpreted to generate an image" [11, 12].

Although the scientific principles of these two technologies are different, they have one significant mathematical property: both of them obtain an image by the measurement of its Fourier spectrum. Because of the spatial limitation of an image, an imaging machine is needed for the sampling of the frequencies in Fourier space which is at a higher rate than the Nyqvist rate, i.e. the minimum sampling rate which is supposed to guarantee that there are no aliasing effects. Therefore if we assume that it is feasible to sample at the Nyqvist rate, then reconstructing the image by utilising an inverse Fast Fourier Transfer (IFFT) is a trivial matter. Unfortunately, it is not always very practicable to obtain all these samples as CT scanners and MRI [14] devices tend to be slow, loud, claustrophobic, and in general not comfortable for the patients. Therefore, the medical community is trying to search for other options to obtain high quality medical images that utilise the fewest Fourier Transform coefficients that are possible. Fortunately, the images used by user were found to exhibit the property of being sparse in gradient. So basically, the images are consisting of large, nearly constant-valued regions which are separated by edge-discontinuities. So it is these redundancies in these images that offer a possible dimensionality reduction that should allow for Fourier sampling at sub-Nyqvist rates. Figure 3 below, shows the example of a sparse gradient image along with an image of its edges.

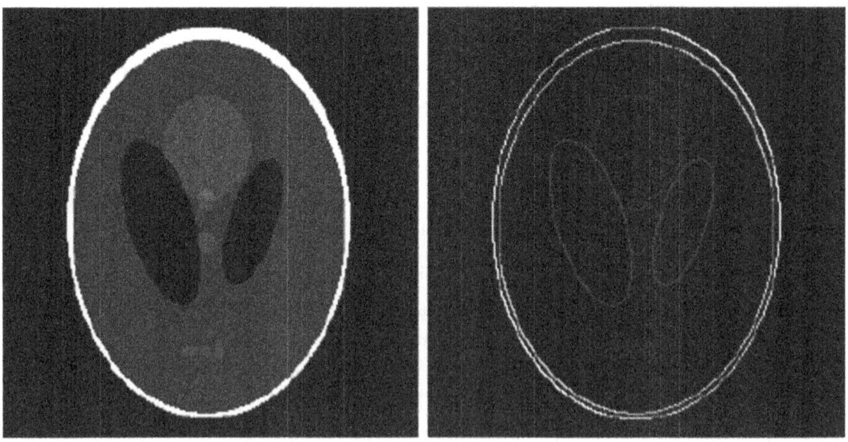

Fig. 3 The famous Shepp-Logan phantom image: a classical example of a sparse gradient image

When a sparse representation is found by using a large dictionary and greedy algorithms, it provides high quality approximations of X-Ray images. The resulting framework was proved to produce approximations that were much more sparser as compared to the ones that arose from the traditional transformations like the Cosine and Wavelet Transforms. However, if the approximations are to be useful in the areas of automatic and remote healthcare systems and reporting, we need to make sure that the high sparsity levels that were achieved do not get affected, when we save the reduced data in a small file [5, 6].

Although normally X-Ray images are found to be sparser if the approximation is performed in the wavelet domain, sometimes the approximations in the pixel intensity domain can be required for the purposes of analysis.

In the course of acquisition of medical ultrasound images [13] they quite often get corrupted by the noise, which is known as speckle. The removal of speckle noise is a very crucial step in the processing of medical ultrasound images. Because of this ill-posed feature of image denoising, there are quite a few regularisation methods that have been used effectively. The sparse dictionary learning and regularisation methods can collaborate for removing the speckle noise. An efficient dictionary learning algorithm is used by the method to train a redundant dictionary, and it is subsequently used in an image prior regularisation model for the recovery of the obtained image.

7 Conclusion

In this chapter we have seen that medical images play a vital role in assisting doctors for various purposes, like making accurate diagnoses, to devise future forms of treatment for a patient, progress of disease. etc. The accuracy of these images is crucial in delivering more accurate diagnoses. However creating accurate and high resolution images usually mean higher volume of data size and it can lead to a strain on the storage resources. Therefore storing them for long-term retrieval and consultation becomes infeasible unless there are more economic ways to store them. Moreover, sometimes remote monitoring or analysis of these images may be needed for a faster diagnosis. In such cases transferring files of large volumes becomes unviable over networks. It has been shown that if a sparse representation of that type of data is encapsulated in a small file it does affect the quality of the image that is recovered. In addition, when there are huge volumes of data to be classified or tested manually, it can become very time consuming. If sparse representation of medical images is applied in machine learning algorithms, it can help in making the training data lightweight as well as making the classification process much faster. So in this chapter we have presented some of the various sparse learning algorithms that can be applied for the efficient and lightweight restructuring of medical images and how sparse representation can help in creating a more efficient healthcare system. They can also be used for machine learning algorithms to make the classification and analysis of medical images automatically and faster, in the absence of human intervention.

References

1. Candes, E.J., Romberg, J., Tao, T.: Robust uncertainty principles: exact signal reconstruction from highly incomplete frequency information. Submitted (2004)
2. Candes, E.J., Romberg, J., Tao, T.: Stable signal recovery from incomplete and inaccurate measurements. Comm. Pure Appl. Math. **59**, 1207–1223 (2006)
3. Donoho, D.L., Tsiang, Y., Drori, I., Starck, J.: Sparse solution of underdetermined linear equations by stagewise orthogonal matching pursuit (2006)
4. Maleh, R., Gilbert, A.C., Strauss, M.J.: Sparse gradient image reconstruction done faster. ICIP Proc. (2007)
5. Mallat, S.: A wavelet tour of signal processing, 2nd edn. Academic Press (1999). Maggioni, M., Katkovnik, V., Egiazarian, K., Foi, A.: Nonlocal transform-domain filter for volumetric data denoising and reconstruction. IEEE Trans Image Proc. **22**(1), 119–133 (2013)
6. Fang, L., Li, S., McNabb, R.P., Nie, Q., Kuo, A.N., Toth, C.A., Izatt, J.A., Farsiu, S.: Fast acquisition and reconstruction of optical coherence tomography images via sparse representation. IEEE Trans. Med. Imaging **32**, 2034–2049 (2013)
7. Fang, L., Li, S., Nie, Q., Izatt, J.A., Toth, C.A., Farsiu, S.: Sparsity based denoising of spectral domain optical coherence tomography images. Biomed. Opt. Express **3**, 927–942 (2012)
8. Wright, J., Ma, Y., Mairal, J., Sapiro, G., Huang, T.S., Yan, S.: Sparse representation for computer vision and pattern recognition. Proc. IEEE **98**(6), 1031–1044 (2010)
9. Barchiesi, D., Plumbley, M.D.: Learning incoherent dictionaries for sparse approximation using iterative projections and rotations. IEEE Trans. Signal Process. **61**(8), 2055–2065 (2013)
10. Cheng, J., Zhang, Z., Tao, D., Wong, D.W.K., Liu, J., Baskaran, M., Aung, T., Wong, T.Y.: Similarity regularized sparse group lasso for cup to disc ratio computation. Biomed. Opt. Express **8**(8), 3763–3777 (2017)
11. Xu, Y., Duan, L., Wong, D.W.K., Wong, T.Y., Liu, J.: Semantic reconstruction-based nuclear cataract grading from slit-lamp lens images. Med. Image Comput. Comput.-Assist. Interv., 458–466 (2016)
12. Yousufi, M., Amir, M., Javed, U., Tayyib, M., Abdullah, S.: Ultrasound compressive sensing using BCS-FOCUSS. In: Proceedings of the IEEE 4th International Conference on Computer and Communications (ICCC), pp. 174–178, Chengdu, China (2018)
13. Kim, J.H., Basarab, A., Hill, P.R., Bull, D.R., Kouame, D., Achim, A.: Ultrasound image reconstruction from compressed measurements using approximate message passing. In: Proceedings of the 24th European Signal Processing Conference, Budapest, Hungary, September (2016)
14. Boydev, C., Demol, B., Pasquier, D., Saint-Jalmes, H., Delpon, G., Reynaert, N.: Zero echo time MRI-only treatment planning for radiation therapy of brain tumors after resection. Physica Med.: Eur. J. Med. Phys. **42**, 332–338 (2017)
15. Bora, A., Jalal, A., Price, E., Dimakis, A.G.: Compressed sensing using generative models. arXiv preprint arXiv:1703.03208 (2017). Finn, C., Abbeel, P., Levine, S.: Model-agnostic metalearning for fast adaptation of deep networks. arXiv preprint arXiv:1703.03400 (2017)
16. Dhar, M., Grover, A., and Ermon, S.: Modeling sparse deviations for compressed sensing using generative models. In: International Conference on Machine Learning, pp. 1222–1231 (2018)

Optimal Analysis of Brain MRI Using Bio-Inspired Computing Techniques

Lambodar Jena, Saumendra Kumar Mohapatra, and Mihir Narayan Mohanty

Abstract Modern world demands intelligent devices and intelligent techniques in different platforms. The area of health care units uses such techniques to improve the analysis and diagnosis of diseases accurately. This chapter provides the insights to bio-inspired intelligent techniques for current and future research. The chapter is verified with biomedical images. The application of fuzzy logic provides the brain magnetic resonance imaging (MRI) detection and segmentation. Further the bio-inspired optimization technique, ant colony optimization (ACO) technique, is considered to optimize the fuzzy techniques for enhancing the performance. The chapter also investigates the state-of-art related to this work. The obtained results by application of the proposed technique found excellent in terms of noise reduction, accuracy as compared to earlier results. The result section exhibits each of the parameters to meet the challenges of current problem.

Keywords Biomedical image processing · Brain MRI · Fuzzy clustering · Bio-inspired algorithms · PSO · Clustering · ANN

1 Introduction

Segmentation of image is one of the essential image preprocessing step in computer vision research. The object and background in an image is separated by applying different image segmentation techniques. There are many applications of image

L. Jena · S. K. Mohapatra
Department of Computer Science and Engineering, ITER, Siksha 'O' Anusandhan (Deemed to be University), Bhubaneswar, India
e-mail: jlambodar@gmail.com

S. K. Mohapatra
e-mail: saumendramohapatra@soa.ac.in

M. N. Mohanty (✉)
Department of Electronics and Communication Engineering, ITER, Siksha 'O' Anusandhan (Deemed to be University), Bhubaneswar, India
e-mail: connectmihir68@gmail.com

H. K. Tripathy et al. (eds.), *Technical Advancements of Machine Learning in Healthcare*, Studies in Computational Intelligence 936,
https://doi.org/10.1007/978-981-33-4698-7_14

segmentation in computer vision such as locating the objects in a satellite image, recognition of finger print and face, medical image analysis, agriculture image analysis, etc. Accuracy in image segmentation has a big impact in successive image processing. Though several researchers are working on image segmentation for several years, still it is a open research area due to different characteristics of images [1, 2].

In segmentation an image is distinguished to many sections or pixel sets. These partitions include different objects of the image having same color and texture. In a particular region all these pixels are same with respect to the characteristics or different possessions such as texture, intensity, or color of the image. The main challenging stage in interpreting an image is dividing the image into background and image. In segmentation an image is subdivided into its ingredient regions or objects. It can also be defined as the process of partitioning one image into set of non-overlapping regions. In Fig. 1 the difference between original and segmented image is displayed [3–5].

There are some rules for image segmentation. These are:

- The separations need to be uniform and standardized with respect to some properties.
- Neighboring regions should have considerably dissimilar values with respect to the properties on which they are standardized.
- Every segment should have easy boundaries, and accurately separated from each other.

Segmentation isolates a picture to its segment sections. The level at which the detachment is conveyed relies upon the issue being explained. Segmentation calculations for images commonly dependent on the intermittence and likeness of the intensity values of the respective image. The discontinuity approach of image segmentation separates an image dependent on unexpected changes in power and similitude depends on apportioning an image into districts that are comparative as indicated by

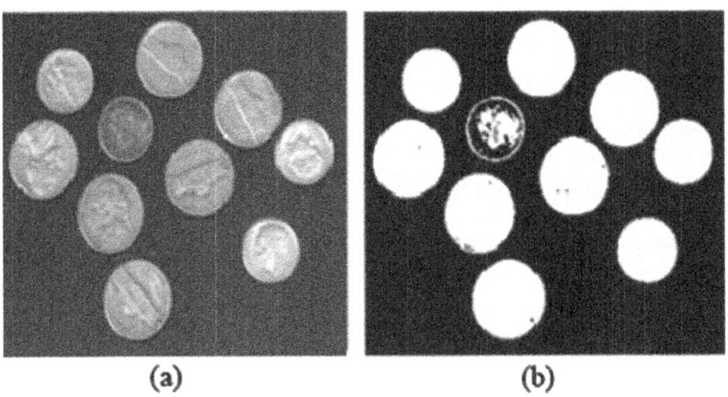

Fig. 1 Original image (**a**) and segmented image (**b**)

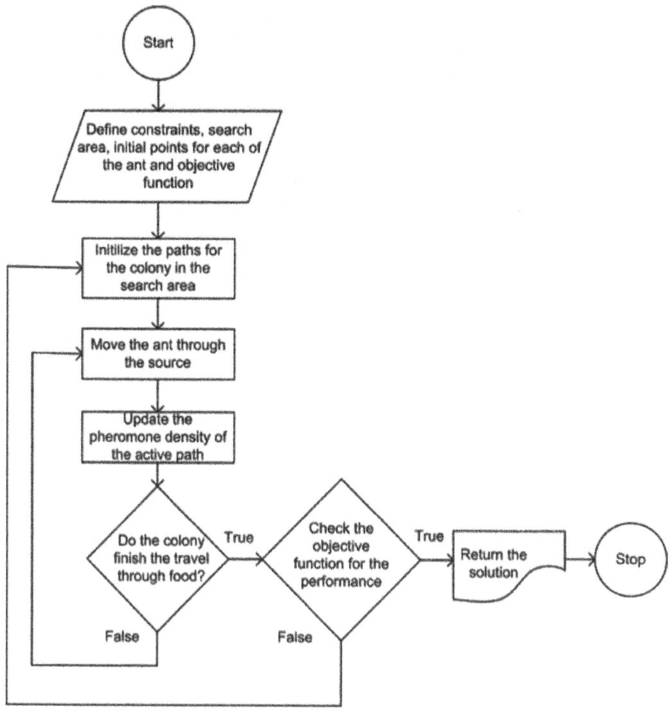

Fig. 2 Flowchart of ACO technique

a lot of predefined criteria. In this manner the decision of picture division strategy relies upon the issue being considered [6].

Distinguishing explicit organs or different highlights in biomedical images requires a lot of skill concerning the shapes and areas of anatomical features. Such division is normally performed physically by expert doctors as a major aspect of treatment arranging and finding [7]. Because of the expanding amount of accessible data and the intricacy of highlights of intrigue, it is getting important to create computerized image segmentation strategies to help and accelerate the diagnosis process [8, 9].

In this chapter, the image segmentation is done by applying fuzzing c-means clustering technique by modifying its objective function by genetic algorithm approach. The proposed model minimizes the objective function more effectively as compared to the conventional FCM, and it provides a better quality of image segmentation. Then the segmented image is smoothened with a Gaussian filter which reduces the noise occurred through the segmentation process. Then the neural network has been evaluated for measures like performance, training state and error histogram. We have considered a bio-medical image preferably an MRI image by using MATLAB software.

Fig. 3 ACO algorithm

procedure $ACO(\pi')$
  input: *problem instance* $\pi' \in \Pi'$
  output: *solution* $\hat{s} \in S'(\pi')$ **or** $\emptyset$

  $sp := \{\emptyset\}$;
  $\hat{s} := \emptyset$;
  $f(\hat{s}) := \infty$;
  $\tau := initTrails(\pi')$;
  while not $terminate(\pi', sp)$ **do**
    $sp := construct(\pi', \tau, h)$;
    $sp' := localSearch(\pi', sp)$;
    if $f(best(\pi', sp')) < f(\hat{s})$ **then**
      $\hat{s} = best(\pi', sp')$;
    end
    $\tau := updateTrails(\pi', sp', \tau)$;
  end
  if $\hat{s} \in S'$ **then**
    return $\hat{s}$
  else
    return $\emptyset$
  end
end *ACO*

2 State of Art

In the previous two decades numerous techniques were created to remove the shape of homogeneous locales inside digitalized images. A few algorithms were introduced to separate the form of similar regions inside computerized images. A great deal of consideration is engaged to edge recognition calculations. Traditionally, the main phase of edge identification is the assessment of subsidiaries of the image intensity. The regularization procedures such as smoothing channel and surface fitting were utilized to make separation progressively invulnerable to noise.

In [10], authors have been calculated the performance of the Prewitt edge finder for noisy image and exhibited that the Prewitt edge identifier works very well for noisy images. The segmentation was done by using Gaussian preconvolution method in [11]. The main reason behind adopting this filter was that, the traditional Gaussian smoothing filters are capable of removing the important high frequency features from the original image. It also emphasizes on the components with high frequency in a digital image. Due to these reasons, it performs poorly in case of low SNR images. A great deal of the consideration is engaged to edge identification, being a vital part

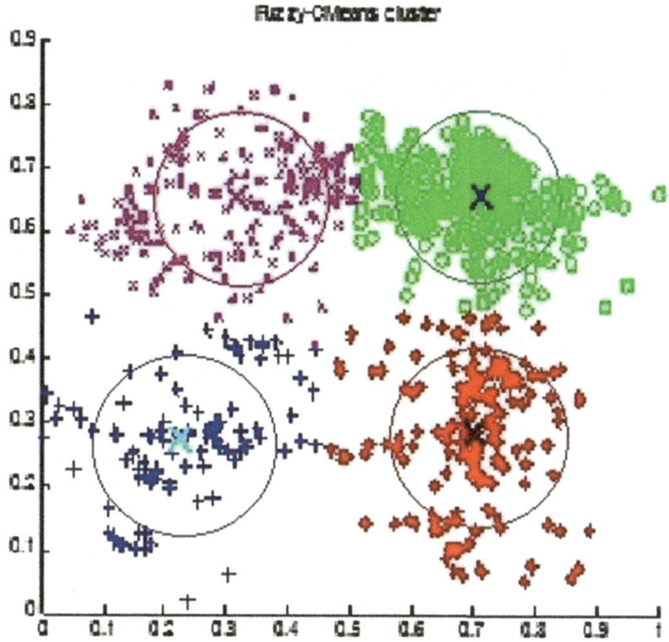

Fig. 4 Fuzzy optimized clusters

in a large portion of the algorithms. Traditionally, the primary phase of edge recognition is the assessment of subsidiaries of the image intensity. Smoothing filter and surface fitting were taken as regularization procedures to make separation increasingly resistant to noise. Authors in [12] have proposed Gaussian preconvolution for segmentation purpose. Be that as it may additionally evacuate real high recurrence edge features, corrupt restriction and debase the location of low differentiate edges during smoothing out the commotion. The old style operators underline the high frequency segments in the picture and along these lines demonstration ineffectively in instances of moderate low SNR or potentially low spatial goals of the imaging gadget. This attention has led to new methodologies in which adjusted exchange offs are looked for between clamor concealment, picture deblurring and the capacity to determine meddling edges, inside and out bringing about administrators acting like band-pass channels for example Vigilant [13]. The comparison of these techniques was presented in the result section. In [14], authors have displayed an assessment of edge locator execution utilizing a structure from movement task. It is found that Canny indicator had the best test execution and the best vigor in union and is one of the quicker executing identifiers. It plays out the best for the undertaking of structure from movement. The original image was segmented into two orthogonal orientations and local maxima were extracted from the section curve in [11]. From their work it can be observed that their proposed model can provide better performance for detecting the edge and improving the noise intensity. A new mathematically morphological algorithm was proposed for detecting the lungs from the CT scan image in [15]. They have shown that their approach is more effective for biomedical image denoising and edge detection as compared to the traditional methods. For detecting the edges from the MRI image authors in [16] applied one of the most popular bio-inspired optimization techniques in their work. They have used ant colony optimization (ACO) for detection of the edges. In ACO based edge detection model, a matrix pheromone was created which displays the information available on the edge pixel location. It is created by analyzing the movements of number of ants in the original image. Further the ant movement was created by applying the local fluctuations of image intensity value. In their work, they have used neural network with momentum for improving ACO based edge detection. Results have shown that by using neural network they were getting very effective results in edge detection based on ACO. Another novel edge detection technique was taken by the authors for detecting the lungs in a CT image having salt-and-pepper noise [17]. They have also compared their obtained result with some earlier works and it was observed that their model is performing more effectively as compared to other traditional algorithms used in image segmentation. A novel boundary edge detector algorithm was proposed by the authors in [18]. They have considered four boundary detector algorithms such as Sobel, Prewitt, Roberts and Canny in their work and Canny method is providing better result as compared to other three methods. An ACE-net model was developed for enhancing the effective features for utilizing in the contracting and expansive paths [19]. Particularly they have proposed ASSP, dense connection and deep supervision mechanisms method for connecting directly to the expansive site of the raw image. The features were considered from multiple sources like scale and reception fields.

Image reconstruction is an exceptionally helpful technique given by numerical morphology. The reproduction change is generally notable in the twofold case, where it just concentrates the associated segments of a picture which are "set apart" by another picture [20]. In [21], the work has three significant objectives: firstly it gives a proper meaning of gray scale reproduction in the discrete case. Two comparable definitions are proposed:

First depends on the limit superposition rule and the subsequent one depends on dark scale geodesic enlargements. Second piece of the work outlines the utilization of paired and particularly dark scale reproduction in picture examination applications: models demonstrating the enthusiasm of dim scale remaking for such undertakings as picture sifting, outrageous vaults and bowls extraction in dim scale pictures, "top-cap" by recreation, double and dim scale division, and so on., are talked about.

3 Proposed Method

Clustering is a procedure for grouping the patterns or objects so that the samples inside a class are more like each other than tests having a place with different classes. As a rule, a clustering procedure can be ordered as either a one-shot parcel or a various leveled segment. One-shot segment clustering technique can be known as a worldwide segment process that produces an ideal parcel in one stage to finish design arrangement, while a progressive segment grouping strategy can be alluded to as a neighborhood segment process that disintegrates a segment method into various stages with the goal that the two most comparable groups are blended locally in one phase [22]. At that point, all privately consolidated bunches in various stages are progressively sorted out into a settled arrangement of gatherings. There have been numerous applications dependent on bunching ideal models, a portion of these applications incorporate picture division, discourse acknowledgment, and information pressure. Many clustering methodologies have likewise been utilized, for example, the strict (hard) clustering calculation and the delicate (fuzzy) clustering calculation, every one of which has its own uncommon qualities. For instance, the issue with the hard clustering calculation, c-means clustering is that it will make the target work combine into a neighborhood least. Instead of doling out an example to one and only one class, the fuzzy-clustering technique allots the example with a number n somewhere in the range of zero and one portrayed as an enrollment work. The fuzzy set hypothesis has been used in an assortment of areas, for example, biomedical image analysis. Hypothesis of fuzzy logic gives a mathematical model to catch the vulnerabilities related with human cognizance forms [23–25].

Originally Dunn has introduced the fuzzy c-means clustering algorithm and earlier it was formulated by [26]. A fluffy c-segment of X is one which portrays the enrollment of each example point in all the groups by a participation work which goes somewhere in the range of zero and one. Moreover, the entirety of the participations for each example point must be solidarity.

Let $X = \{x_1, x_2, \ldots, x_N\}$ be an example of N perceptions in D^n (n-dimensional Euclidean space); x_k is the k-th include vector; y_k is the jth highlight of y_k. In the event that C is a whole number, $2 \le c < n$, a customary (or "hard") c-segment of X is a c-tuple $(x_1, x_2, \ldots, x_C)$ of subsets of X that fulfills three conditions:

$$x_j \neq \phi, \le j \le c; \tag{1}$$

$$x_j \cap x_j \neq \phi; \; i \neq i \tag{2}$$

$$\bigcup_{j=1}^{c} X_i = x \tag{3}$$

where ϕ is the empty set, and $(\cup, \cap)$.

The FCM calculations are better portrayed by revaluating conditions (condition 1) in terms of matrix theoretic. Toward the end, consider U be a genuine $c \times N$ matrix, $U = [u_{ik}]$. U is the network portrayal of the parcel $\{y_j\}$ in condition (1) in the circumstance.

$$u_i(x_k) = u_{ik}\{1; x \in x \tag{4}$$

$$0;\ \text{otherwise}\} \tag{5}$$

$$\sum_{i=1}^{N} u_{ik} > 0 \quad \text{for all } i; \tag{6}$$

$$\sum_{i=1}^{N} u_{ik} = 1 \quad \text{for all } K \tag{7}$$

Summing up this thought, we allude to U as a fluffy c-parcel of X when the components of U are numbers in the unit interim [0, 1] that keep on fulfilling the two conditions (2b) and (2c). The reason for this definition is c functions $u_i : X \rightarrow [0,\ 1]$ whose values $u_i(x_k) \in [0,\ 1]$ are deciphered as the evaluations of enrollment of the x_k s in the "fluffy subsets" u_i of X.

Appropriately, the fuzzy-set, and, thus, fuzzy parcel, were presented as methods for adjusting the fundamental sayings hidden bunching and order models with the point of accommodating this need. By this gadget, a point y_k may have a place completely with a solitary group, however as a rule, can appreciate incomplete enrollment in a few fluffy bunches. We indicate the arrangements of all hard and fluffy c partitions of X by:

$$Mc = \{U_{C\times N} | u_{ik} \in [0,\ 1] \tag{8}$$

$$Mfc = \{U_{C\times N} | u_{ik} \in [0,\ 1] \tag{9}$$

A few clustering techniques have been proposed for recognizing optimized fuzzy c-parcels in X. Among them, the most famous and well-considered technique is related with the summed up least-squared error utilitarian.

$$h_m(V, u) = \sum_{i=1}^{N} \sum_{j=1}^{c} \left(u_{ji}\right)^{w} \|x_{i^-} \cdot V_j\|_A^2 \tag{10}$$

where,

$x = \{x_1,\ x_2, \ldots, x_n\} \subset R^n$ = the data,
c = total amount clusters in X; $2 \leq c < n$,
w = weight parameters; $1 \leq w < \infty$,
V = fuzzy partition of X; $V \in M_{fc}$,
$U = (u_1,\ u_2, \ldots, u)$ = vectors of centers,
A = weight matrix (5 h).

The weight appended to each squared error is $\left(v_{jk}\right)^{w}$, the mth intensity of $x_j s$ s participation in group I. The vectors $\{v_i\}$ in condition (5f) are seen as "bunch focuses" or focuses of mass of the apportioning subsets. On the off chance that $w =$ 1, it very well may be indicated that i_w limits just at hard V's $\in Wc$, and comparing

x_i s are only the geometric centroid of the Iris. By considering these perceptions, we can break down its fundamental components to perceive what property of the focuses $\{x_j\}$ it measures:

d_{ij}^2 = squared distance from point x_j to centre of mass v_i.

$(u_{ij})^w d_{ij}^2$ = squared_error earned by representing x_i by v_i weighted parameters.

Weighting type m controls the relative loads set on each of the squared_errors d_{ij}^2. As $w \to 1$ from prior conversation parcels that limit i_w become progressively hard (and, as referenced previously, at $w = 1$, are essentially hard) [27]. Alternately, every section of ideal for $J|_w$ approaches $(1/c)$ as $w \to 1$. Subsequently, expanding m will in general corrupt participation toward the fuzziest state. Optimized fuzzy clustering for X is defined as the pair of $\hat{V}, \hat{u}$, which minimizes the i_m. The basic required condition for weight $w = 1$ is known. For $w > 1$, if $x_j \neq \hat{u}_J$ for all i and j, $\left(\hat{V}, \hat{u}\right)$ may be locally optimal for I_m only if

$$\hat{u}_i = \sum_{i=1}^{N} (\hat{u}_{ij})^w x_i v \sum_{i=1}^{N} (\hat{u}_{ij})^w;\ 1 \le i \le C; \tag{11}$$

$$\hat{u}_{ij} = \left(\sum_{j=1}^{C} \left(\frac{\hat{d}_i i}{\hat{d} ji} \right)^{2v(w-1)} \right)^{-1};\ l \le k \le N;\ l \le j \le c \tag{12}$$

3.1 Ant Colony Optimization

Depending upon the technique followed by the ants to reach their nest from food using shortest way, the Ant Colony Optimization (ACO) is developed. The way in which ants solve most of their problems is an important point of research for long time. Even the ants are known to be blind they are capable of finding the shortest path from food to nest is also another point which attracts most of the biologist to study this activity. A volatile item named pheromones is used by the ants to mark their path from the nest to the location of food. They use this technique so that at the time of returning after getting the food they can easily reach back at the nest. These substances are traced by the ants through their receiver antenna present on their head. The pheromones dropped by an ant is also traced by other ants to follow the path to food. If on the route an ant finds two paths with pheromones they select the path with more concentrated pheromones. Since the longer path will take more time in comparison to the shorter one the majority of the ants will follow the shorter path after some time [28–30]. The steps followed in ACO are as follows:

1. To point out the optimization problem a group with certain number of ants are selected. In the optimization problem a pool of ants is defined with a decision

variable which consists of some required values that can be taken. Each ant is assigned to a decision variable.
Estimate preliminary pheromone quantity (τ_0) as $\tau_0 = 1/Z_{\min}$, where $Z_{\min}$ is the least value of the objective function without any penalty violation. For every decision variable pheromone and visibility parameters are calculated by:

$$\tau_{ij} = 1/\tau_0,\ v_{ij} = 1/x_{ij}, i = 1, 2, \ldots, nv \quad j = 1, 2, \ldots, n_{\text{pool}} \tag{13}$$

where.
x_{ij} = Design variable value.
n_v = Design variables used for optimization purpose.
n_{pool} = Values in the pool.

2. A design variable is selected by each ant in the colony. Then specific values are selected by the ants for their decision variable from the pool. These collections are done with the help of a decision mechanism that is liable on probability computation and it can be derived as follows:

$$P_{ij}(t) = \left(\tau_{ij}(t)\right)^{\alpha}.\left(v_{ij}\right)^{\beta} / \sum_{j \in \text{allowed}}^{n_{\text{div}}} \left(\tau_{ij}(t)\right)^{\alpha}.\left(v_{ij}\right)^{\beta}$$
$$i = 1, 2, \ldots, nv \quad j = 1, 2, \ldots, n_{\text{pool}} \tag{14}$$

   where $P_{ij}(t)$ jth is the pool value probability.
   i = decision variable.
   t = time.
   α and β are constraints which are considered for influencing the local trail values and visibility.
   This procedure carries on until all ants consigned values for their first design variables.

3. At the end of each tour a local update rule is applied. The amount of pheromone for values selected by each ant from the given pool is decreased so that it will promote examination in the process of searching the best path. Then the pheromones are evaporated because of their volatile nature. The mathematical term for this is given by:

$$\tau_{ij}(t) = \zeta \cdot \tau_{ij}(t) \tag{15}$$

   where ζ is the local-update coefficient with its value ranges from 0 to 1.
   If this parameter is selected very close to 1, then there occurs a fast convergence which results to the end of the process to the local optimum. If the value of ζ is chosen very close to 0 then a problem arises in converges faster to that of 1.

4. In the next step a value is assigned for the next decision variable from the pool. The process of assigning values to decision variables is continued until all the ants present in the colony are assigned. Then Local updated rule is applied at the end of each tour. Then each ant becomes a part of the solution for the optimization

problem. If anyone of the candidate solutions can not convince any constraint, that candidate solution is punished by using the equation $Z_p = Z(1+C)^{\varepsilon}$, where Z_p is the penalized objective function value of the candidate solution, C is the total constraint violations, and ε is the penalty coefficient.

5. Apply global update scheme using Eq. 16:

$$\tau_{ij}(t+n) = \rho \cdot \tau_{ij}(t) + \Delta\tau_{ij}(t) \tag{16}$$

where ρ = constant chosen between 0 and 1.
$(1-\rho)$ = evaporation amount of pheromone.
$\Delta\tau_{ij}$ = change in pheromone amount.
$\Delta\tau_{ij}$ is represented by:

$$\Delta\tau_{ij} = \sum_{k=1}^{m} \Delta\tau_{ij}^{k} \tag{17}$$

where ρ = any ant from 1 to m.
m = number of ants.
$d\ \Delta\tau_{ij}^{k}$ = pheromone change for ant k.
$\Delta\tau_{ij}$ term is calculated by;

$$\Delta\tau_{ij}^{k} = 1/Z_k \tag{18}$$

where Z_k = penalized objective.
It shows the end of one process in ant colony algorithm. For starting another process, every ant is returned back to their original decision variables and earlier steps are simulated again.

6. Repeat steps 2 to 5 since the termination criteria is fulfilled, which is normally occupied as the highest number of iterations (Figs. 2 and 3).

Here, *best*(π′, *sp*′) denotes the individual from population *sp* with the best objective function value. The use of the procedure *localSearch* (π′, *sp*′) is optional (Fig. 4).

3.2 Artificial-Neural-Network (ANN)

An artificial neural network (ANN) is a generalized mathematical model which is based on biological nervous systems. The fundamental elements of neural networks are artificial neurons. Input, output, and hidden are three basic layers of a simple neural network as presented in Fig. 5.

In neural network the output of the hidden layer h and output layer y can be calculated as:

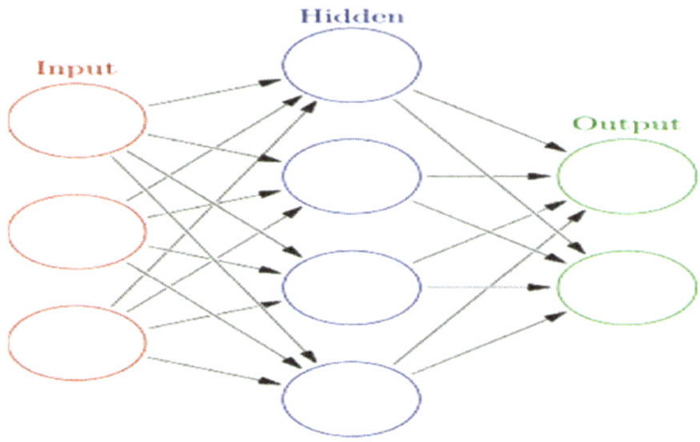

Fig. 5 Standard MLP structure

$$h = \sigma(W_1 x + b_1) \tag{19}$$

$$y = \sigma(W_2 h + b_2) \tag{20}$$

where W_1 and W_2 are the weights of neuron and x is the input. b_1 and b_2 are the bias. σ is the activation function [31].

3.3 Algorithm for Image Segmentation

The proposed steps for segmenting the digital image is described as follows;

The segmentation is done for biomedical image. Therefore the brain MRI image is considered as the inputted image.

1. Since the original image is a color image, later it is transformed to the gray image. Conversion of input image into gray scale image is done as follows;

$$\text{Gray}(i, j) = (\text{Red factor} * 0.3) + (\text{Green factor} * 0.59) + (\text{Blue factor} * 0.11)$$

2. Focal point is a specific region inside a cerebrum image. Therefore, the ROI was removed for investigation of the image. ROI is assessed in factual strategy commencing the pixel by thinking about limit.
3. For denoising purpose Gaussian filter was adopted for smoothing purpose. The smoothing is done as follows;

   (a) Original image of size $a * b$ is considered.
   (b) Two parameters K and L were gained for padding, where $K = 2 * a$ and $L = 2 * b$.
   (c) Size of the padded image is $K * L$ and was constructed through applying necessary amount of zeros to the image inputted to the model.

(d) Mathematical formula for generating smoothing filter with Gaussian model is

$$S(u, y) = e^{-s^2(u,y)\nu 2s_0^2}$$

4. Image matrix was subsequently changed over to power matrix of values extending starting 0 to 1 for clustering.
5. Preliminary image segmentation was conducted by applying the following fuzzy c-means clustering mechanism:
6. a. The amount of clusters C and $V(t)$ were finalized and fuzzification factor w with $(1 < w < \infty)$, value, $\in > 0$, and $t = 0$ were set.
   b. The cluster center matrix $W^{(i)} = [w_1, w_2, \ldots, w_s]$ was measured:

$$w = \frac{1}{\sum_{y=1}^{n} (\mu_{y,i})^{w}} \sum_{y=1}^{n} (\mu_{y,j})^{w} z_y, \quad \text{for every } j \tag{21}$$

   c. The membership function matrix is calculated as:

$$[\mu_{y,j}] = \left[\sum_{i=1}^{s} \left(\frac{|z_x - w_j|}{|z_y - w_i|} \right)^{2\nu(w-1)} \right]^{-1}, \quad \text{for every } y \text{ and } j; \tag{22}$$

   d. Parameter $\mu = \max[|V^{(t+1)} - Y^{(t)}]$ was calculated. If $\mu > \varepsilon$.

The preliminary image segmentation was conducted by applying the following fuzzy c-means clustering mechanism:

This optimized result value is utilized as an underlying incentive for the instatement of FCM, and the procedure was completed as portrayed in stage 6. At that point edge identification was performed utilizing notable "sobel" administrator and undesirable limit was evacuated. At last the segmented form image was acquired by utilizing a Gaussian channel as depicted in stage 4. At that point the new clustering centers were prepared with various ANN algorithm.

The input and output of the neural network was first initialized. One feed forward ANN was designed by mentioning the particular amount of hidden layer. In the hidden layer the activation function tan-sigmoid and in the output layer the linear activation function is used. The neuron size is defined by keeping the accurate balance between overfitting problem. The separation of input and target data vector was defined with previously defined ratio for training and testing data set. The training of the network is done by Gradient descent algorithm. In this training algorithm the main aim is to update the network weights in such a direction that combine the gradient error surface with previous training error. After successfully completing the training stage different performance measuring parameters were measured.

4 Results and Discussion

Here, successfully the proposed methodology is implemented to extract boundaries of both the T2 brain MR images. Both the T2 MR images are obtained from the Department of Neurosurgery at SCB Medical College and Hospital. The T2 MR image showing colloid cyst is obtained from a 34 year old male patient who has a history of 10 year of headaches while the other image showing occipital edema is obtained from a 46 year old male patient with complaints like headaches, lack of coordination, and changes in personality. The first algorithm based on the complementary pair of structuring elements is used to extract the boundary of the T2 MR image of colloid cyst. The second algorithm which is based on Fuzzy morphology is used to extract boundary of the T2 MR image of occipital lesion. In Fig. 6 MRI T2 scanned image is displayed.

For the colloid cyst, the results obtained with modified morphological model are compared with traditional boundary detecting methods. The performance is evaluated on basis of Mean Square Error and Peak Signal to Noise Ratio which is calculated as follows

$$MSE = \sum_{i=1}^{m} \sum_{j=1}^{n} (f_1(i, j) - f_2(i, j))^2 \tag{23}$$

$$PSNR = 10 \log(255^2 / MSE) \tag{24}$$

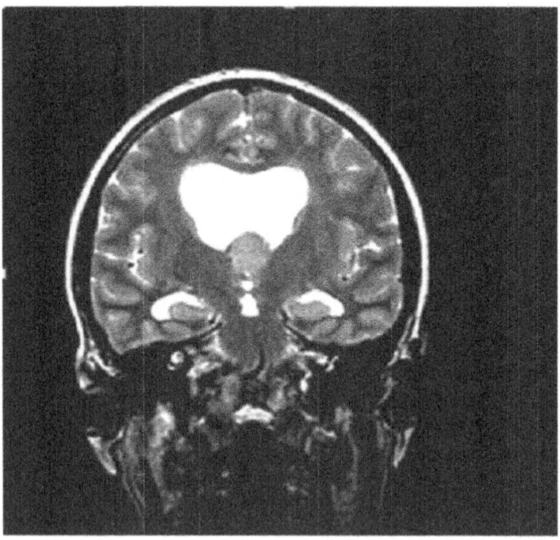

Fig. 6 Brain MRI image

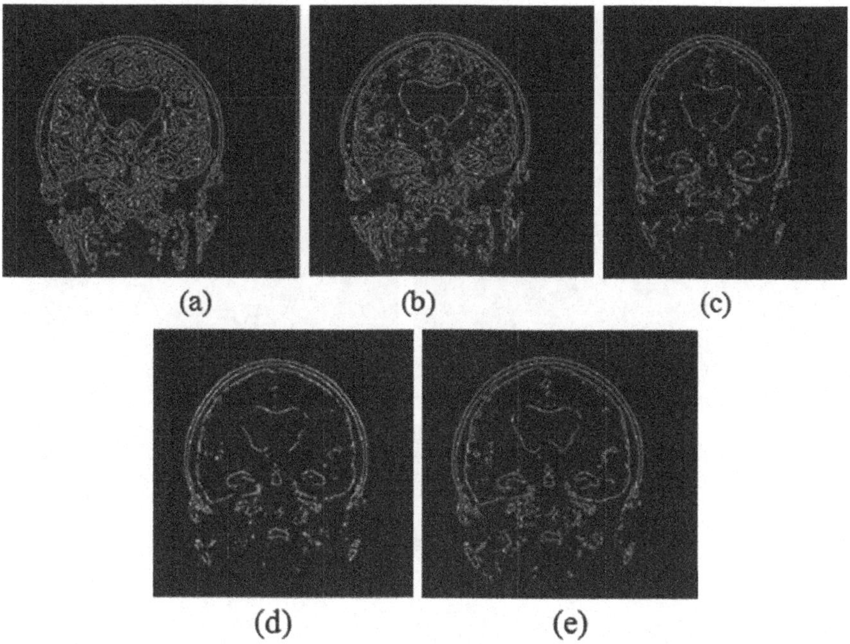

Fig. 7 Segmented image obtained through traditional methods **a** Canny, **b** Log, **c** Prewitt, **d** Roberts, **e** Sobel

where f_1 is the input image and f_2 is the output image of size $m \times n$. The results obtained through traditional image segmentation algorithm are displayed in Fig. 7.

The Boundary extracted using the modified morphological model is continuous and better than the traditional methods as shown in the following Fig. 8.

The mean square error for proposed morphological model is presented in Fig. 9 and the SNR peaks are displayed in Fig. 10. In Table 1 the mean square error and SNR obtained from the proposed morphological model is presented.

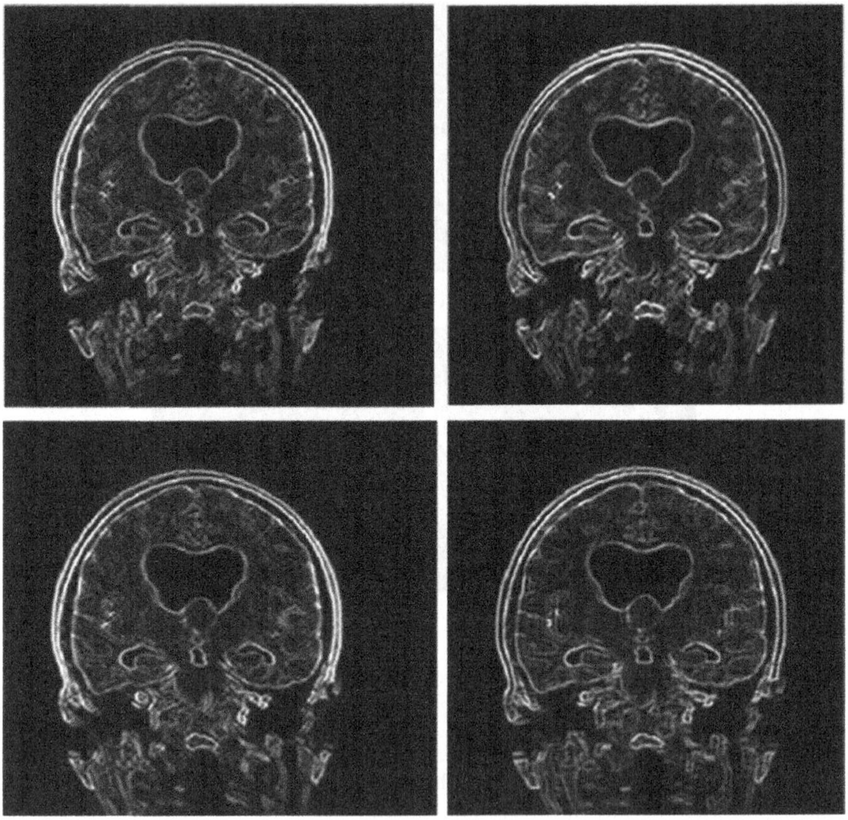

Fig. 8 Extraction of boundary with different angles by applying the modified morphological algorithms

The above table shows the modified morphological yields less noisy images in comparison to the traditional methods as they have comparatively high Peak Signal to Noise Ratios. Then the fuzzy gradient operation was performed upon the filtered image for different values of *e* (neutralizing parameter) and a (scaling parameter) of the structuring element. The original and filtered image is displayed in Fig. 11. After applying the fuzzy gradient the obtained result is shown through Figs. 12, 13, 14, 15, 16 and 17. The graphical analysis from the graph shown below interprets that for **e** = **0.99** for any value of "**a**" well detected boundaries are extracted and noise is removed to a greater extent which is shown in the bellow figures.

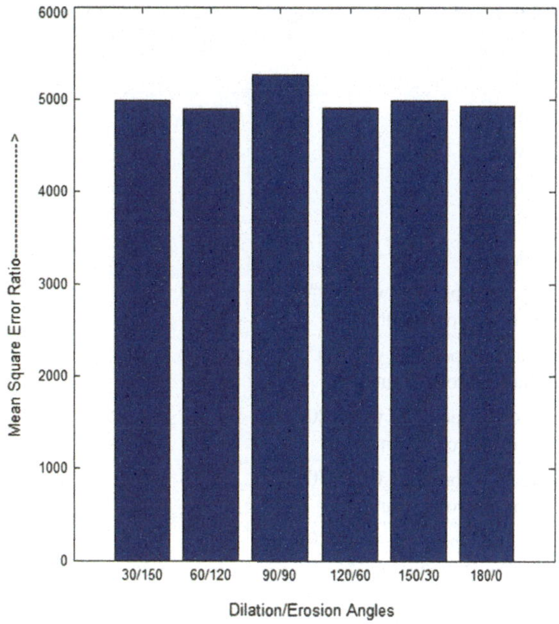

Fig. 9 Mean square error for the proposed model

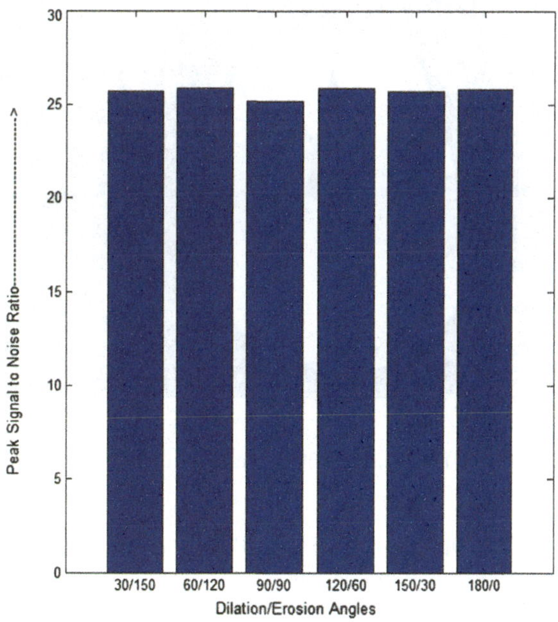

Fig. 10 SNR ratio for the proposed model

Table 1 MSE and PSNR values obtained through morphological methods

Operators	Mean square error(MSE)	Peak signal to noise ratio (PSNR in dB)
Canny	7635.1	21.4202
Prewitt	7641.8	21.4113
LOG	7635.8	21.4192
Roberts	7641.3	21.4120
Sobel	7645.7	21.4115
Gradient operators with 60°/120° (dilation/erosion) angles	4893.0	25.8697
Gradient operators with 90°/90° (dilation/erosion) angles	5264.2	25.1383
Gradient operators with 120°/60° (dilation/erosion) angles	4903.5	25.8482
Gradient operators with 150°/30° (dilation/erosion) angles	4990.6	25.6721
Gradient operators with 180°/0° (dilation/erosion) angles	4929.0	25.7964

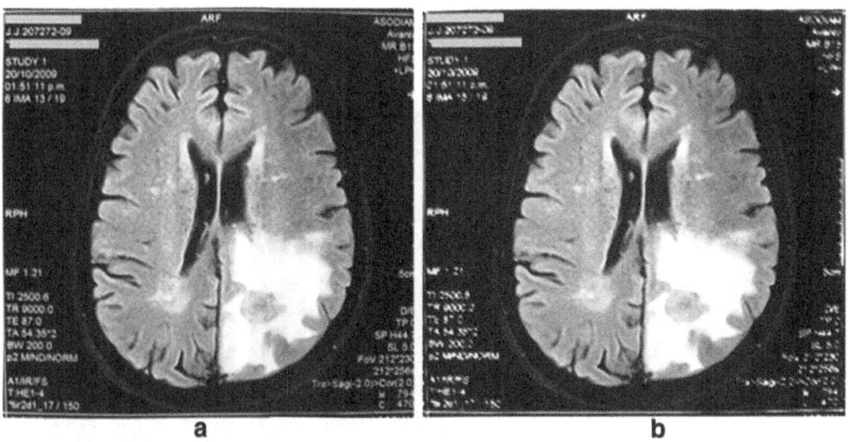

Fig. 11 A Original and **b** filtered brain MRI image

The graphical Analysis for PSNR versus Neutral element for Uniform (e) for a = 1 to 5 is shown in Fig. 18.

Peak Signal to Noise Ratio for different values of '**a**' and '**e**' is shown is Table 2.

The original acquired image is shown in Fig. 19 and after finding the Region of Interest (ROI) it is displayed in Fig. 20. The denoised ROI is shown in Fig. 21. The segmented image is shown in Fig. 22. The finalized smoothed image is displayed in Fig. 23.

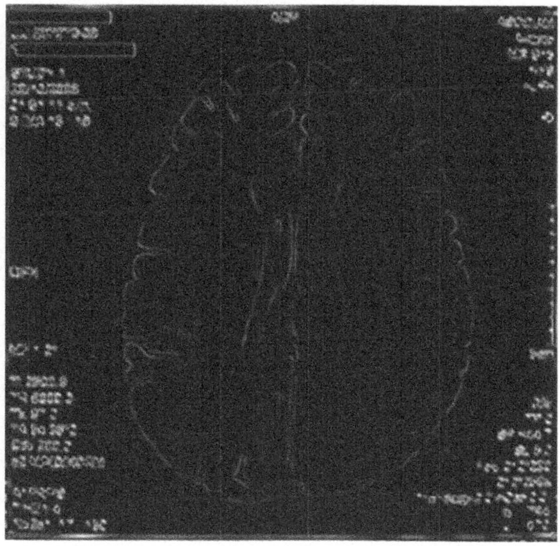

Fig. 12 Fuzzy gradient image for e = 0.9, a = 1

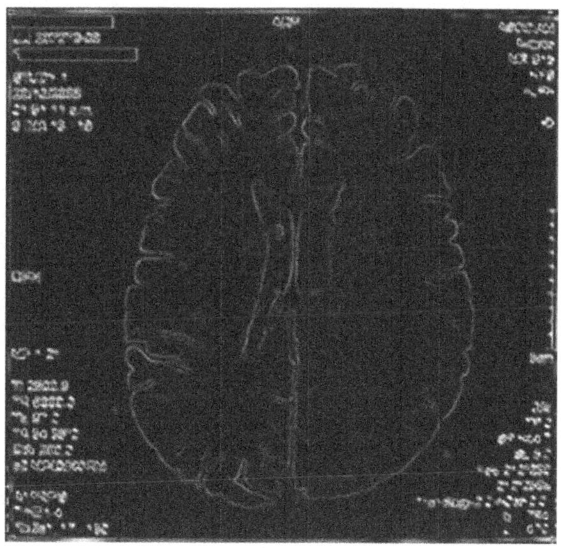

Fig. 13 Fuzzy gradient Image for e = 0.96, a = 1

After completing all these preprocessing steps the clustering is done with conventional FCM and modified GA-based FCM. The obtained clustering result is shown in Figs. 24 and 25. The objective function parameters for both conventional FCM and modified GA-FCM are presented below.

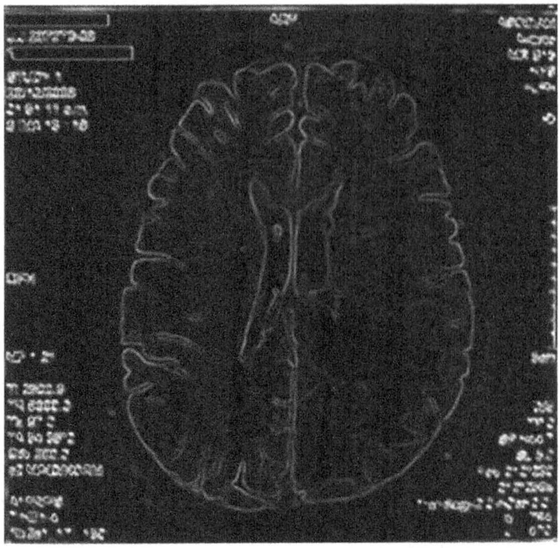

Fig. 14 Fuzzy gradient image for e = 0.99, a = 1

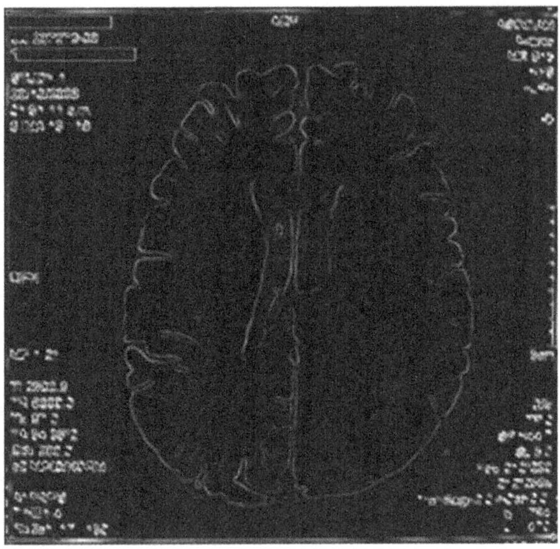

Fig. 15 Fuzzy gradient image for e = 0.96, a = 2

For conventional FCM

Iteration = 29, obj. objective function = 8.75146.

For modified GA-FCM

Iteration = 19, objective function = 6.36258.

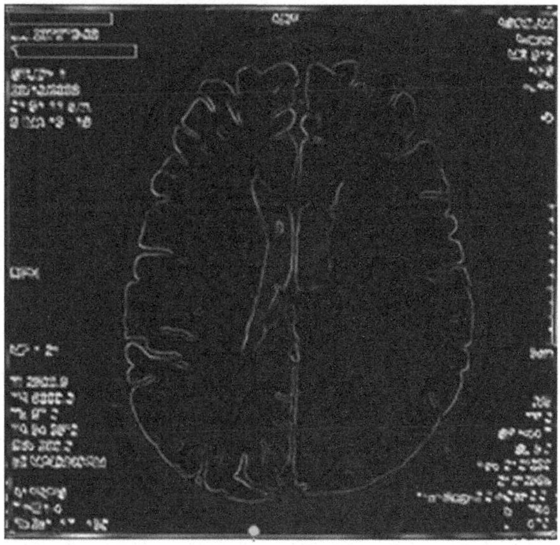

Fig. 16 Fuzzy gradient image for e = 0.96, a = 5

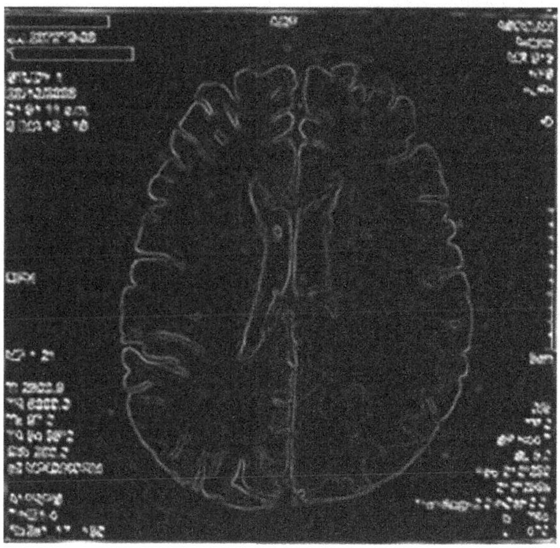

Fig. 17 Fuzzy gradient image for e = 0.99, a = 5

After successfully completing the clustering steps the clusters are fitted with the neural network model. The number of hidden layer in the neural network is ten and it is trained with gradient descent momentum algorithm. The respective performance of the proposed neural network is shown in Figs. 26, 27, and 28.

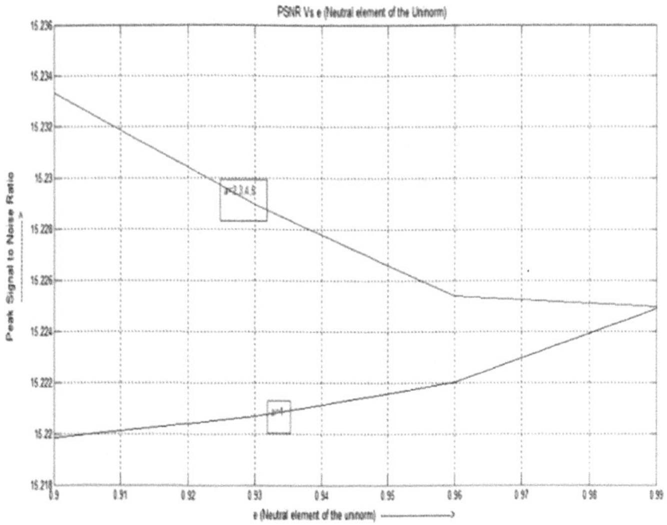

Fig. 18 PSNR versus neutral element for uniform (e) for a = 1 to 5

5 Future Prospect

The boundary extraction method using modified morphological model is found to be more efficient than the traditional methods. It detects continuous boundaries and is also suitable for boundary extraction of noisy images. Also the method is very simple and easy to implement. The results obtained from the Fuzzy algorithm indicate that the method is a novel contribution toward boundary extraction for biomedical images. The fuzzy method is simple and easier on the user to implement. The fuzzy method also has an advantage of removing noise to a greater extent for higher values of scaling parameter "a." Even boundaries become more prominent for higher values of the "e", i.e. the neutralizing element for the norm. The results also indicate that this is a good starting point to develop more complex algorithms such as boundary detection either based on directional structuring elements or adaptive structuring elements or both. The developed methods can also be extended for image segmentation and registration for biomedical images. The efficiency can be enhanced by the use of optimization techniques.

Table 2 Peak signal to noise ratio (in dB) for values of $a = 1$ to 5 and $e = 0.9$ to 0.99

PSNR (in dB)	e = 0.9	e = 0.91	e = 0.92	e = 0.93	e = 0.94	e = 0.95	e = 0.96	e = 0.97	e = 0.98	e = 0.99
a = 1	15.2198	15.2200	15.2203	15.2206	15.2210	15.2214	15.2220	15.2227	15.2236	15.2249
a = 2	15.2330	15.2318	15.2303	15.2289	15.2276	15.2264	15.2253	15.2246	15.2243	15.2249
a = 3	15.2333	15.2318	15.2303	15.2289	15.2276	15.2264	15.2253	15.2246	15.2243	15.2249
a = 4	15.2333	15.2318	15.2303	15.2289	15.2276	15.2264	15.2253	15.2246	15.2243	15.2249
a = 5	15.2333	15.2318	15.2303	15.2289	15.2276	15.2264	15.2253	15.2246	15.2243	15.2249

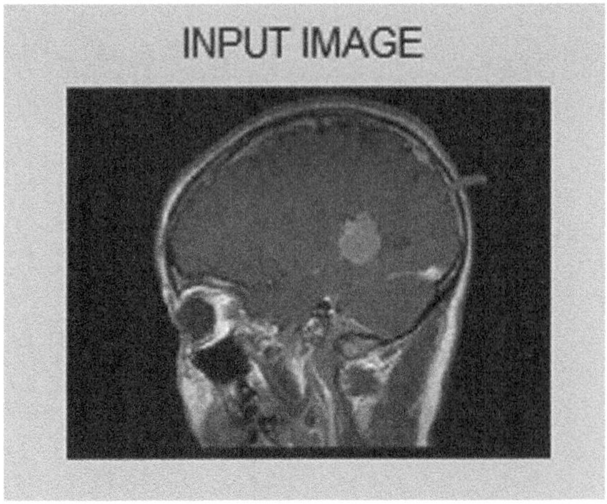

Fig. 19 Original input image

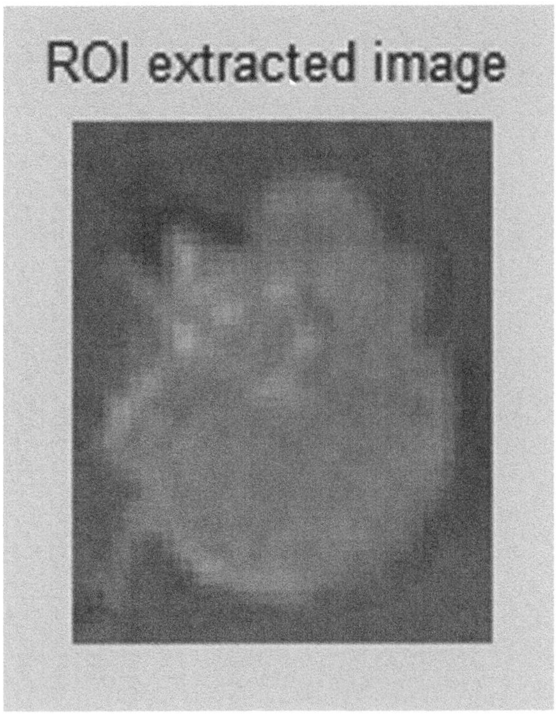

Fig. 20 After extracting the RO

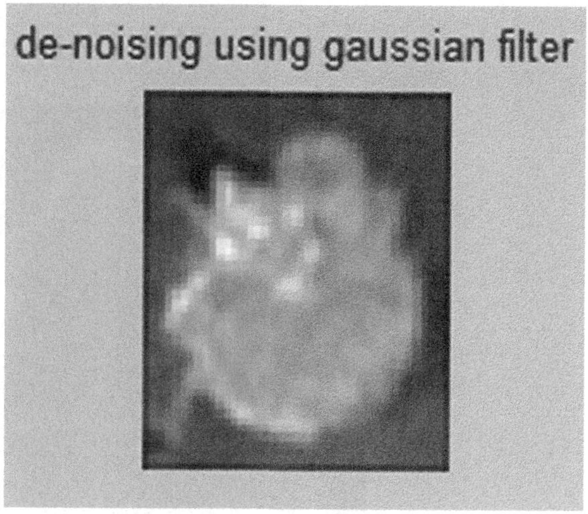

Fig. 21 Filtered image

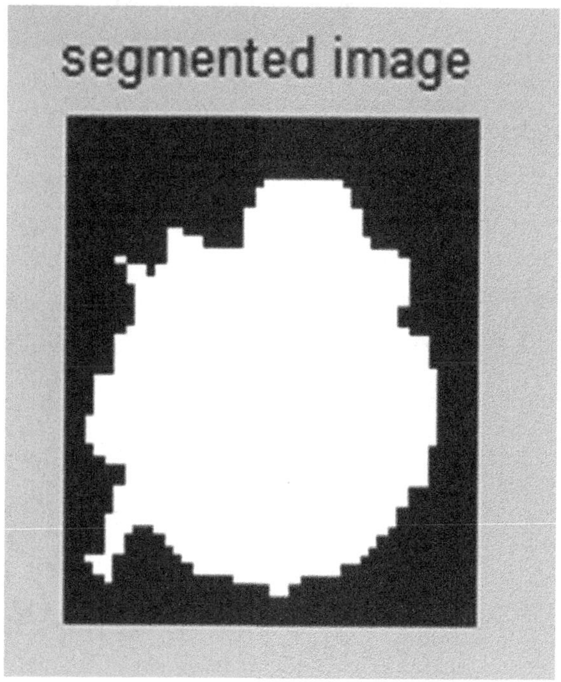

Fig. 22 Segmented image

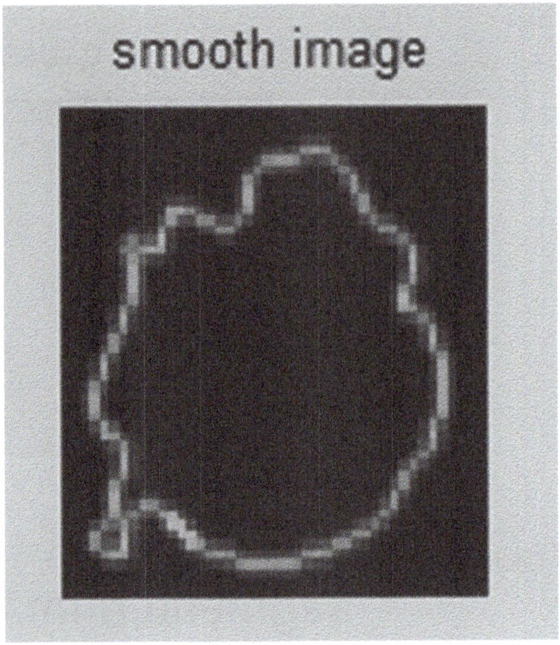

Fig. 23 Image after smoothening

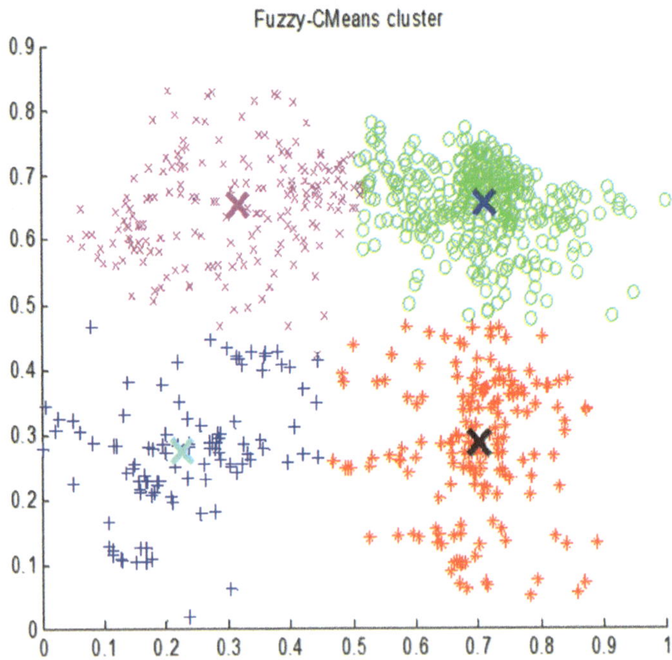

Fig. 24 Conventional FCM cluster

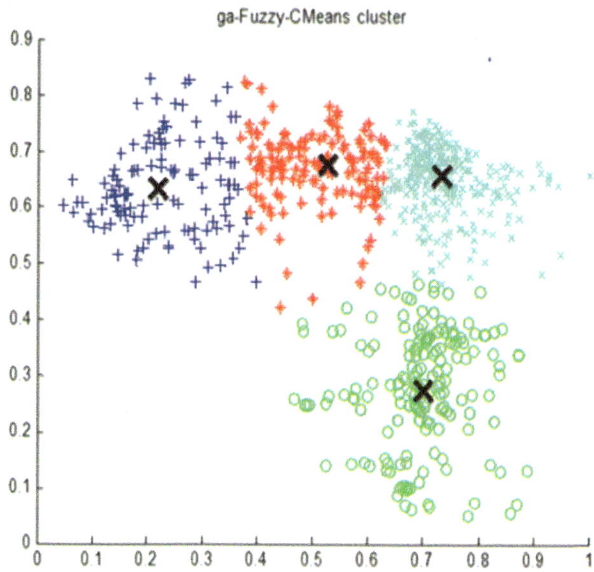

Fig. 25 Clusters obtained through modified GA-FCM

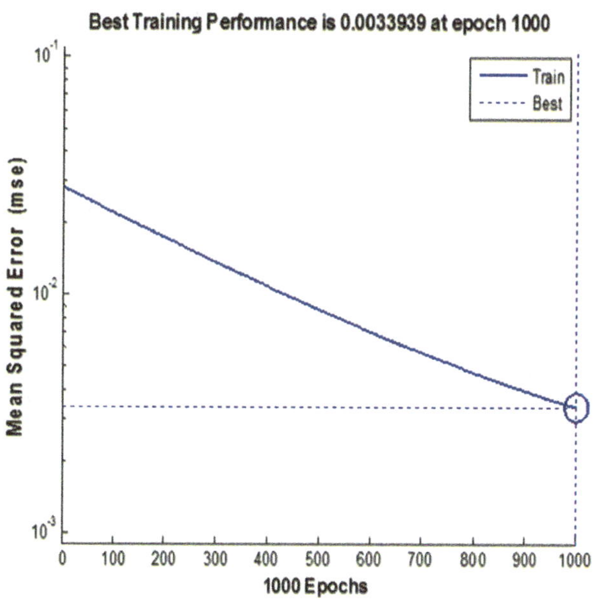

Fig. 26 Overall performance of the ANN

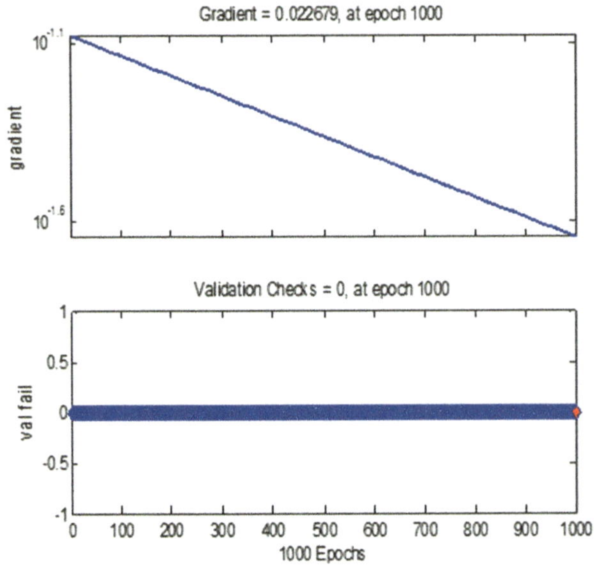

Fig. 27 Training performance of the ANN

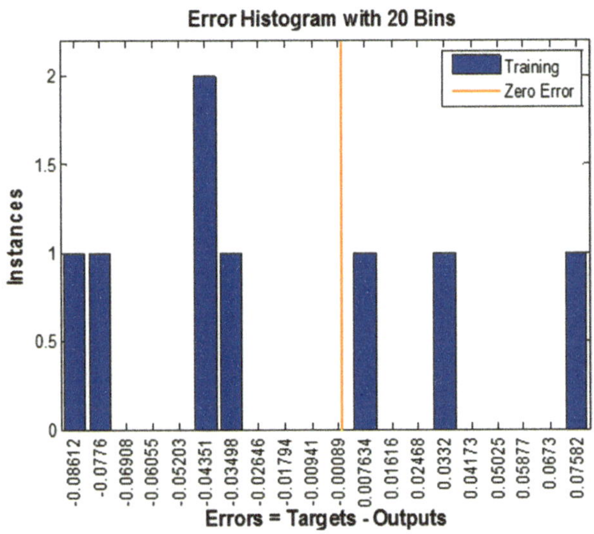

Fig. 28 Error histogram of the ANN

References

1. Haralick, R.M., Shapiro, L.G.: Image segmentation techniques. Comput. Vis. Graph. Image Process. **29**, 100–132 (1985)
2. Pal, N.R., Pal, S.K.: A review on image segmentation techniques. Pattern Recogn. **26**, 1277–1294 (1993)
3. Arbelaez, P., Maire, M., Fowlkes, C., Malik, J.: Contour detection and hierarchical image segmentation. IEEE Trans. Pattern Anal. Mach. Intell. **33**, 898–916 (2010)
4. Chen, L.-C., Papandreou, G., Schroff, F., Adam, H.: Rethinking atrous convolution for semantic image segmentation. arXiv:1706.05587 (2017)
5. Liu, C., Chen, L.-C., Schroff, F., Adam, H., Hua, W., Yuille, A.L., Fei-Fei, L.: Auto-deeplab: hierarchical neural architecture search for semantic image segmentation. In: Proceedings of the IEEE Conference on Computer Vision and Pattern Recognition, pp. 82–92 (2019)
6. Mallick, P.K., Mohanty, M.N., Kumar, S.S.: White patch detection in brain MRI image using evolutionary clustering algorithm. In: Research Advances in the Integration of Big Data and Smart Computing, pp. 323–339. IGI Global (2016)
7. Jyoti, A., Mohanty, M.N., Kumar, M.P.: Morphological based segmentation of brain image for tumor detection. In: 2014 International Conference on Electronics and Communication Systems (ICECS), pp. 1–5. IEEE (2014)
8. Mallick, P.K., Satapathy, B.S., Mohanty, M., Kumar, S.S.: Intelligent technique for CT brain image segmentation. In: 2015 2nd International Conference on Electronics and Communication Systems (ICECS), pp. 1269–1277. IEEE (2015)
9. Mallick, P.K., Ryu, S.H., Satapathy, S.K., Mishra, S., Nguyen, G.N., Tiwari, P.: Brain MRI image classification for cancer detection using deep wavelet autoencoder-based deep neural network. IEEE Access **7**, 46278–46287 (2019)
10. Zhang, D.-Q., Chen, S.-C.: A novel kernelized fuzzy c-means algorithm with application in medical image segmentation. Artif. Intell. Med. **32**, 37–50 (2004)
11. Chuang, K.-S., Tzeng, H.-L., Chen, S., Wu, J., Chen, T.-J.: Fuzzy c-means clustering with spatial information for image segmentation. Comput. Med. Imaging Graph. **30**, 9–15 (2006)
12. Chen, S., Zhang, D.: Robust image segmentation using FCM with spatial constraints based on new kernel-induced distance measure. IEEE Trans. Syst. Man Cybern. Part B (Cybern.) **34**, 1907–1916 (2004)
13. Cheng, T.W., Goldgof, D.B., Hall, L.O.: Fast fuzzy clustering. Fuzzy Sets Syst. **93**, 49–56 (1998)
14. Pham, D.L.: Spatial models for fuzzy clustering. Comput. Vis. Image Underst. **84**, 285–297 (2001)
15. Nascimento, S., Mirkin, B., Moura-Pires, F.: A fuzzy clustering model of data and fuzzy c-means. In: Ninth IEEE International Conference on Fuzzy Systems. FUZZ-IEEE 2000 (Cat. No. 00CH37063), pp. 302–307. IEEE (2000)
16. Rahebi, J., Tajik, H.R.: Biomedical image edge detection using an ant colony optimization based on artificial neural networks. Int. J. Eng. Sci. Technol. (IJEST) **3**, 8211–8218 (2011)
17. Yu-Qian, Z., Wei-Hua, G., Zhen-Cheng, C., Jing-Tian, T., Ling-Yun, L.: Medical images edge detection based on mathematical morphology. In: 2005 IEEE Engineering in Medicine and Biology 27th Annual Conference, pp. 6492–6495. IEEE (2005)
18. Thanh, D.N., Hien, N.N., Prasath, V.S., Hai, N.H.: Automatic initial boundary generation methods based on edge detectors for the level set function of the Chan-Vese segmentation model and applications in biomedical image processing. In: Frontiers in Intelligent Computing: Theory and Applications, pp. 171–181. Springer (2020)
19. Zhu, Y., Chen, Z., Zhao, S., Xie, H., Guo, W., Zhang, Y.: ACE-Net: biomedical image segmentation with augmented contracting and expansive paths. In: International Conference on Medical Image Computing and Computer-Assisted Intervention, pp. 712–720. Springer (2019)
20. Behera, S., Mohanty, M.N., Patnaik, S.: A comparative analysis on edge detection of colloid cyst: a medical imaging approach. In: Soft Computing Techniques in Vision Science, pp. 63–85. Springer (2012)

21. Chabrier, S., Rosenberger, C., Emile, B., Laurent, H.: Optimization-based image segmentation by genetic algorithms. EURASIP J. Image Video Process. **2008**, 842029 (2008)
22. Karypis, M.S.G., Kumar, V., Steinbach, M.: A comparison of document clustering techniques. In: Text Mining Workshop at KDD2000 (2000)
23. Gómez-Skarmeta, A.F., Delgado, M., Vila, M.A.: About the use of fuzzy clustering techniques for fuzzy model identification. Fuzzy Sets Syst. **106**, 179–188 (1999)
24. Langari, R.K., Sardar, S., Mousavi, S.A.A., Radfar, R.: Combined fuzzy clustering and firefly algorithm for privacy preserving in social networks. Expert Syst. Appl. **141**, 112968 (2020)
25. Zhou, J., Lai, Z., Miao, D., Gao, C., Yue, X.: Multigranulation rough-fuzzy clustering based on shadowed sets. Inf. Sci. **507**, 553–573 (2020)
26. Bezdek, J.C., Ehrlich, R., Full, W.: FCM: The fuzzy c-means clustering algorithm. Comput. Geosci. **10**, 191–203 (1984)
27. Clark, M.C., Hall, L.O., Goldgof, D.B., Clarke, L.P., Velthuizen, R.P., Silbiger, M.S.: MRI segmentation using fuzzy clustering techniques. IEEE Eng. Med. Biol. Mag. **13**, 730–742 (1994)
28. Dorigo, M., Birattari, M., Stutzle, T.: Ant colony optimization. IEEE Comput. Intell. Mag. **1**, 28–39 (2006)
29. Dorigo, M., Blum, C.: Ant colony optimization theory: A survey. Theoret. Comput. Sci. **344**, 243–278 (2005)
30. Karnan, M., Logheshwari, T.: Improved implementation of brain MRI image segmentation using ant colony system. In: 2010 IEEE International Conference on Computational Intelligence and Computing Research, pp. 1–4. IEEE (2010)
31. Haykin, S.S.: Neural Networks and Learning Machines/Simon Haykin. Prentice Hall, New York (2009)

Pandemic Drone with Thermal Imaging and Crowd Monitoring System (DRISHYA)

Shivam Pandey, Rahul Kumar Barik, Somya Gupta, and R. Arthi

Abstract The idea proposed here is the introduction of an Unmanned Aerial Vehicle (UAV) named "Drishya" to tackle the situation of the spread of novel coronavirus. The UAV has been equipped with all the necessary technologies to cater to such adverse situations. Drishya's main objective is to monitor social distancing and trace COVID-19 infected suspects with the help of two cameras, one for normal vision and the other for high range thermal optimization. The thermal camera will be able to detect any suspect with a temperature higher than normal and hence can be sent for screening. With such technology least human intervention is required on the field which makes it more safe. This process is a better alternative due to its high efficiency and least human involvement. It is most applicable for high transmission areas or rather the areas symbolized as a red zone. It also acts as a helping hand for the medical teams out for screening person to person.

Keywords UAV · Novel coronavirus · Social distancing · Suspects · Thermal optimization · Screening · Red zone

S. Pandey (✉) · R. K. Barik · S. Gupta · R. Arthi
Department of ECE, SRM Institute of Science and Technology, Ramapuram Campus, Chennai, India
e-mail: pandeyshivam305@gmail.com

R. K. Barik
e-mail: rahulbarik004@gmail.com

S. Gupta
e-mail: somyag00@gmail.com

R. Arthi
e-mail: arthir2@srmist.edu.in

H. K. Tripathy et al. (eds.), *Technical Advancements of Machine Learning in Healthcare*, Studies in Computational Intelligence 936,
https://doi.org/10.1007/978-981-33-4698-7_15

1 Introduction

With the proliferation of Unmanned Aerial Vehicles (UAV's) in the twenty-first century, the near future is all set up to welcome the use of UAVs in a far more dynamic way with more support and interest from individuals. With the pandemic hitting hard globally this 2020, the world felt rather helpless in tackling COVID-19. With lives lost, economies crumbling the unemployment rate rising like never before, the pandemic has left no stone unturned to put a pause to this world. The maximum one can do is contain the virus and stop it from spreading. Hence various Governments are following social distancing norms and lockdown measures wherein minimum human interactions are involved. In a country such as India accounting to 17.7% of the world population, i.e. 1.3 billion approximately, it is tough to confine the spreading of the virus. The most prominent symptoms of the coronavirus are high fever, itchy throat and nausea, hence self-quarantine has been suggested. This global pandemic is spreading at a higher rate than expected, but with the use of technology things can get a bit handy and more safe.

Drones have emerged as one of the best technologies in many aspects. In the early 1980s the United States started to deploy drones for military purposes, with time and advancements they started adding sophisticated systems and versatile weapons to their drone artillery making themselves more advanced than before. Besides military usage, drones were also used commercially. Military usage included surveillance of territories and borders whereas commercial usage included the civilians, with public and private organization.

Drones have only evolved from then, known as the "Evolution of Drone Information Technology". In the initial stage, reliable controls and stable flight capability was the target wherein the development took place in maintaining handy controls and stability of the drone. Next stage saw the advancement of on-board the drone body wherein there was an overhaul done to the cameras and sensors on the leading group of the automation, making it increasingly programmed and exuberant. After that the stage came where accuracy and precision were taken into account. With so many advancements, the accuracy of the drone was one of the main aspects, hence scalability of drone usage was done. Now, with proliferations in technology and with the introduction of Artificial Intelligence (AI) to this World, it was no far when it would be introduced to the UAVs. The drones saw a drastic change after the development with respect to the addition of AI to their systems.

With all such technologies, various integration was made possible, hence making it vulnerable to many new systems that can be used for various applications. One such example being when the drone was introduced as a delivery medium by Amazon. Now, the proposed work is an example of the various integration that could form a useful solution for this world. The paper portrays a true sense of credibility wherein the perfect usage of cameras and sensors are put to the right place for the right application. The drone has been just a medium for giving our system aerial manoeuvrability that makes it more productive and efficient. The pandemic seen as the name of Covid-19 can be well tackled in terms of crowd monitoring and thermal sensing with such a system.

Now to understand the spread of novel coronavirus first we need to get a rough idea of what R0 (R-naught) value is. R0 actually explains how many persons can be infected further from one single infected person. R0 receives more attention than any other metrics with respect to the depiction of the spread of such a disease. Practically, the R0 value is never fixed, but during the initial outbreak in China it was expected to be 5.7 which is strategically very high with respect to other diseases. Later on it was also found to be ranging from 2 to 2.5. These values change according to the conditions and precautions we take, that is with time. Any R0 value less than 1 signifies a decrease in the spread whereas R0 value more than 1 signifies increase in the spread of infection.

The best solution for such a contagious disease is social distancing. With the social distancing norms into action the transmission numbers can be brought down strategically. The proposed work suggests a solution to monitor social distancing norms and identify suspects carrying the symptoms in commercial areas where there is a high risk of the spread of the virus.

A quad-copter can be used for manoeuvring through crowded regions with a stabilized thermal video output wherein it can detect people with high temperature and make a record of it. The quad-copter can be stationed at the local police station with a control room equipped with all the technical necessities needed for the operation as shown in Fig. 1. The frequency of surveillance can depend on the areas prioritized under red, orange and green zones, respectively. During the relief period for the people which corresponds to the relaxation time given to the people for buying basic essentials a drone can be sent off to hover around market places, roads, etc., where there is a chance of any gathering formation, and cover a maximum area from above, glancing through the activities carried out by the people. If a person with a high temperature has been sensed by the drone, an inbuilt speakers enable themselves and create an awareness in that area so that people follow social distancing and avoid any contact with anyone and also the person on himself goes for a test.

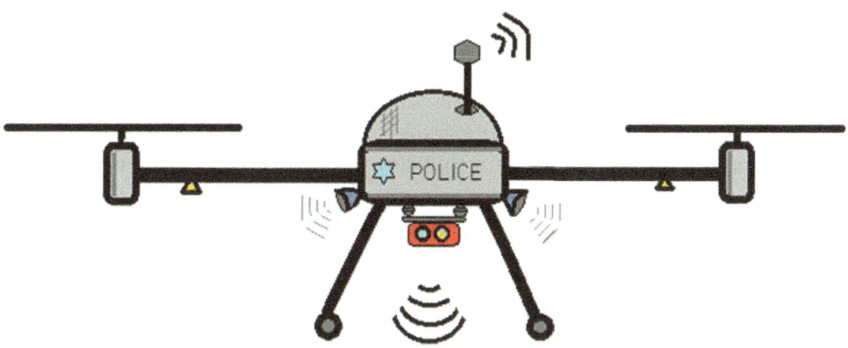

Fig. 1 Schematic of pandemic drone

With the help of point-to-point tracing the distance between any two persons can be calculated through various algorithms using digital image processing, helping us to see if or if not social distancing has been being followed. Whenever the drone detects the minimum distance between any two persons to be less than 3 feet, it initiates the warning protocol and creates awareness through inbuilt speakers in it, and if in case it is too much crowded, it can also send in a red alert to the base station that will further involve police intervention.

With such technology and such a system, it is made sure that the human involvement is minimum, and that no human lives are put into danger. The specifications of the drone enable it to carry a payload of 2 kg with a flight time of 25 min. The main problem faced today while using an UAV is to worry about the fight time, but with various advancements in drone technology, it is getting better day by day.

The paper contains the introduction to "the pandemic drone with thermal imaging and crowd monitoring system" where we come to know about the implementation of this drone technology. Section 2 lists out all the related works that are used in this paper. Section 3 contains the methodology and lists out the various hardware components, software used in the system. Section 4 shows the results and discussions where the end result of our implemented drone has been shown. Section 5 concludes the proposed work.

2 Related Work

In [1], the author discusses about using an UAV (Unmanned Aerial Vehicle) in surveillance, for monitoring areas and also for peacekeeping activities, it also highlights an efficient means of using drones for surveillance. In [2], the paper discusses about using multiple drones together in co-ordination and to do that in a more convenient way. The paper [3] uses drones for military-based surveillance of borders making it easy to cover a large perimeter of area. In [4], a paper on using drones to find out parking lots which helps in reducing the search time for people in finding parking spots, thereby effectively manage parking spaces and avoid long queues. The paper [5] uses drones for surveillance and heat leakage detection in civilian areas using high resolution thermal detection cameras. In [6], a paper on using drones for detecting and tracking the subjects or individuals with fever using various algorithms, the detection is done using infrared thermography. The paper [7] uses CNN, i.e. Convolutional Neural Networks for detecting human crowd so as not to fly drones over that area and declaring it as no fly zone.

In [8], the author uses drones for detecting a crowd and counting the people via fast algorithms with high accuracy. The paper [9] introduces about IR imaging for getting colour-guided thermal images using high resolution cameras. In [10], the paper discusses about using drones for visual surveillance to detect objects and run analysis to exactly identify the object. In [11], the author uses drones for motion detection via visual surveillance and to monitor people, events, etc. In [12], the author uses amateur drones for surveillance using cognitive Internet of Things (IOT) making it more efficient and overcoming the difficulties generally faced in amateur drone based surveillance. In [13], the author suggests a vision drone-based system to analyse crowds gathered using an efficient colour histogram technique, mainly to monitor any riot like situation. In [14], the paper discusses about drones being used by the police for surveillance and monitoring of areas, for crime check and security.

In [15], the work implements an automatic fever system to monitor the temperature of humans using an IR thermal camera, which captures the thermal image of the person and measures the temperature. The paper [16] uses a system to monitor the temperature of a driver in a car so as to be aware if the driver feels drowsy, to avoid accidents. In [17], the author implements a system to monitor the temperature of students in classrooms to avoid large spread of viral diseases or influenza, if a fever like temperature is detected, the system sends a warning thereby controlling the spread of a disease. The paper [18] processes infrared images to detect and track people with abnormally high temperature, especially at large gatherings to avoid a wide spread of a flu. The paper [19] uses IR thermography to detect leakage of any gas or harmful substances in various places especially in factories to avoid any kind of mishaps.

In [20], the paper discusses about using a IR camera to detect the temperature of senior citizens at homes and a wireless system to communicate about it to medical experts, thereby providing an easy way of monitoring their health. The paper [21] uses a histogram-based technique to predict the fall of a patient from bed using thermal IR imagery, it is mainly implemented to monitor the safety of critical patients. In [22], the work uses thermal camera to monitor the temperature of an open TEM—cell that has been used for calibrating small antennas. In [23], the author uses a drone-based system along with Deep Learning algorithm to detect humans in forest areas, mainly for monitoring and surveillance purposes. The paper [24] implements an automatic human tracking system via high-end cameras placed on the drone for various surveillance purposes.

In [25], the author uses a drone-based system for surveillance and rescue of humans during a natural calamity like floods or cyclones. The system has been mainly used to detect humans stuck under debris so as to ensure quicker help to those people. The work in [26] uses a drone system to track, monitor and survey people in the riverside areas for various safety purposes. In [27], the author has analysed the total flight time of a drone, its efficiency and charge hold up, uses a mathematical framework to analyse semantics like reaction time of drones. It also takes information from the flight controller via gyro and inertial sensor. The paper [28] uses drone for surveillance in an efficient manner and to increase the flight time, the drone will be used to monitor hidden activities using high-end cameras, additionally the prototype is added with transmission in FPV goggles.

In [29], the author has implemented a power-over fibre drones instead of airborne base stations in terms of flight power and flight time. In [30], the work introduces a drone with automated flight control using marker recognition technology, the system maintains a certain amount of distance between the drone and marker in flight, these drones will mainly be used for commercial purposes like food and product delivery. The paper [31] implements automatic landing of drones in a base station using various processing algorithms.

3 Methodology

The very imminent threat of this Covid-19 pandemic is the main motivation behind the making of "Drishya—a multi-functional drone". It is a quad-copter equipped with two cameras, one is a high resolution camera that can be used for surveillance and monitoring of containment areas to ensure whether the various norms are being followed. The other camera is a low resolution thermal IR camera for temperature detection of the people on the roads. The camera is also equipped with image processing power which can identify if there are large crowds gathered at a particular location and are not maintaining the norms of social distancing.

The drone's first and foremost function is to detect a person on the streets with high temperature via the high range thermal camera placed on the drone as shown in Fig. 2. The camera used here is the MLX90640 32 × 24 IR array which is a contactless temperature measurement camera sensor. If a person with an abnormally high temperature is detected via our temperature recognition system, the person's facial identity and the location where the person was found is noted via the GPS module and sent to the police station server for further tracing of the individual.

The drone has been equipped with a high resolution camera for surveillance of areas, the reason for using an UAV for surveillance is that it can monitor small areas where it might be hard for police vehicles to go through and monitor. The drone can also cover wide areas in quick time making it easy for the police to conduct surveillance. The camera has been equipped with image processing power to identify the number of people gathered in an area and if found so, it alerts the base station about the gathering along with the location so that the police can further take care of the situation. Also via the advanced image processing algorithms the distance between two people is noted and if it is found to be less than the specified social distancing norms an alert or announcement is given via the speaker placed on the drone.

Since two cameras are fitted on the drone, a dedicated single module can be used for both the cameras so that both the cameras work in coordination. It will be based on master–slave mechanism wherein the high resolution surveillance camera functions as the master and the thermal IR camera as the slave. So, wherever the high resolution surveillance camera moves and points, the thermal camera also points in the same direction. This coordination is required because when the thermal camera detects an abnormal temperature in an individual, the high resolution camera was intended to see and store the facial identity of the individual.

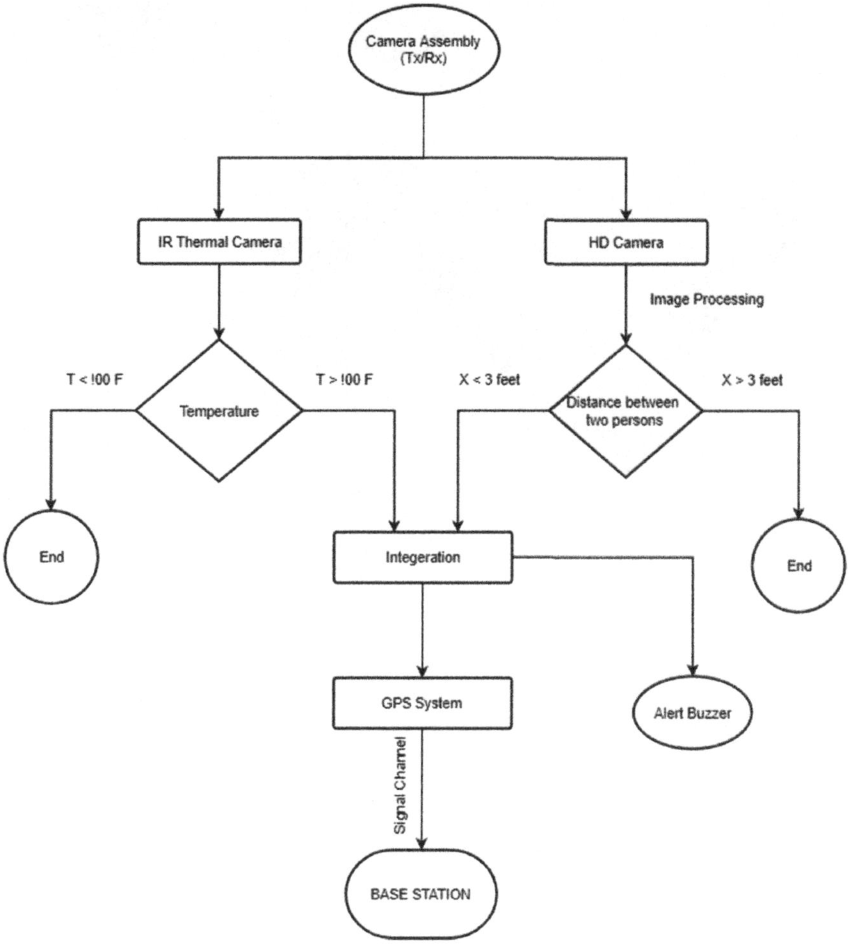

Fig. 2 Flow diagram of Drishya—a multi-functional drone

The speaker on the UAV can be used by the surveillance team to make announcements in cases of large crowd gatherings or when the social distancing norms are not being followed. The speaker will be attached along with an amplifying module to make the sound louder and clear with no interference of noise.

3.1 Hardware Required

Drone Frame: It is the base of the drone that is made up of carbon fibres as shown in Fig. 3. The carbon fibre material is preferred as it is strong and at the same time light in weight which will make the drone fly better and will consume less power.

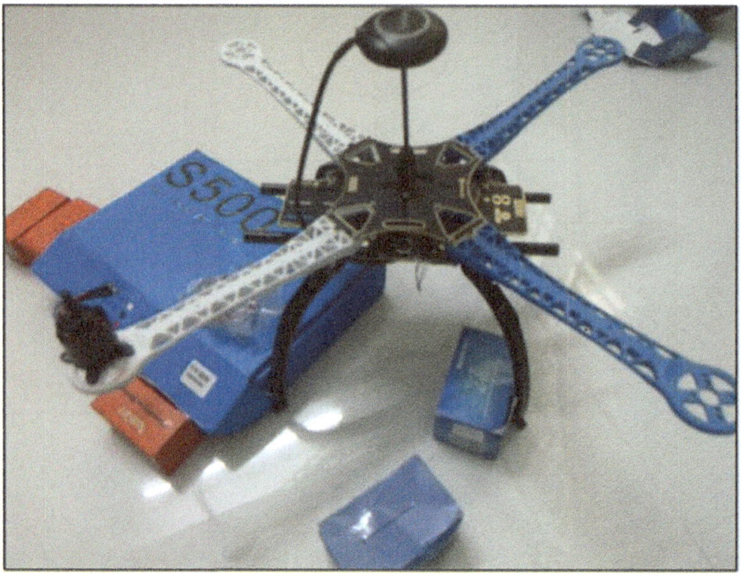

Fig. 3 Drone frame

Drone Propeller: It is attached on top of each brushless motor, giving it flight.

Brushless Motor: These are AC motors which give enables the drone to fly, in the quad-copter four motors are connected to the four propellers. The brushless motors used here is the Turnigy Multistar 2216–800 Kv Multi-Rotor Motor V2, these provide great thrust power for the drone.

ESC: It is known as Electronic Speed Controller which controls the speed of the brushless motors as shown in Fig. 4. Each brushless motor is connected to an ESC. The ESC used specifically for this drone is the 80 A ESC 2-6S Brushless.

PDB: This is the Power Distribution Board, which distributes the power coming from the flight battery to the different components attached to the drone. The power distribution board ensures safe transfer of power distributed among the brushless motors that are connected to the propellers.

Flight Controller: The flight controller is the brain of the drone system as shown in Fig. 5. The entire functionality of the drone is processed by this unit, which is placed on top of the Power Distribution Board. The flight control algorithm sends an output to the speed controllers (ESC) and in turn these speed controllers send an output to the motors.

GPS Module: The module used here is the NEO 8M GPS module. It gives the exact latitudinal and longitudinal coordinates to the server. It is very accurate and has less power consumption. It is required so as to know the exact location where an individual with a high temperature is detected and also if there are any large gatherings in a particular area.

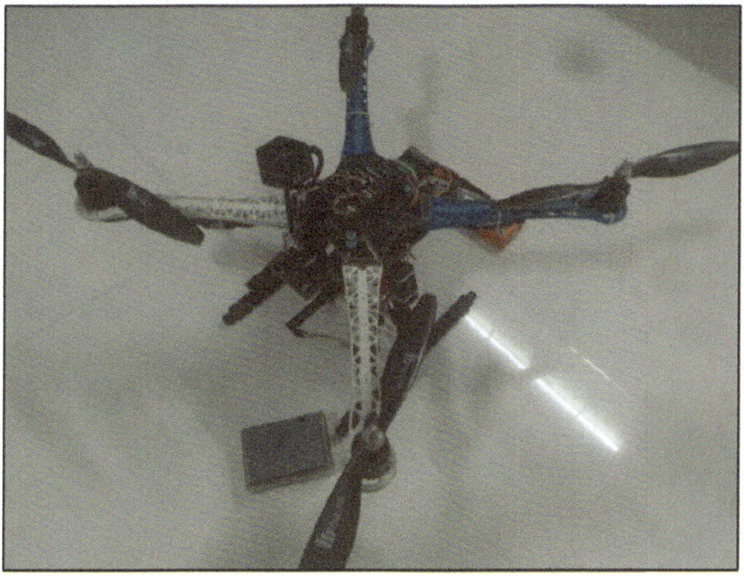

Fig. 4 Structure of the drone with drone propeller, brushless motors, ESC and Li-Po battery

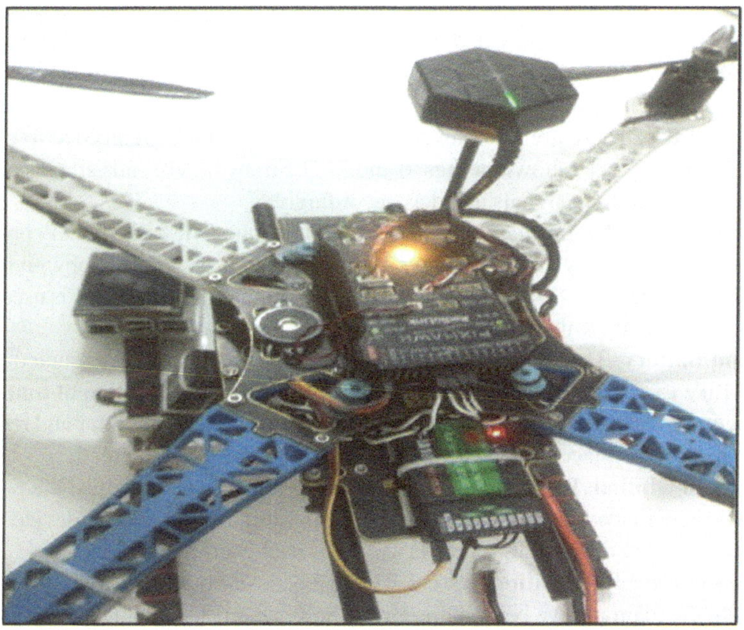

Fig. 5 Flight Controller and GPS module

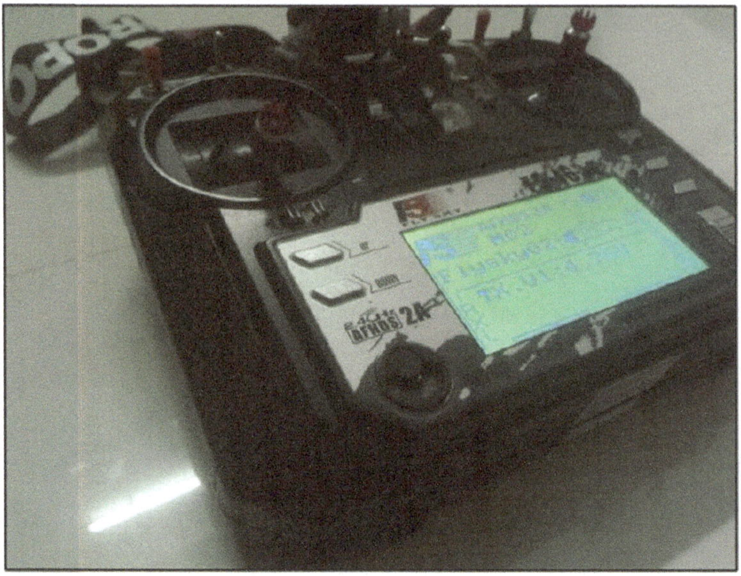

Fig. 6 Transmitter

VTX: It is known as the video transmitter. The video transmitter takes the feed from the camera and sends it over a wireless medium, this feed can be picked by goggles or screen on the receiver end.

TX and RX: These are the transmitter and receiver which are needed to control the flight of a drone as shown in Figs. 6 and 7. The transmitter sends signals and the receiver receives these signals and acts accordingly.

Li-Po Battery: It is the main power supply of the drone. The Li-Po battery provides a durable power supply and at the same time it is light in weight, thereby giving the drone more flight time. 8000 mAh 6S 25C/50C Lithium polymer battery is used here, which gives a flight time of about one hour.

Li-on Battery: This gives the power to the sensors and cameras mounted on the drone. Like Li-Po, it is light in weight and can run for a long duration of time.

Telemetry TX and RX: It used to transmit data from the transmitter and receiver. The transmitter is placed on the drone and the receiver can be a screen.

Camera Gimbal: It is a 3-axis brushless motor driver used to adjust the position of the camera placed on the drone. It is a 3-axis camera stabilization device which can adjust the up, down, left, right, forward and backward movements.

Temperature Recognition System: This is the most important part of the Drishya and fulfil the main motive behind this idea. The system is used to detect the temperature of people in the areas of surveillance. This temperature check is possible by using MLX90640 32 $\times$ 24 IR array which is a thermal IR camera which identifies the temperature of humans as shown in Fig. 8. It is a low resolution thermal camera.

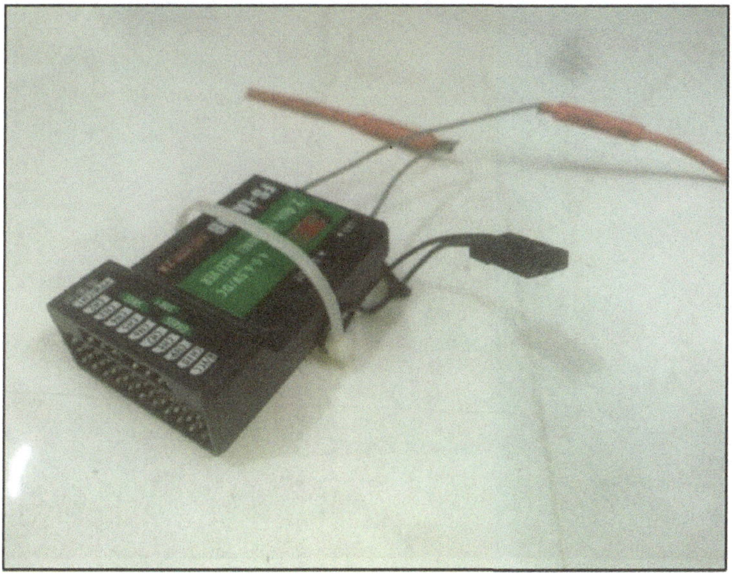

Fig. 7 Receiver

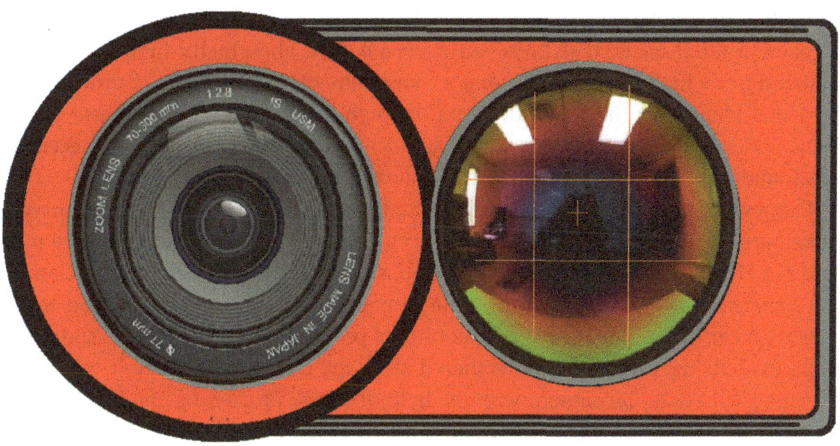

Fig. 8 A thermal IR camera and a high resolution camera module setup

Normally, high-end thermal cameras are high cost and use micro bolometer technology. But this IR camera uses a thermal file technology which has a lower SNR (Signal to Noise Ratio) and is most effective in determining the abnormalities in the temperature of an individual.

The test with other IR thermal cameras has been done, one is the MLX90614 and the other is the MLX90641, but MLX90640 has turned out to be the most accurate

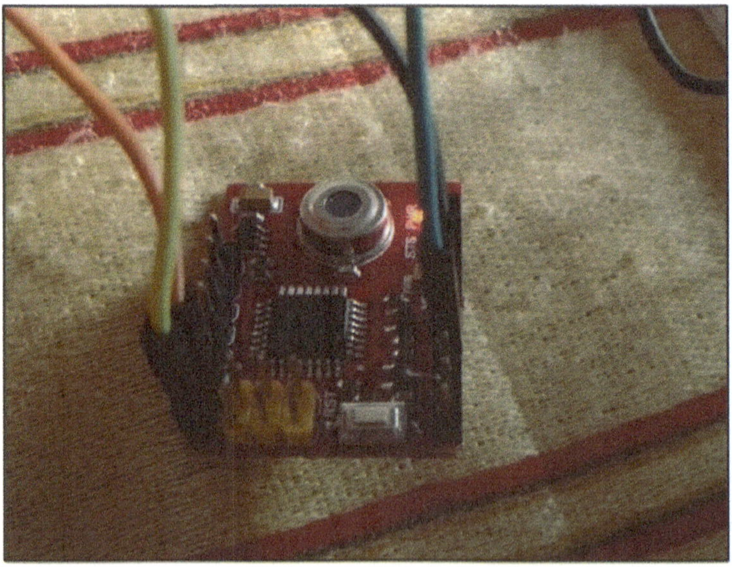

Fig. 9 A thermal IR camera and a high resolution camera module setup

of the three. Now when the drone is surveying any area and by using the thermal IR camera fitted on it, if it finds out a person with abnormally high (fever like) temperature, which is one of the major symptoms of COVID-19, the drone stores the facial identity of that individual via the high resolution camera present on the drone and simultaneously marks the exact location where the respective individual was found out and is sent to the server as shown in Fig. 9.

Camera: A high resolution camera is fitted on the drone which is used for surveillance purposes. It gives live feed of the occurence and incidents. The camera used here is a High Definition 1200TVL CMOS Camera with 2.8 mm Lens FPV Camera that enables crystal clear viewing. Using image processing algorithms fed to the camera, it can count and analyse the number of people gathered in an area and if that count exceeds the described norms then it alerts the base station about it.

Along with that, the camera with the help of image processing can calculate the distance between two individuals and if the distance to be found is less than the mentioned social distancing norms (1 m) it sends an alert to the base station.

Speaker: The drone is fitted with an audio system to make important announcements in areas under surveillance. The speaker is integrated with LM1875 which amplifies the sound output coming from the audio system and reduces noise interference, thereby enabling crystal clear audio while making important announcements. The main purpose of installing a speaker on the drone is to give alerts in case people are not following the social distancing norms or if there is a large crowd gathered in a certain area.

3.2 *Software Required*

Mission Planner: The machine planner software has been used to program the entire transmitter–receiver module so as to enable the flight control mechanism of the drone as shown in Fig. 10 and the design configuration as shown in Fig. 11.

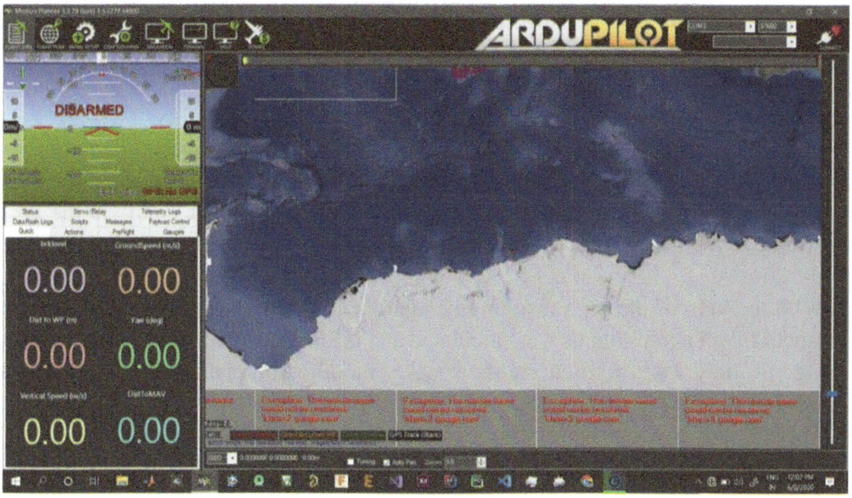

Fig. 10 Mission planner interface

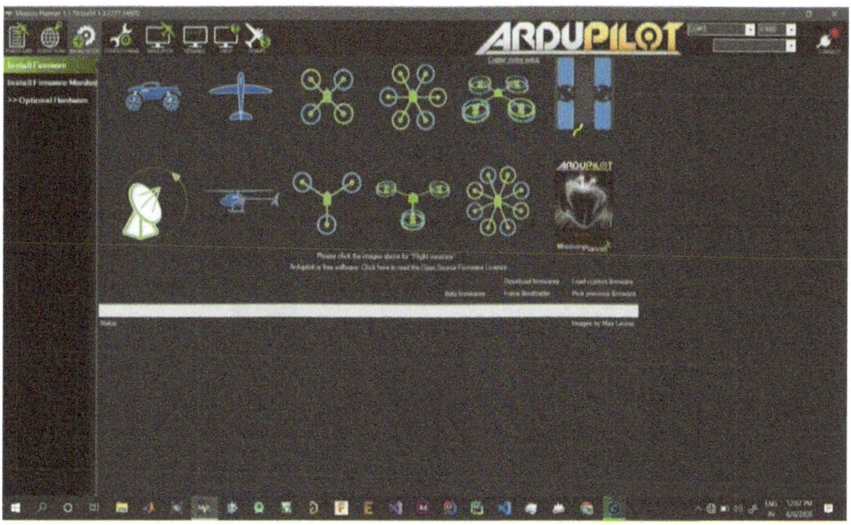

Fig. 11 Design configuration

Google Earth: As there is use of telemetry, Google earth has been a viable tool that was used tracking and tracing through the Google maps.

4 Results and Discussions

Our drone "Drishya" was capable of carrying the weight of all the cameras and speaker module. It recorded a flight time of 25 min via the available power supply of the battery. As shown in the Fig. 12 it was able to successfully survey and monitor market areas where a crowd formation has the maximum possibility.

The thermal IR camera was able to detect and monitor the heat signatures of individuals in an area and if a temperature above 96° Fahrenheit was detected, that particular body is indicated in orange colour as shown in Fig. 13 and via the high resolution camera an image of the individual's face and the location was sent to the base station.

With the help of the high resolution camera and image processing algorithm the distance between individuals was calculated and if found to be less than 3 feets shown in Fig. 14. they were notified via the speaker module and distanced themselves as shown in Fig. 15.

The following results were observed after the trial run of the overall module and recordings are as shown in Table 1.

- The recorded flight time of 25 min in a decent altitude which could be extended by supplying external battery was achieved.
- All the components worked perfectly during the time of testing.

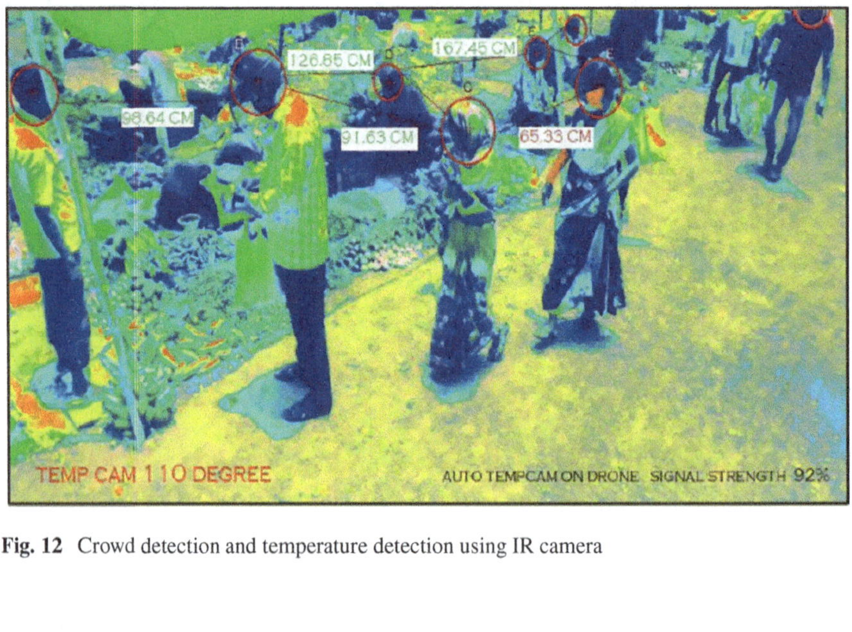

Fig. 12 Crowd detection and temperature detection using IR camera

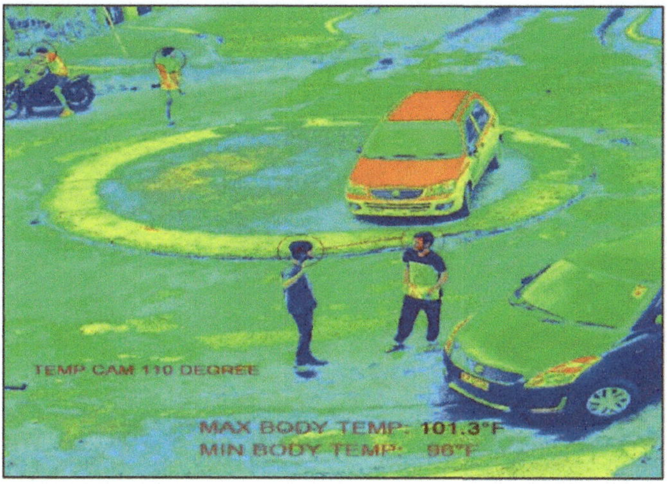

Fig. 13 Temperature detection

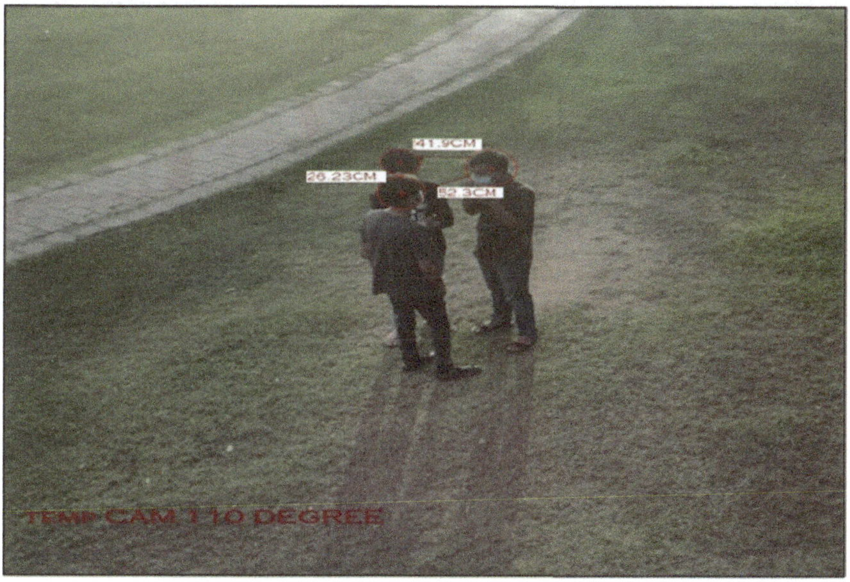

Fig. 14 Distance calculation using image processing

- Control from the base station was very easy and effective with no signal loss.
- The cameras had a good response and perfect picture quality video.
- Accuracy in crowd monitoring.

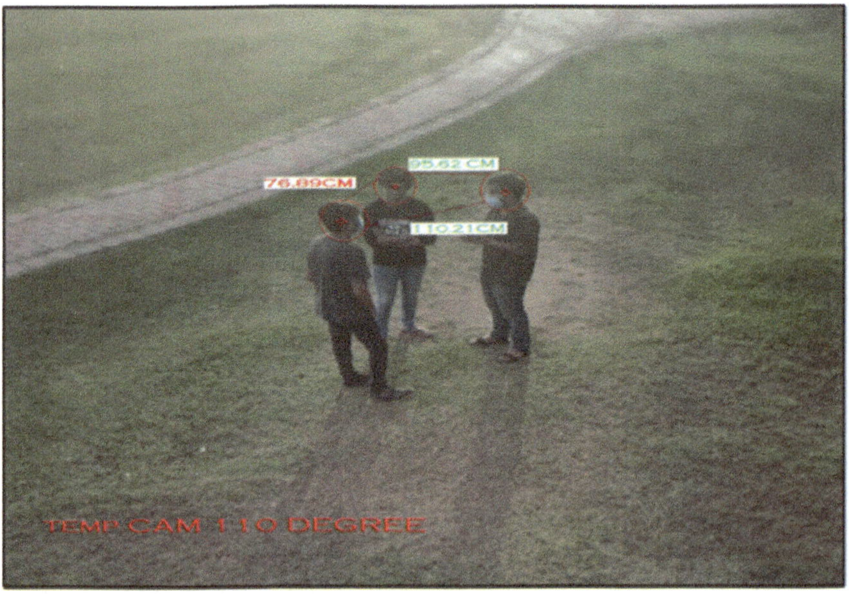

Fig. 15 Maintaining distance after alert

Table 1 Shows the flight time (min) with respect to the weight load (g) and distance travelled

S. no	Weight (g)	Flight time (min)	Distance (km)
1	500	66.9	53
2	750	44.6	36
3	1000	33.4	22
4	1500	22.3	13
5	1750	19.1	8

The load in terms of weight with respect to Time is shown in Fig. 16. It has been clearly understood that as the weight in grams increases, the flight time and distance gets decreased justifying the drone concept.

5 Conclusion

Considering the ongoing pandemic caused by the novel coronavirus, implementation of this drone-based tracking and surveillance system will help out the police in monitoring and managing the pandemic in order to avoid the spread of this virus. Our drone "Drishya" when implemented has the capability of detecting an individual with fever, which is one of the primary symptoms of this virus using a high accuracy thermal camera. This drone is also capable of determining the number of people in

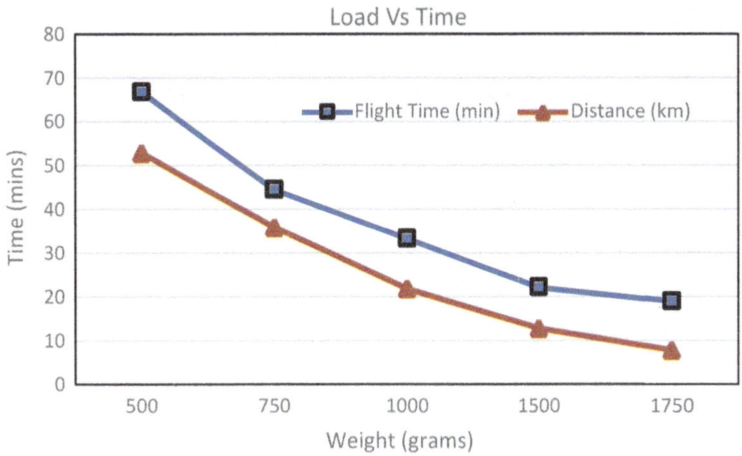

Fig. 16 Load over time

an area and if it exceeds the specified amount it notifies the base station, thereby breaking the chain so as to avoid forming of a cluster which is highly responsible for the spike in the number of cases. In addition to these, the proposed work and the drone can measure the distance between individuals so as to monitor whether the social distancing norms are being followed.

As drone technology will be ever-enduring and boundless, our proposed work can be modified and implemented from numerous points of view. In the event that in future a pandemic like the crown infection emerges, this drone technology can be applied with the necessary changes which will help mankind in battling future pandemics. At present the drone technology has just one charging station present at the base, however sooner rather than later there can be energizing stations set at different spots to charge the drones without any problem. With the consistently developing field of man-made consciousness, drones can be furnished with AI so that if the charge left in the automaton is less, it would itself be able to go to the closest charging station.

Our drone Drishya equipped with all technological advancements can prove to be revolutionary in our fight against the deadly coronavirus and other kinds of pandemic in the future. The drone can prove to be revolutionary in our fight against this deadly virus and also help out the corona warriors who are working day in and day out to eliminate this deadly virus from the world.

References

1. Zaheer, Z., Usmani, A., Khan, E., Qadeer, M.A.: Aerial surveillance system using UAV. In: IEEE Thirteenth International Conference on Wireless and Optical Communications Networks (WOCN), pp. 1–7 (2016)
2. Alwateer, M., Loke, S.W., Fernando, N.: Enabling drone services: drone crowdsourcing and drone scripting. IEEE Access **7** (2019)
3. Kim, S.J., Lim, G.J.: Drone-aided border surveillance with an electrification line battery charging system. J. Intell. Robot. Syst. **92**(3–4), 657–670 (2018)
4. Sarkar, S., Totaro, M.W., Elgazzar, K.: Intelligent drone-based surveillance: application to parking lot monitoring and detection. In: Unmanned Systems Technology XXI, vol. 11021, p. 1102104. International Society for Optics and Photonics (2019)
5. Kayan, H., Eslampanah, R., Yeganli, F., Askar, M.: Heat leakage detection and surveillance using aerial thermography drone. In: IEEE 26th Signal Processing and Communications Applications Conference (SIU), pp. 1–4 (2018)
6. Fallah-Haghmohammadi, H., Necsulecsu, D.-S.: Fever detection for dynamic human environment using sensor fusion. In: IEEE International Conference on Optimization of Electrical and Electronic Equipment (OPTIM) and 2017 International Aegean Conference on Electrical Machines and Power Electronics (ACEMP), pp. 881–886 (2017)
7. Tzelepi, M., Tefas, A.: Human crowd detection for drone flight safety using convolutional neural networks. In: IEEE 25th European Signal Processing Conference (EUSIPCO), pp. 743–747 (2017)
8. Küchhold, M., Simon, M., Eiselein, V., Sikora, T.: Scale-adaptive real-time crowd detection and counting for drone images. In: 25th IEEE International Conference on Image Processing (ICIP), pp. 943–947 (2018)
9. Chen, X., Zhai, G., Wang, J., Hu, C., Chen, Y.: Color guided thermal image super resolution. In: 2016 Visual Communications and Image Processing (VCIP), pp. 1–4 (2016)
10. Savitha, C., Ramesh, D.: Motion detection in video surveillance: a systematic survey. In: IEEE 2nd International Conference on Inventive Systems and Control (ICISC), pp. 51–54 (2018)
11. Hu, W., Tan, T., Wang, L., Maybank, S.: A survey on visual surveillance of object motion and behaviours. IEEE Trans. Syst. Man Cybern. Part C (Appl. Rev.) **34**(3), 334–352 (2004)
12. Ding, G., Wu, Q., Zhang, L., Lin, Y., Tsiftsis, T.A., Yao, Y.-D.: An amateur drone surveillance system based on the cognitive Internet of Things. IEEE Commun. Mag. **56**(1), 29–35 (2018)
13. Müller, T., Müller, M.: Vision-based drone flight control and crowd or riot analysis with efficient color histogram based tracking. In: Airborne Intelligence, Surveillance, Reconnaissance (ISR) Systems and Applications VIII, vol. 8020, p. 80200R. International Society for Optics and Photonics (2011)
14. Engberts, B., Gillissen, E.: Policing from above: drone use by the police. In: The Future of Drone Use, pp. 93–113. TMC Asser Press, The Hague (2016)
15. Somboonkaew, A., Prempree, P., Vuttivong, S., Wetcharungsri, J., Porntheeraphat, S., Chanhorm, S., Pongsoon, P. et al.: Mobile-platform for automatic fever screening system based on infrared forehead temperature. In: IEEE Opto-Electronics and Communications Conference (OECC) and Photonics Global Conference (PGC), pp. 1–4 (2017)
16. Vasudevan, S.K., Kowshik, G., Anudeep, J.: Driver feedback system with white line fever detection. In: IEEE International Conference on Vision Towards Emerging Trends in Communication and Networking (ViTECoN), pp. 1–6 (2019)
17. Van, L.P., De Praeter, J., Van Wallendael, G., De Cock, J., Van de Walle, R.: Machine learning for arbitrary downsizing of pre-encoded video in HEVC. In: IEEE International Conference on Consumer Electronics (ICCE), pp. 406–407 (2015)
18. Haghmohammadi, H.F., Necsulescu, D.S., Vahidi, M.: Remote measurement of body temperature for an indoor moving crowd. In: IEEE International Conference on Automation, Quality and Testing, Robotics (AQTR), pp. 1–6 (2018)

19. Manekiya, M.H., Arulmozhivarman, P.: Leakage detection and estimation using IR thermography. In: IEEE International Conference on Communication and Signal Processing (ICCSP), pp. 1516–1519 (2016)
20. Medjeldi, T., Guillemette, S.: Wireless system for detecting human temperature. In: IEEE Science and Information Conference, pp. 156–159 (2013)
21. Song, K.-S., Nho, Y.-H., Kwon, D.-S.: Histogram based fall prediction of patients using a thermal imagery camera. In: IEEE 14th International Conference on Ubiquitous Robots and Ambient Intelligence (URAI), pp. 161–164 (2017)
22. Malarić, K., Malarić, R., Herceg, J.: Measurement of temperature inside open TEM-cell with thermal camera. In: 25th International Conference on Software, Telecommunications and Computer Networks (SoftCOM), Split, pp. 1–5 (2017)
23. Yong, S.P., Yeong, Y.-C.: Human object detection in forest with deep learning based on drone's vision. In: IEEE 4th International Conference on Computer and Information Sciences (ICCOINS), pp. 1–5 (2018)
24. Krishna, S.L., Chaitanya, G.S.R., Reddy, A.S.H., Naidu, A.M., Poorna, S.S., Anuraj, K.: Autonomous human detection system mounted on a drone. In: IEEE International Conference on Wireless Communications Signal Processing and Networking (WiSPNET), pp. 335–338 (2019)
25. Tariq, R., Rahim, M., Aslam, N., Bawany, N., Faseeha, U.: Dronaid: a smart human detection drone for rescue. In: IEEE 15th International Conference on Smart Cities: Improving Quality of Life Using ICT and IoT (HONET-ICT), pp. 33–37 (2018)
26. Kim, S., Lee, W., Yim, J., Park, Y.-S., Lee, Y.-T.: Human monitoring system using drones for riverside area. In: IEEE International Conference on Information and Communication Technology Convergence (ICTC), pp. 1054–1057 (2017)
27. Cheng, Z., West, R., Einstein, C.: End-to-end analysis and design of a drone flight controller. IEEE Trans. Comput. Aided Des. Integr. Circuits Syst. **37**(11), 2404–2415 (2018)
28. Saha, A., Kumar, A., Sahu, A.K.: FPV drone with GPS used for surveillance in remote areas. In: IEEE Third International Conference on Research in Computational Intelligence and Communication Networks (ICRCICN), pp. 62–67 (2017)
29. Yazawa, R., Matsuura, M.: Flight demonstration of power-over-fiber drone for airborne base stations. In: IEEE 23rd Opto-Electronics and Communications Conference (OECC), pp. 1–2 (2018)
30. Kim, J., Lee, Y.S., Han, S.S., Kim, S.H., Lee, G.H., Ji, H.J., Choi, H.J., Choi, K.N.: Autonomous flight system using marker recognition on drone. In: IEEE 21st Korea–Japan Joint Workshop on Frontiers of Computer Vision (FCV), pp. 1–4 (2015)
31. Venugopalan, T.K., Taher, T., Barbastathis, G.: Autonomous landing of an unmanned aerial vehicle on an autonomous marine vehicle. In: IEEE Oceans, pp. 1–9 (2012)

Development of Algorithm for Precise Movement Controller for Robotic Arm

S. Lalithakumari and R. Pandian

Abstract Robotics and automation play a vital role all around and it emerges in the medical field also. Movement control of the robot moved well beyond its conventional uses in manufacturing. Medical devices, automotive robotics electronic gadgets benefited from motion control subsystems due to the advantages such as less cost, power saving. The critical elements are complexity of the electronics and embedded software for motion control. It is very essential to care about the proper accuracy and precision. Many research works have been implemented in order to achieve the accuracy and precision. But maintaining the precision of the movements of medical robotic arm controller is a challenging task. This work addresses this problem and enumerates a suitable proposed work in order to overcome this. The suitability of the proposed work, which employs Image processing, Deep learning network is well authenticated by developing a hardware model.

Keywords Robot · Medical image · Deep learning · End effector · Sensors

1 Introduction

Robots are automated machines which can be programmable, and they can be made to carry out complex tasks with minimal human interventions. Many robotic arm-based scanning devices are used in industries in order to achieve the automatic scanning process. Robotics and automation play a vital role all around and it emerges in the medical field also. Movement control of the robot moved well beyond its conventional uses in manufacturing. Medical devices, automotive robotics electronic gadgets benefited from motion control subsystems due to the advantages such as less cost, power saving. The critical elements are complexity of the electronics and embedded software for motion control. It is very essential to care about the proper accuracy and precision. As per the recent report by Credence Research, the global medical robotics market costing \$7.24 billion in 2015 and is expected to elevate

S. Lalithakumari (✉) · R. Pandian
Department of EIE, Sathyabama Institute of Science and Technology, Chennai, India
e-mail: lalithavengat@gmail.com

H. K. Tripathy et al. (eds.), *Technical Advancements of Machine Learning in Healthcare*, Studies in Computational Intelligence 936,
https://doi.org/10.1007/978-981-33-4698-7_16

$20 billion by 2023. This is due to the heavy demand in the usage of robots in minimally invasive surgeries, especially for neurologic, orthopedic, and laparoscopic procedures. Wide variety of robots are used in human treatment include surgical robots and rehabilitation robots. Usage of Assistive and therapeutic robotic devices rapidly increasing. Robots can also be used for telemedicine, surgical assistances, Rehabilitation, Medical Transportation, and to make Sanitation and Disinfection. This proposed work aims to design and fabricate robotic arm to complete an automatic scanning. For example, Ultrasonic NDT is used in many industries for checking the material discontinuity and weld defects. Automatic scanning is only done in the ultrasonic method in order to avoid manual scanning, this proposed work aims to develop automated ultrasonic scanning robot is to reduce the human interaction in the scanning process which can be a time taking process for acquiring signals. Similarly, many fabrication industries require such an automatic scanning robot. Different kind of scanning devices has been used, but end effector is present in all the devices, in order to carry any device like probes, cutting tool, assembly tool. The robotic end effector must be designed such a way of moving across the object, automatically. The control of movement and direction is provided by an Arduino based on robotic arm control system. To achieve the task, it is necessary to move the probe across the platform.

Many works have been done in the past regarding automatic movement. Wu et al. [1] have proposed an automatic model-based path planning method for surface inspection on a robot-based scanning system. The scanning system consists of a 6 degree of freedom robot and a coded structured light scanner. The method which has been used in this paper consist of four steps: model framework extraction, scan region segmentation, viewpoint generation, and scan path generation. The method which has been used in this paper can achieve high-precision and efficiency for surface inspection on a robot-based scanning system. The planned path has been linked by a group of viewpoints from which the scanner can detect the full features of the object. The scanning system which has been used in this paper consist of 6 degree of freedom. The scanner is mounted on the end of the robot. The followed four coordinate systems, i.e. robot base coordinate system, robot end coordinate system, scanner coordinate system, and object coordinate. Appelgren et al. [2] have proposed a standard six-axis industrial robot. The test for metal deposition has been done with automated ET and UT through a standard robot. In this paper evaluation of UT test has been performed by sending the ultrasonic signal and robot position into MATLAB and calculated a C-scan image. This paper has mainly focused, if standard six-axis robot can replace linear axis type and which method to be used for metal deposition. Polikar et al. [3] have proposed method of analysis of ultrasonic NDE signals obtained during weld inspection of piping in boiling water reactors. Ultrasonic method of non-destructive testing has been used in weld inspection of boiling water reactor piping for detecting corrosion cracking in this paper. Two different databases namely LMT database and EPRI database of ultrasonic weld inspection signals that have been used to evaluate the performance of the overall signals. Stubbs et al. [4] have proposed a traditional x, y, z immersion C-Scan system which is similar to most traditional ultrasonic immersion C-scan systems. They have proposed a standard six-axis industrial robot with

UDRI improvements. In this paper digital camera has been picked up by the robot in order to image the test object. A new, unique, automated ultrasonic inspection system has been designed that incorporates new, off-the-shelf technologies and components. These components have been developed for other applications but can be integrated into NDT systems. They have designed and constructed a fully automated ultrasonic inspection system for the detection of embedded defects in rotating gas turbine engine components. The improvements which have been done to the components compared to previous one is six-axis robot as the mechanical manipulator. Movement speed is more per second compare to previous one. Graphical user interface, accuracy has been improved. Mineo et al. [5] have proposed an industrial six-axis robot positioner to perform c-scanning of two test coupons one steel, and other CFRP. An application of a six degree of freedom robotic positioner (KUKA KR5 Arc HW) for automated NDT by means of multiple inspection techniques has been present. A PC has been used to interface and control both ultrasonic data acquisition, and an industrial robot controller. For inspection of smaller components, conventional industrial six-axis robotic positioner has been used. Ultrasonic scanning of simple geometry has been demonstrated. A post-processing MATLAB script has been developed to evaluate the amplitude and/or the time-of-flight (TOF) of the acquired UT waveforms. Solis et al. [6] have proposed ultrasound probe manipulator WTA-1RII which composed by master–slave robotic system for assuring a precise positioning of the probe also they have introduced an automated scanning algorithm by the feedback control based on ultrasound image processing in real time. The probe holding robot contains 6 degree of freedom parallel link manipulator which hold ultrasonic probe, 6 degree of freedom serial link passive arm which holds whole manipulator, and master controller. Mineo et al. [7] have proposed industrial 6-axis manipulators through an external pc, running the developed software, to generate NDT path-tools. A KUKA KR16 L6-2 robot has been used for the purpose of inspecting surface. They have developed NDT robot toolbox which ultimately assist NDT technicians to move from a component CAD file to the actual physical inspection, without the need to use multiple pieces of software not optimized for robotic NDT inspections. Xiao et al. [8] have proposed a six degrees of freedom industrial robot in order to hold the non-destructive testing (NDT) probe normal to the test surface, and also ultrasonic time-domain reflectometry (UTDR) which has been used to identify the flaw echo. NDT data has been acquired at a scanning speed of up to 50 mm/s. The ultrasonic signals have been acquired synchronously with positional data regarding the robot. Mineo et al. [9] have proposed a 6-axis robot for deployment of NDT probes for inspection purpose. They have developed a high-level custom toolbox that utilizes external control of industrial 6-axis manipulator to achieve complex path planning and provide synchronization of the employed ultrasonic phase array inspection system. For inspection system two KUKA KR16 L6-2 robot arm has been used which has payload capacity of 6 kg, with maximum speed of 2 m/s.

Reshamwala et al. [10] applied a thought behind fabricating the robot for teaching human exertion. Basically, a two-sectioned robot arm is proposed with haptic glove and a robot arm. Haptic gadgets must be littler so they are lighter, more straightforward and simpler to utilize. Szabo et al. [11] proposed a technique for a 5 DoF automated arm. The automated arm has 5 servomotors and designed with an additional servo motor to rotate the gripper. The automated arm has an SSC-32 control board, which could control every one of the engines. The control board has employed an ATmega168 microcontroller which directions on RS-232 interface with a PC will control the engines. The microcontroller gets explicit directions which can be deciphered and can control the engines along these lines to move the mechanical arm. Huang et al. [12] proposed and control of the automated arm, whose framework is joined with a binocular vision framework for the holding plate. Utilizing 8052 MCU of Atmel arrangement controls particularly all the axes of the robotic arms. Their experimental results reveal that the developed system of dual robotic arms can get organizes from binocular vision and hold the payload. Szabo et al. [13] designed an automated arm control technique with stereo vision, with two cameras. They adopted a stereo separation computation to realize how much development does the automated arm needs at the base joint. Bassily et al. [14] elucidated a build up of a human–machine correspondence interface between the Leap Motion controller and the 6-DOF Jaco automated arm. An algorithm was also proposed to map between the client hand developments, followed by the Leap Motion controller. The framework ought to take into account a progressively regular human–PC association and a smooth control of the automated arm. From these literatures, it is understood that a proper hardware must be associated with a dedicated control system in order to achieve a perfect robotic arm controller. Chapter 2 explains a suitable hardware and software requirements. Results and discussion are explained in Chap. 3 and this research work is concluded in Chap. 4.

2 Hardware Requirements

In this proposed system, an ultrasonic signal acquirement, using the robotic arm scanner is proposed. The hardware requirements of the proposed system essentially consisting of a robotic end effector is used with 5 degrees of freedom. Each movement is associated with 5 servo motors. One servo motor is dedicated to the circular motion up and down movements are controlled by 2 motors. Arm and gripper are actuated by one motor individually. Driver control units are also assembled in order to provide proper control of motors. Arduino Uno is used for the control of the movements. The entire platform is moved with the help of L298 motor driver. Two position sensors are also used for beginning and endpoints, respectively. The gripper is designed in such a way that, it can hold camera or ultrasonic probe at one particular instant of time. A Raspberry pi is used to send and receive the acquired images and video remotely. Provision has been given to acquire the data from both Ethernet cable and Wi-Fi. Two SMPS are used to energize the hardware module. Once the UT signals are acquired from the automated scanning system, they are undergone signal analysis techniques.

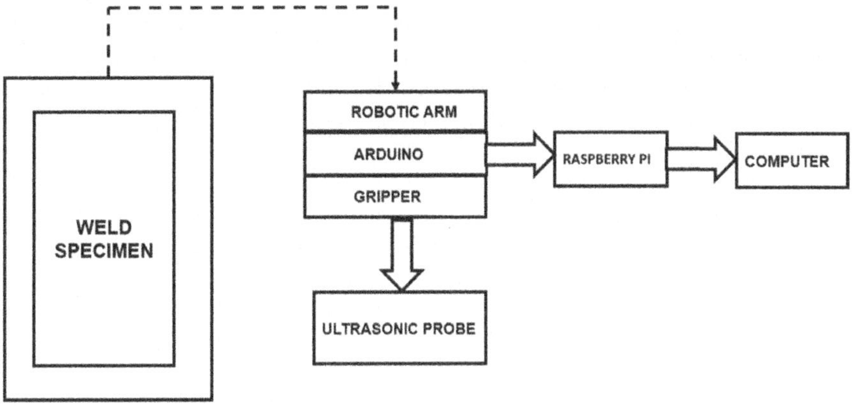

Fig. 1 Block diagram of proposed work

The proposed circuit diagram is shown in Fig. 1. The speed of automated arm for scanning can be controlled by two switches. The scanning direction can also be controlled by another two switches. These switch inputs are given to Arduino. The logical output from Arduino is given to the motor driver circuit and thus the motor's movements are being controlled. The gripper is designed in such a way that the UT probe is also connected to it and the ultrasonic signals can be acquired.

The end effector is shown in Fig. 5. It is capable of rotating five different joints. Five servo motors are connected to achieve the operation. The joints of the end effector perform the rotations in circular motion, up-down movements, arm rotation, and gripper. Servo motors used in this work has inbuilt servo controllers. The gripper attached to this end effector is used to hold either the camera or ultrasonic probe. Two position sensors are used in this work, for sensing the beginning and end positions of scanning. A position sensor is any device used for measuring the distance traveled by a body starting from its reference positions. It measures linear or angular position in reference to a fixed point or arbitrary reference. The sensor can also be used to detect the presence or absence of an object. Here, the signals from the beginning position sensor and activate the end effector. The type of position sensor also dictates its working principle. The Arduino Uno R3 is a microcontroller board based on a removable, dual in-line-package (DIP) ATmega328 AVR microcontroller. It has 20 digital input/output pins (of which 6 can be used as PWM outputs and 6 can be used as analog inputs). Programs can be loaded on to it from the easy-to-use ARDUINO computer program. The ARDUINO has an extensive support community, which makes it a very easy way to get started working with embedded electronics. The R3 is the third, and latest, revision of the ARDUINO UNO.

The ARDUINO UNO is a microcontroller board based on the ATmega328. It has 20 digital input/output pins (of which 6 can be used as PWM outputs and 6 can be used as analog inputs), a 16 MHz resonator, a USB connection, a power jack, an in-circuit system programming (ICSP) header, and a reset button. It contains everything needed to support the microcontroller; simply connect it to a computer with a USB cable or power it with a AC to DC Adapter or battery to get started. The UNO differs from all preceding boards in that it does not use the FTDI USB-to-serial driver chip. Instead, it features an ATmega16U2 programmed as a USB-to-serial converter. This auxiliary microcontroller has its own USB boot loader, which allows advanced users to reprogram it. The ARDUINO has a large support community and an extensive set of support libraries and hardware add-on "shields" (e.g. you can easily make your Arduino wireless with our Wixel shield), making it a great introductory platform for embedded electronics. Note that we also offer a Spark Fun Inventor's Kit, which includes an Arduino Uno along with an assortment of components (e.g. breadboard, sensors, jumper wires, and LEDs) that make it possible to create a number of fun introductory projects. This is the 3rd revision of the UNO (R3), which has a number of changes: The USB controller chip changed from ATmega8U2 (8 K flash) to ATmega16U2 (16 K flash). This does not increase the flash or RAM available to sketches. Three new pins were added, all of which are duplicates of previous pins. The I2C pins (A4, A5) have also been brought out on the side of the board near AREF. There is a IOREF pin next to the reset pin, which is a duplicate of the 5 V pin. The reset button is now next to the USB connector, making it more accessible when a shield is used. The execution of the proposed work is elucidated in chapter.

3 Result and Discussion

The proposed work is executed as per the process flow diagram, which is shown in Fig. 2. The gripper and the camera are connected to the end effector and the corresponding ultrasonic signal values and the captured images are acquired and transmitted in wireless mode through Raspberry pi. The image and signals are read and it can be processed in MATLAB if needed.

Linear Movement Of the Robot Flow Chart is shown below, which describes the movement of the robot (Fig. 3).

The selection of limit switch enables the start and endpoint for scanning. The forward and backward movements are carried over as per the On and Off positions of the switches. If we need to have some delay at the source and destination points can also be achieved by the delay set option. The Robotic Arm Movement flow chart is shown in Fig. 4. The arm movements of the robot can be precisely controlled by the proper control of motors, which are explained in the chart.

The end effector and gripper are shown in Fig. 5.

It is capable of rotating five different joints. Five servo motors are connected to achieve the operation. The joints of the end effector perform the rotations in circular motion, up-down movements, arm rotation, and gripper. Servo motors used in this work has inbuilt servo controllers. The gripper attached to this end effector is used to hold either the camera or ultrasonic probe.

Two position sensors are used in this work, for sensing the beginning and end positions of scanning. A position sensor is any device used for measuring the distance traveled by a body starting from its reference positions. It measures linear or angular

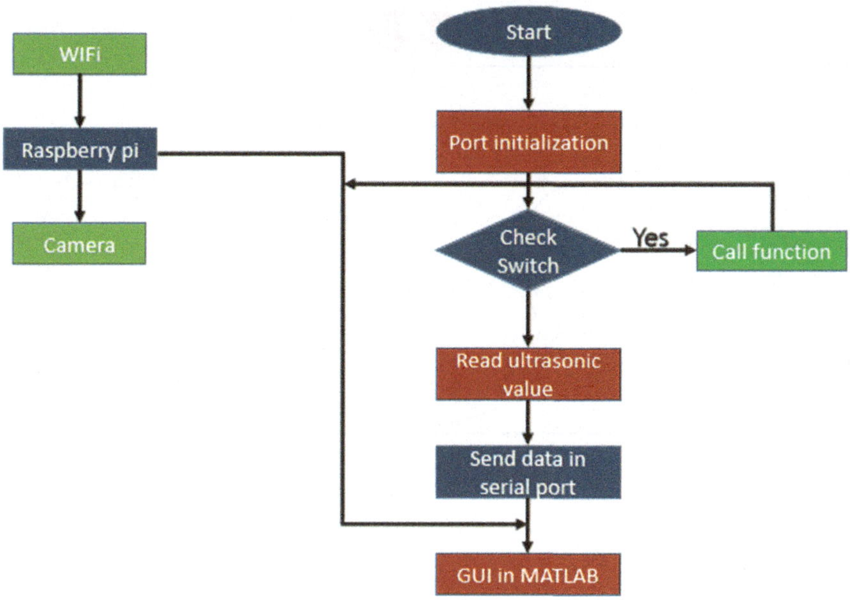

Fig. 2 Process flow diagram

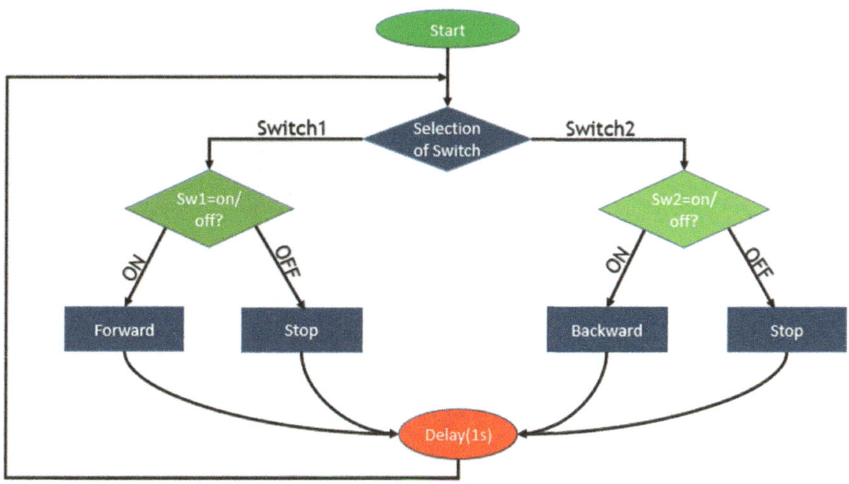

Fig. 3 Linear movement of the robot flow chart

position in reference to a fixed point or arbitrary reference. The sensors can also be used to detect the presence or absence of an object. Here, the signals from the beginning position sensor and activate the end effector. The type of position sensor also dictates its working principle. They are shown in Fig. 6.

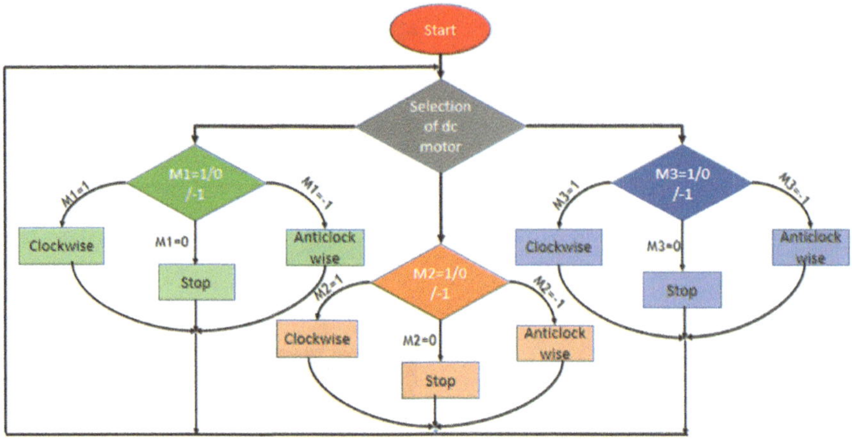

Fig. 4 Robotic Arm movement flow chart

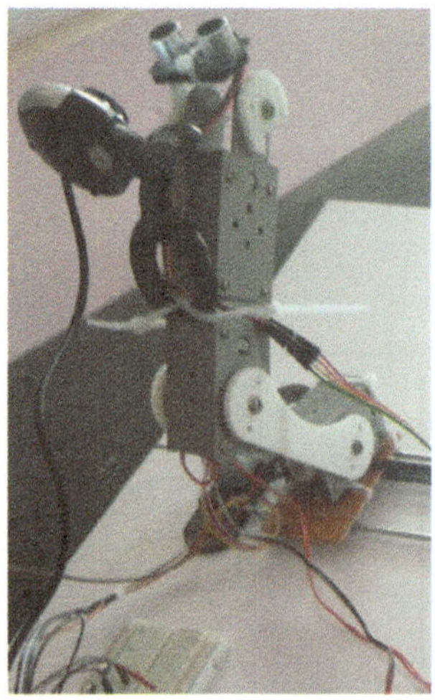

Fig. 5 End effector and gripper

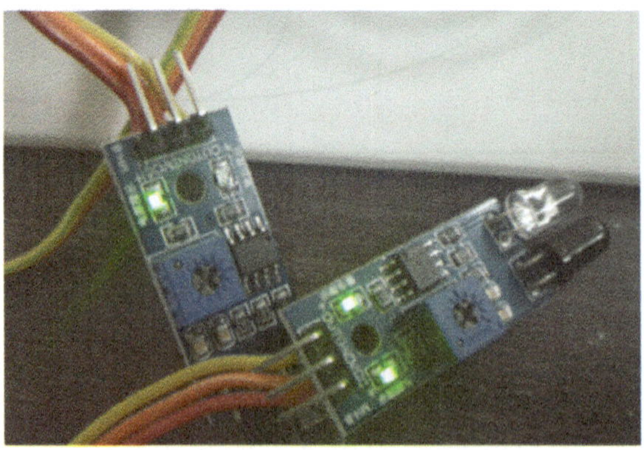

Fig. 6 Position sensors

Fig. 7 Platform

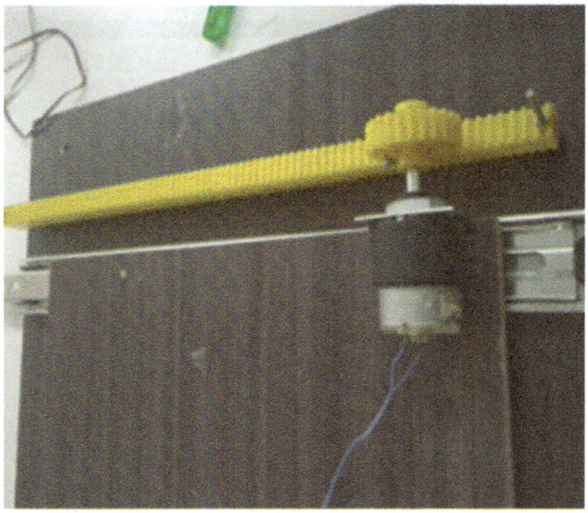

The end effector is designed in such a way to move on the platforms. It is a gear drive-based platform which is shown in Fig. 7.

The model of the robot is shown in Fig. 8.

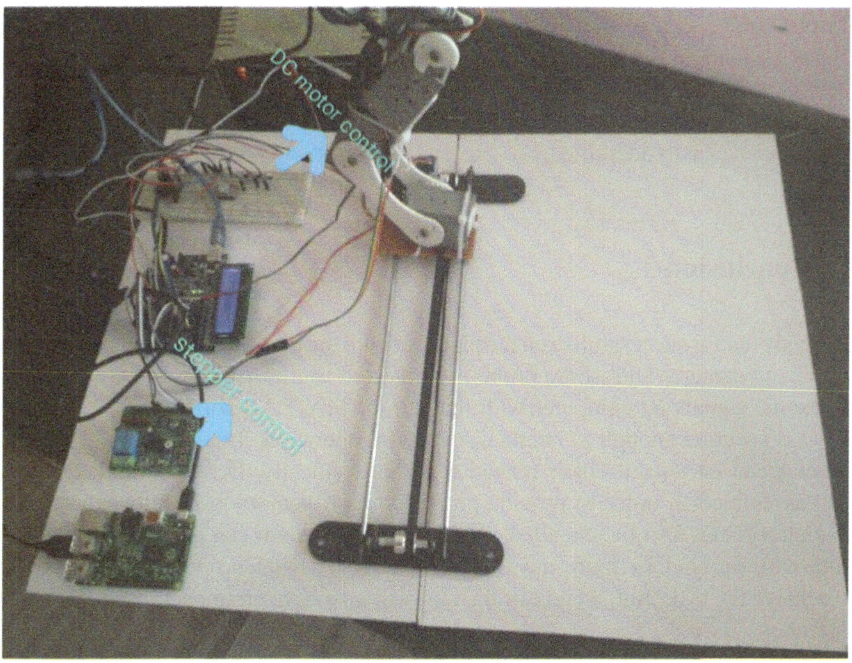

Fig. 8 Model of the robot

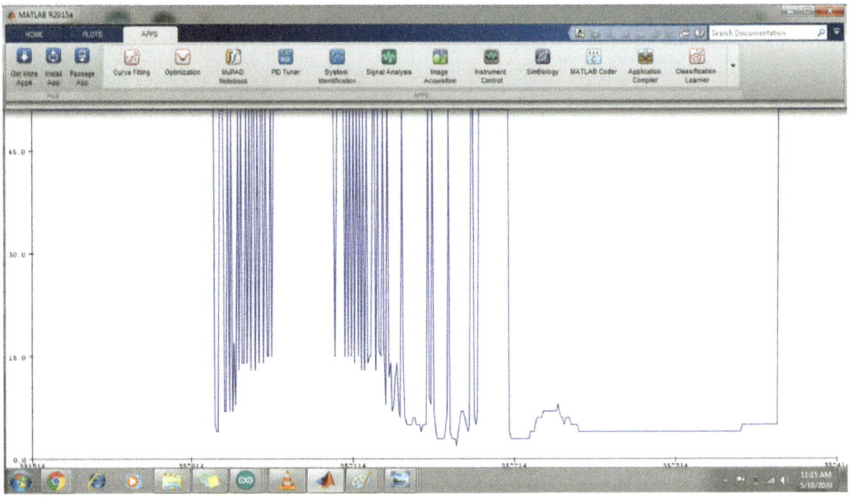

Fig. 9 Ultrasonic signal acquired from automatic robot scanner

After the completion of the hardware fabrication, the robotic arm is moved in the platform. The ultrasonic probe is fixed in the gripper and the arm is moved across the surface, which is to be inspected. The acquired signal is transmitted through the Raspberry pi and it is visually displayed in the computer. The acquired ultrasonic signal is shown in Fig. 9.

The acquired ultrasonic signal can be further analyzed using any suitable computer-based analysis techniques. The discontinuity in the inspected surface or object can be easily identified.

4 Conclusion

The end effector successfully run the platform with the gripper carrying the ultrasonic probe and camera. Ultrasonic probe is connected to the Arduino board to acquire ultrasonic signals on computer with the help of MATLAB software. The Arduino UNO is accurate enough to obtain a successful operation. The positions of the end effector can be altered either manually or automatically. Driver control units are also assembled in order to provide proper control of motors. In future the length of platform can also be extended, and degree of freedom can also be increased to improve the model. In future, any tool can be attached to the proposed model in order to achieve the task. But, weight of the tool will also have an impact of the design of the robot.

References

1. Wu, Q., Lu, J., Zou, W., Xu,D.:Path planning for surface inspection on a robot-based scanning system. In: 2015 IEEE International Conference on Mechatronics and Automation (ICMA), Beijing, pp. 2284–2289 (2015)
2. Appelgren, A. et al.: Automatic ultrasonic testing for metal deposition. In: 18th World Conference on Nondestructive Testing, 16–20 April 2012, Durban, SouthAfric
3. Polikar, R., Udpa, L., Udpa, S. S., Taylor, T.:Frequency invariant classification of ultrasonic weld inspection signals.In: IEEE Transactions on Ultrasonics, Ferroelectrics, and Frequency Control, vol. 45, no. 3, pp. 614–625
4. Stubbs, D. et al.: An automated ultrasonic system for inspection of aircraft turbine engine components. University Of Dayton, OH, USA (2005)
5. Mineo, C. et al.: Robotic non-destructive inspection. Bndtiseptember, 2012, University of Strathclyde, UK.Proceedings of a Meeting Held 11–13 September 2012, Northamptonshire, UK, Red Hook
6. Solis, J. et al.: Develoment of the ultrasound probe holding robot wta-1RII and an automated scanning algorithm based on ultrasound image effect. CISM **524**
7. Mineo, C. et al.: Robotic path planning for non-destructive testing-a custom matlab toolbox approach. **37** (2016)
8. Xiao, Z. et al.: An optimized robotic scanning scheme for ultrasonic ndt of complex structures. Exp. Techn. **41** (2017)
9. Mineo, C. et al.: Robotic path planning for ndt of complex shaped surfaces. QNDE Conf. U.S.A. (2014)
10. Reshamwala, A., Singh, R.: A review on robot Arm using haptic technology. In: Internationa-Journal of Advanced Research in Electrical, Electronics and Instrumentation Engineering, vol. 4, Issue. 4 (2015)
11. Szabo, R., Gontean, A.: Remotely commanding the lynxmotion AL5 type robotic arms. Telecommun. Forum (TELFOR), pp. 889–892 (2013)
12. Huang, G.-S., Chen, X.-S., Chang, C.-L.: Development of dual robotic arm system based on binocular vision. In: Automatic Control Conference (CACS), CACS International, pp. 97–102 (2013)
13. Szabo, R., Gontean, A.: Robotic arm control in 3D space using stereo distance calculation. In: International Conference on Development and Application Systems (DAS), pp. 50–56 (2014)
14. Bassily, D., Georgoulas, C., Güttler, J., Linner, T., Bock, T.: TU Munchen and Germany, Intuitive and Adaptive Robotic Arm Manipulation Using the Leap Motion Controller. Conference ISR ROBOTIK, pp. 1–7 (2014)

Scope of Medical Bots in Clinical Domain

Deep Mukherjee, Hrudaya Kumar Tripathy, and Sushruta Mishra

Abstract There is no question that Medical Science has come very far over the past 5 years but still when any human treats any patient there is always a chance of human error. This lead to the use of artificial intelligence combined with medical robots to make them smarter and error-free to reduce the mishaps caused by the doctors. Now not only getting health care has become safer but also has solved the problem of hospitals being understaffed. The chapter consists of a basic introduction of medical bots about why they came into existence and their features. It also gives a vivid description about what is artificial intelligence and how it is being used together with machines to make them perform better. The chapter then explains the types of medical bots available out there in the world and we have made a broad classification of the types of medical bots. Discussion of the types with examples and their need is thoroughly explained in the later part of the chapter. We then discuss the ongoing projects and current development going on in this field with examples. We further discuss the key technologies used or present in the world which are helping to make better bots for this industry. Lastly we discussed the major challenges faced by the scientists in this challenging field which makes it even difficult to achieve.

Keywords AI · Medical bots · Machine learning · Medical bots

D. Mukherjee (✉) · H. K. Tripathy · S. Mishra
B. Tech in Computer Science and Systems Engineering-2021, KIIT University,, Bhubaneswar, India
e-mail: deep.mukherjee02@gmail.com

H. K. Tripathy
e-mail: hktripathyfcs@kiit.ac.in

S. Mishra
e-mail: sushruta.mishrafcs@kiit.ac.in

H. K. Tripathy et al. (eds.), *Technical Advancements of Machine Learning in Healthcare*, Studies in Computational Intelligence 936,
https://doi.org/10.1007/978-981-33-4698-7_17

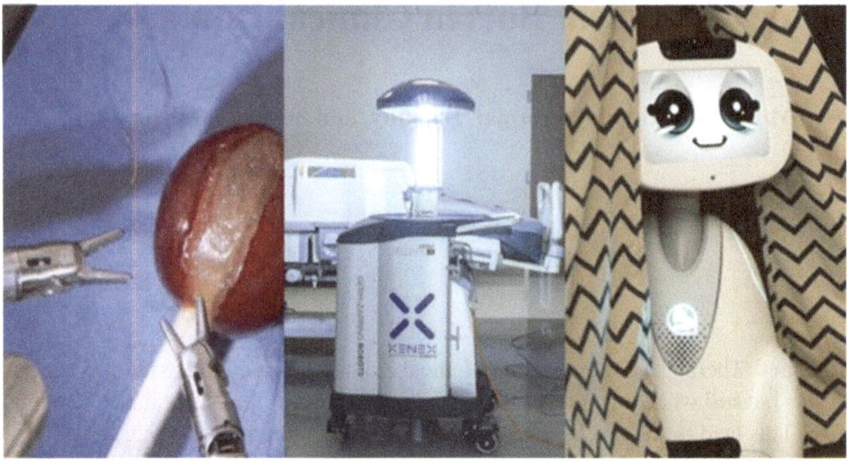

Fig. 1 A sample illustration of bots in the market

1 Introduction

Medical bots, devices in the medical field which has revolutionized the way we look forward to hospitals. They are not only one of the most extreme field in Medical Science but also undoubtedly one of the hardest. They have allowed the doctors to operate from a remote location, predict epidemics, and to increase the efficiency and accuracy of the way things work in this field. They are being also used in drug discoveries and have made available to quick need of professional medical expertise.

This field was introduced to the science of medicine during the early 1980s. This started with the introduction of robotic arms to perform surgeries with uncanny precision but due to lack of proper imaging technology this field was constrained until this decade where unimaginable technological advancements has made medical bots fairly easier to experiment with.

This field is still being constantly upgraded with the far more advance equipment to achieve the perfect bot which can one day sure to replace the humans as doctors. Figure 1 shows a sample illustration of medical bot.

2 Current Robotic Perception Trend

The current scenario is now prioritizing the use of networks to learn models with a huge amount of data with a single hidden layer and the sigmoid activation function to train the model to provide a boundary for the other models with a deeper network to compare them for improvements. Other functions like tanh or leaky rectifiers can be used to improve the training time and accuracy by reducing the effect of one of the major problems of deeper networks-diminishing gradient by using simpler monotonic derivatives [1]. Another major problem with the deeper networks is their tendency to overfit. To tackle this problem another technique has been developed—regularization. This method helps to make the models become robust against promotion sparsity and also weight saturation [2].

There are many regularization techniques that were specifically made to tackle the problems of the autoencoders. A common method to tackle is to use alternating layers of pooling and convolution layers. The pooling layers help to reduce the dimension and the number of trainable parameters which in return helps to regularize the model [3]. This is also known as implicit regularization which is by default present in any network. Another effective method is Batch Normalization which helps to significantly improve the rate of convergence. Residual networks like Resnets also helps to travel deeper into the network without facing the diminishing gradient problem [4].

3 Machine Learning Usage in Training Robotic System Perception

One of the most important differences between machine learning and deep learning is that although deep learning is a subset of machine learning deep learning is better when it comes to think rather than act like an algorithm. Deep learning is generally better when it comes to making sense of the data provided using the multilayers for feature extraction. Deep learning can automatically extract features and can easily find patterns in the data be it sound or image. This is the only reason why deep learning is leading when it comes to image processing and natural language processing [5]. Deep learning has reduced the cost by half when it comes to the use of sensors and ML to study and form a meaning of the data and give us a prediction. This method of study is also known as supervised learning.

Another field of study is unsupervised learning in which the data is studied and looked for a pattern with no insight [6]. This method can be utilized to scan and decode the data from the environment and make a decision [7]. Now robots can move around more rationally using deep learning and sensors which are driven by ML algorithms. But they fail to perform well enough when it comes to performing in a congested room. The level of accuracy needed will be exponential. To tackle this challenge we utilize deep convolution networks which will help to gain an advantage when it comes to a sense of perception [8].

4 Deep learning in Robotic Navigation

To make a fully autonomous system using deep learning is not as easy as it seems. It requires optimal perceptual capabilities. The process of perception of a robot's environment and interpreting the information it acquires allows it to understand the condition of its surroundings, devise plans to change the state, and observe how its actions impact its environment. When it comes to an unstructured environment, object recognition/detection is very challenging due to the object variations and the amount of data from the sensors the model has to process like the difference between the types of the road [9]. Deep learning utilizes the capabilities of machine learning to capture the motion as well as optimal perceptual functionalities. The challenge of driving in an environment includes problems of movement of the robot in navigating varied obstacles by pushing and pulling. Even in structured environments, automated driving is difficult due to the complexities of the related state space [10]. This state space comprises of appearance, dimension, a position as well as the weight of objects within the scene. Deep learning and machine learning have made a huge impact and have greatly improved the performance of the robots.

5 Features of Medical Robotics

Physicians control the medical robots using consoles which are independent of their location. They can either be in a completely remote location or nearby where the bot is being used The remote/console has all the arms being under the control of the doctor who is performing the surgery. The form of the arms mainly depends on the type of the surgery that is needed to be performed. All the necessary medical data with respect to the surgery is fed to the bot which helps it to more around during the surgery very easily and with utmost precision.The main reason to use these medical bots are only because they have:-

- Better diagnostic capabilities
- Better precision and less risk
- increased the patient comfort level.

Medical bots are now been used for more complicated surgeries with higher risks as well as to perform simple tasks. They have allowed the doctors to be present in the room to perform surgeries from remote location which has certainly made the world a smaller place. This resulted in the doctors become less fatigue and the patients have access to professional help from the best. Doctors now can relax and perform the surgeries which help them to be at their peak condition to go with the procedure.

5.1 Improving Patient Care [11, 12]

"exchange ideas, encourage innovation, and discuss the importance of technologies like robotic-assisted surgery and therefore the increasing role they are doing and can still play in health-care.", this was beautifully said by Brian Miller, senior vice president and general manager of systems and vision at Intuitive Surgical.

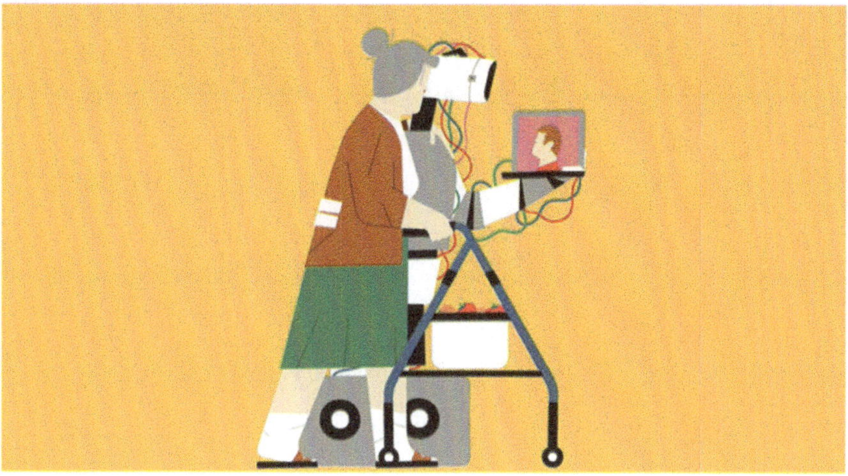

Fig. 2 An illustration of futuristic medical bot

In the near future medical bots assisting/performing surgeries will uplift the medical standards all over the world for less riskier and better diagnosis. The number of applications of these technologies is unimaginable and has far-reaching benefits. This will help to reduce the barrier between man and machine for better collaboration. A futuristic medical bot is shown in Fig. 2.

6 AI(Artificial Intelligence) for Medical Robotics

Artificial Intelligence is the machine trying to mimic the human brain and the way it works to understand a complex problem and analyze it to come up with a solution by learning, correcting, and reasoning.

The current scenario of using AI is not optimal because we are lacking the numbers when it comes to see a bot operating or being used in this industry with confidence. Having strict regulation and procedures not only makes the process more hectic but it is essential to maintain the standard of the medical industry. A comparison between bot and non-bot is highlighted in Fig. 3.

Applications of Medical Robots[13]

Medical bots require more attention because they are going to be future of the medical industry. They with unimaginable precision can perform surgery with minimal infection and error risks. There will not be any area left for human error unless they are duly trained to tackle every possible scenarios which may develop during a surgery. They will not only uplift the standards of the medical industry but will also help for new discoveries.

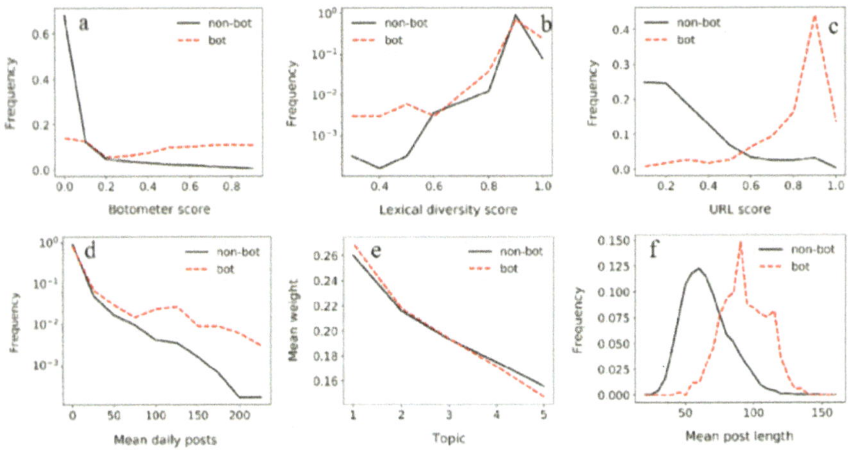

Fig. 3 Comparison between bot and non-bot

- Due to utmost precision and safety medical bots can outperform doctors
- The bots can also work in a very constrained environment thus making it very versatile as it can even perform life saving surgeries while being inside an ambulance.
- Nanites or nano robots are still hypothetical but once implemented they will revolutionize the medical industry. They will be able to cure cancers, increase life span, and also to increase the rate of recovery.
- The applications of robotics are tremendous. They can be used for surgeries, cleaning, basic nursing problems, and also to dispense medicines.

7 Available Bots Changing the World

We can classify the robots in two broader sections such as robots using machine learning and robots without using machine learning to perform other medical jobs.

We can further classify the robots on the basis of their jobs such as there are robots to help people stand after their paralysis and there are robots doing complex surgeries to outperform the doctors in terms of reliability. Doctors will always be needed and nobody can replace the doctors but the truth is they can perform better when both machines and doctors form up a team to do the impossible and reach a new benchmark in medical history.

Let's now classify the robots on the basis of them using machine learning and not using any sort of algorithm to perform their duties. We will list out few of the world-renowned inventions which are working wonders in the medical industry but this is not the end. Research is still going on and many more advanced devices are still available doing wonders for this world. Classification of medical bots is shown in Fig. 4.

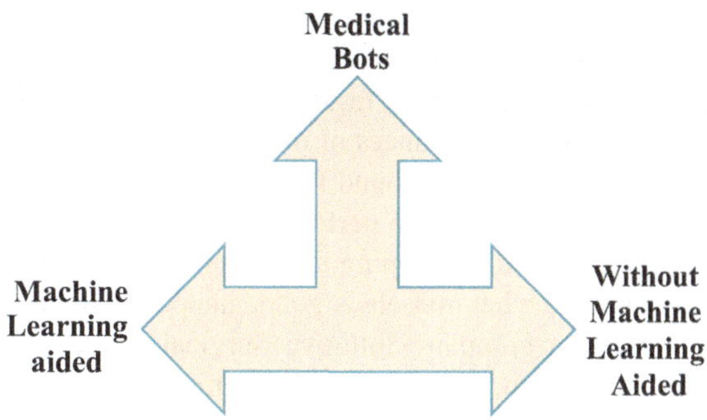

Fig. 4 Classification of medical bots

8 Without Using Machine Learning

There are medical bots which does not require any kind of machine learning algorithm. Their jobs are entirely to increase the doctors efficiency without interfering the doctors ability to do the task. The machines will be either controlled or guided by the doctors from all over the world.

8.1 DaVinci

The elite ubiquitous of medical bots, and the standard for Robot-Assisted Surgery is where we should start exploring.

This machine is the actual miracle that removed the boundary of robot and medical tool because this device is always under the control of the surgeon.

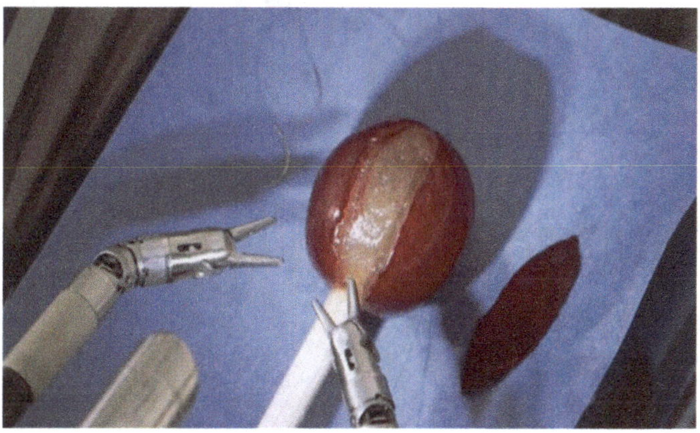

Fig. 5 Da Vinci performing historic surgery on a grape

The most important feature of DaVinci machine as shown in Fig. 5, is that it can get done with an operation with the minimal number of incisions with the extreme precaution and precision which results in less bleeding, faster healing, and less exposure helps to reduce the chances of infection.

DaVinci has been around this medical industry since the last 18 years and it is continuously evolving to perform more delicate operations. But major tech companies have started developing their own advanced systems like DaVinci and we can only imagine what miracle is gonna happen in the upcoming decade.

American company Intuitive Surgical is the one to have developed DaVinci Surgical System, which is a robotic surgical system approved by the Food and Drug Administration (FDA) in 2000. The main purpose of the device is to facilitate surgery using a minimally invasive approach. The bot is constantly controlled by a surgeon from a console which can be present in any remote location. The system is used for prostatectomies, and increasingly for heart valve repair and gynecologic surgical procedures. The name DaVinci System was partially inspired from "Leonardo Da Vinci" because his "study of human anatomy eventually led to the planning of the primarily known robot in history.

This elite bot was used in an estimated 200,000 surgeries in 2012, majorly for hysterectomies and prostate removals. As of September 30, 2017, there was an installed base of 4,271 units worldwide—2,770 within the US, 719 in Europe, 561 in Asia, and 221 in the rest of the globe. This is an expensive bot,the Si version of the system costs on the average just below US$2 million, in addition to many hundred thousand dollars of annual maintenance fees. The system has been hugely criticized because of its maintenance cost and the complications it faces during the surgery. Figure 6 shows the full view.

The Da Vinci System has been utilized in the subsequent procedures:

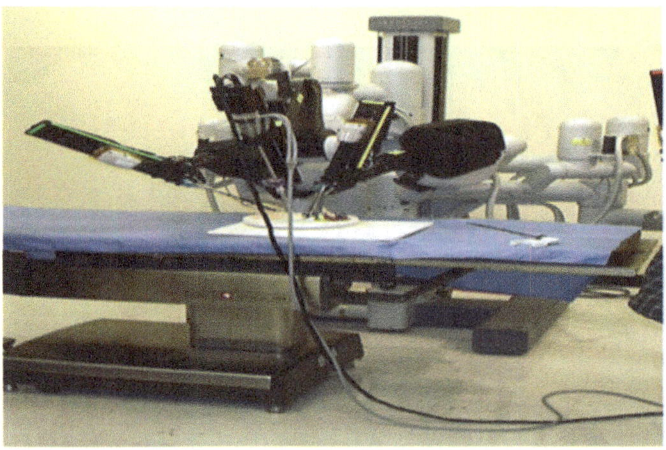

Fig. 6 Da Vinci Bot full view

- Radical prostatectomy, pyeloplasty, cystectomy, nephrectomy, and ureteral reimplantation;
- Hysterectomy, myomectomy, and sacrocolpopexy;
- Hiatal hernia repair.

8.2 Endoscopy-Bot

Inserting a tiny camera or tool on an extended wire into the body through a "natural opening to search for damage, foreign objects, or traces of the disease is known as Endoscopy. This technique may still be a thing of the past and can be uncomfortable but new improvements to the procedure are constantly being added by companies like Medineering make use of the flexible robots as seen in Fig. 7 that can be controlled like an remote-controlled car to the exact spot where the doctor wants it to go. They then can stay there as long as they are needed from taking a biopsy to cauterizing a wound without any risk of human error like unstable hands which may lead to severe damage to sensitive spot.

At present there are "capsule endoscopies" where the procedure is swallowing a pill-sized robot that travels along with your digestive tract gathering data which is to be sent to the doctors.

Endoscopy means to peep inside the human body. This procedure includes using an instrument endoscope to look inside human organs and cavities by inserting the device unlike the other medical imaging techniques.

Endoscopes act as an extra pair of eyes for the doctors to look inside the human body. They are widely used for gastrointestinal diagnostics. There are 3 types of endoscopes:

- Rigid.
- Flexible.
- Capsule endoscopes.

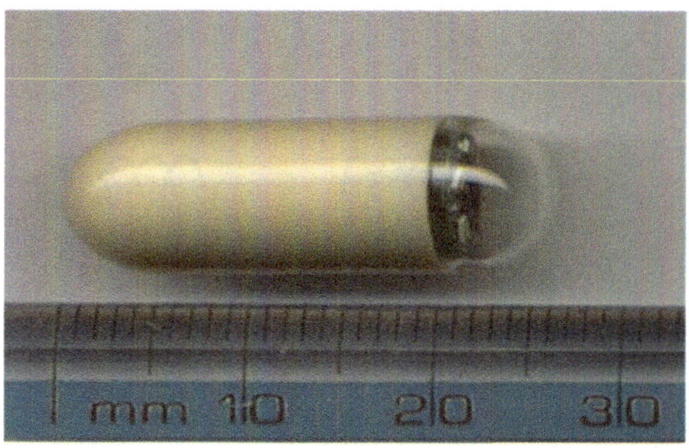

Fig. 7 Endoscopy bot full view

Rigid and versatile endoscopes are used to focus on a particular region of interest. Capsule endoscopes are mainly used for the gastrointestinal. With the advancement of technology, robotic endoscopy has been increasingly developed and accepted.

8.3 Targeted Therapy Micro-robot

This new amazing technology is used to deliver drugs to any specific part of the human body. The major use of this device is to deliver radiation to a tumor, or just to reduce the side effects of drugs by constricting it to the organ where it would be needed.

The most astonishing thing about this bot is the way it navigates. New research in this domain has generated microbots with tiny, helical tails that can be controlled by magnetic fields to spin themselves forward through blood vessels to the specific part of the body. Movement of microbot is highlighted in Fig. 8.

The hardest part to reach in a body is to reach a particular area without affecting the other areas. In such cases, a treatment like surgery or chemotherapy is followed. A pair of researchers in Caltech's Division of Engineering and applied science have been trying to invent a whole new technique to deliver medicine to the target area only by using robots so small that it can find in blood vessels and navigate around using a remote which will be situated outside the human body and controlled by the doctors.

Wang and Wei Gao, assistant professor of medical engineering is the main pioneer behind the development of this astonishing technology. The main intention was to treat tumors which are within the digestive tract.

The bots contain tiny spheres of magnesium coated with thin gold layers and a digestion resisting polymer–parylene. A circular portion of the sphere is left uncovered. The magnesium on the uncovered portion reacts with the fluids which in turn creates small bubbles and that bubble is then projected giving it the thrust needed to push itself around in the digestive tract as seen in Fig. 9.

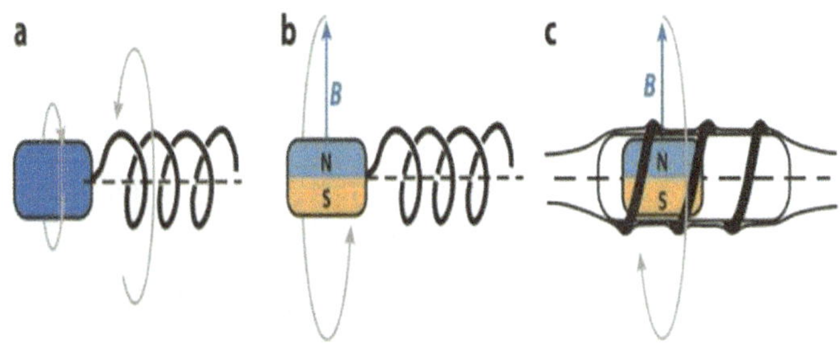

Fig. 8 Illustration of the movement of microbot

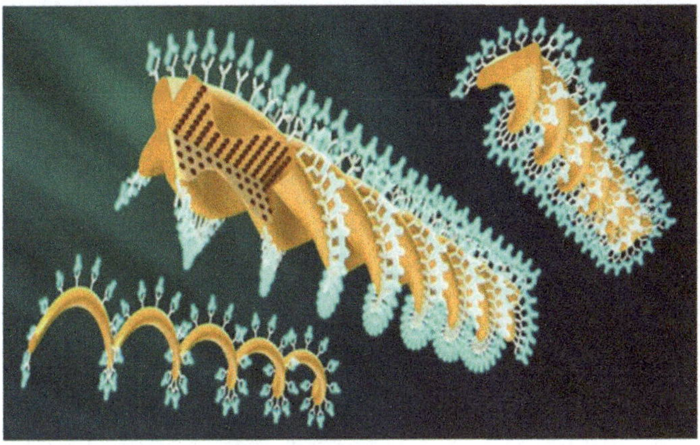

Fig. 9 Illustration of the microbot

The way it delivers medicine is very interesting. The medicine is first sandwiched between each microsphere and the parylene coating. Then a capsule made from paraffin is used to protect the bot from the acidic environment.

At this stage, the spheres are capable of carrying drugs but still lack the crucial ability to deliver them to the desired location. To deliver the drug, Wang and Gao used a new technology which uses the pulse from infrared laser lights. This is also known as photoacoustic computed tomography also known as PACT.

When the bots reach the designated place of interest then a high infrared light is beamed at them. The capsules absorb the infrared light and heat up to melt the paraffin and then the uncovered portion reacts with the acid and forms bubbles which makes them propel forward. They are not steerable but the random propulsion makes it a hit and trial approach where majority of the bots will stick to the infected tissue and start releasing the medicine.

This approach was tested on animals and the results were promising. With new motivation researchers will keep pushing the invention till it full proof for humans.

8.4 Clinical Training Bots

Clinical bots are mainly used to train the upcoming nurses and doctors. They are mainly a robot to mimic the human behavior under certain circumstances. They have been made as real as possible which makes them perfect subjects to work on during the training phase of the doctors.

Hal is a robot boy as seen in the Fig. 10, is designed to vigorously shake its head, and close his eyelids. His mouth is slightly open which has no sound expect the machinery. He was made as a training robot. He can bleed, urinate, has reflexes when light is shone on him, can be controlled to have heart attack or go into shocks.

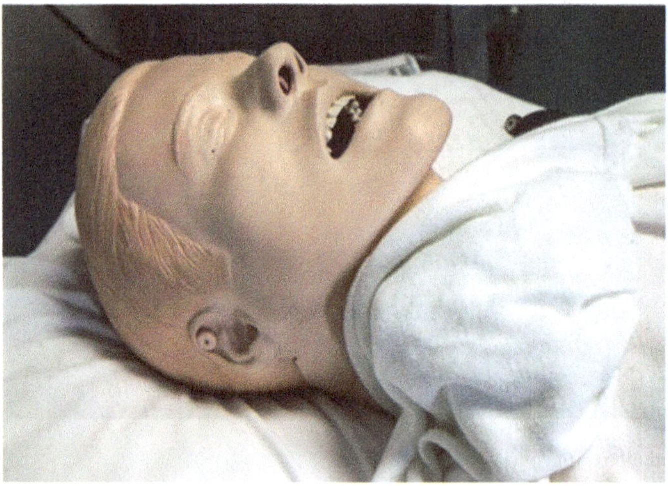

Fig. 10 Hal the robot boy

He can also shed tears. He can be attached to any hospital machines and can be jolted using a defibrillator.

Hal is made up of mechanical pneumatic system which makes it imitate breathing and he exhales CO_2 using a CO_2 tank. His hydraulic system makes him bleed and shed tears. He has a 5-year-old voice and can express his emotions using his face.

8.5 Robotic-Assisted Biopsy

MURAB—MRI and Ultrasound Robotic-Assisted biopsy is a bot designed to scan the patient's body than the 3D image is created exactly where the biopsy is needed of.

This bot is mainly used for minimum invasion for early cancer diagnosis. After the imaging is done the bot just backs out as precisely as possible for least cut needed. The main concept of the bot was developed to improve the biopsy gathering for cancer diagnosis by increasing the precision and the effectiveness.

An innovative technique, called Tissue Active Slam (TAS), is going to be developed within the project to optimally register the intraoperational acquired volume to the preoperational MRI image. Biopsy bot is depicted in Fig. 11.

Once Tissue Active Slam (TAS) is done, all that the doctors have to do is to select the target on the mixed image then the bot will steer itself to the exact position where it is needed. This procedure can significantly increase the medical standards and the workflow which in return will help to save lives by an exact targeting of early stage lesions,visible under MRI.

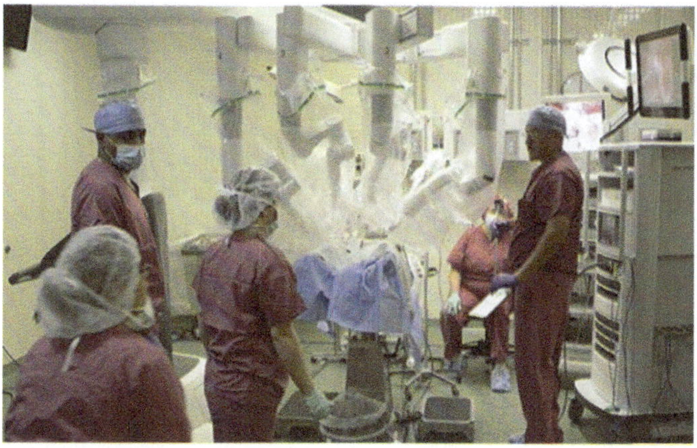

Fig. 11 Full view of the biopsy bot

9 Using Machine Learning

These medical bots use machine learning algorithm to predict/think independently about how to act at a particular moment without any human interactions. Once the device has been setup then the device will continue the task assigned till its service is no longer required [14].

9.1 Exoskeletons

This is a tool which will be greatly used by those who have suffered from paralysis. This is basically a metal frame which we have to wear like a suit. After being strapped to it, the device will act like the substitute of skeletal structure.

They can even be useful for correcting malformations or for rehabilitation after a brain or spinal cord injury by providing weak muscles with the additional help they need to perform movements and begin healing the damage. Figure 12 shows a exoskeleton bot.

They are mainly used to assist the paralyzed. In spite of being developed for a sole purpose this device can also be used to rehabilitate after spinal or brain injury by helping the weaker muscle the proper support they need. This can also act for correcting the severe cases of malformations. They mainly run on user input to the system and soon it is being developed to control it directly using our mind.They also have preregistered moves which uses the Artificial Intelligence to assist the user.

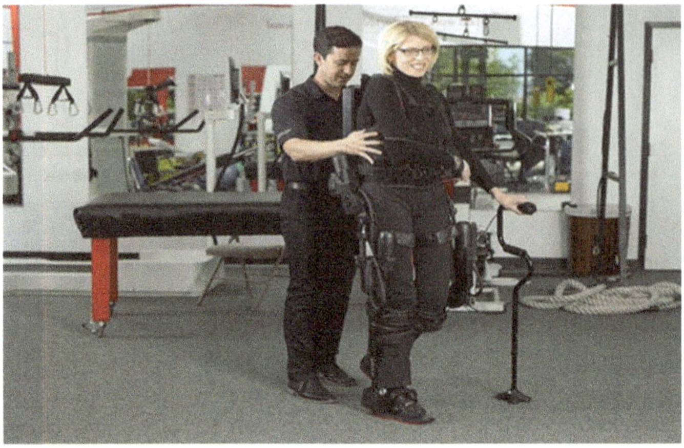

Fig. 12 Full view of the exoskeleton

9.2 Robotic Nurses

The only thing that keeps the hospitals running is the nurses who are working all day and night taking care of the patients. They are like the RBC of the medical department. But in spite of all these they are being pressurized till they break due to the extreme work pressure. This is when robotic nurse revolutionized. They have been programmed to fill out the digital forms, monitor a patient, and also to check for the vital signs when needed. They have also taken over the minor but important jobs which the nurses had to go through everyday like drawing blood and pushing trolly from a room to another. This helps to save a lot of time for the nurses which they can invest to look after any other patients.

They can also help the nurses to transfer the patients from one place to another which will reduce the physical stress and they are also programmed with such efficiency that they can check for the medication of the patients without any possibility of error.

All the information are now being stored on the cloud so as days goes by the robot will only get better and depend less on history to come up with a decision. They can also help a patient to get rid of loneliness and stabilize the mood swings the patients with mental illness go through. Figure 13 shows a demonstration of robotic nurse and Fig. 14 depicts the full view.

Hospitals situated in the West Coast of America are now into a robot named VGo which helps them to break the language barrier between people. RIVA, another bot is now helping the hospitals to prepare the IV syringes and bags. Another bot LUCAS which was built to be used during the emergencies as a chest compression device.

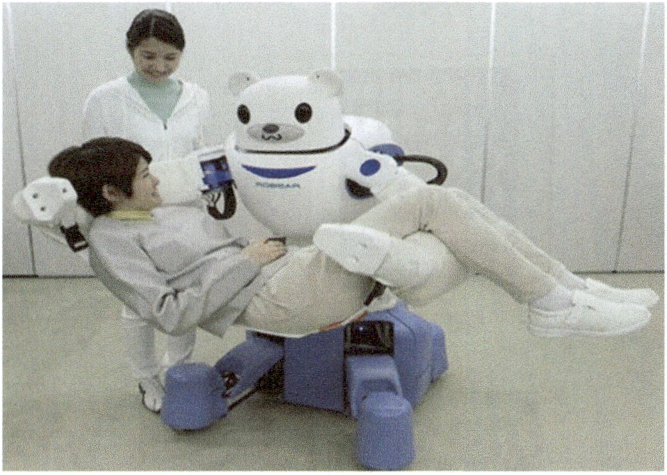

Fig. 13 Robotic nurse demonstration

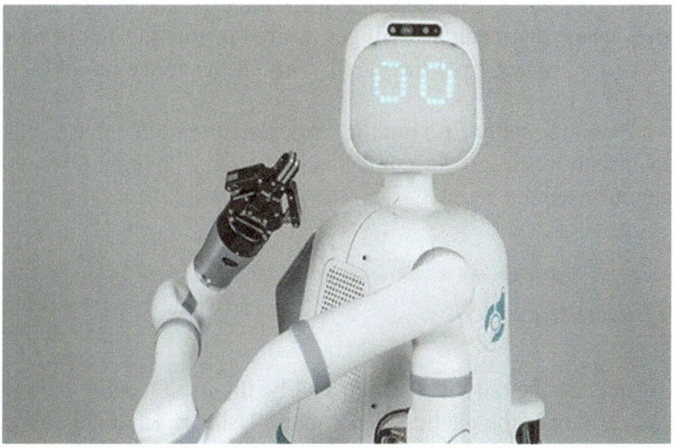

Fig. 14 Illustration of the robotic nurse

9.3 Pharma-Botics

University of California has been developing a concept for the last 5 years and now it has even been approved by the hospitals and has been performing outstanding since the last ten months.

This is an automatic pill dispenser machine built just like vending machines. Based on the user requirements it will dispense the pills. It has its own pill storage. The operation of the bot is pretty simple. It has a scanner to scan the user requirements/prescription and using the servo motors will dispense the medicines as

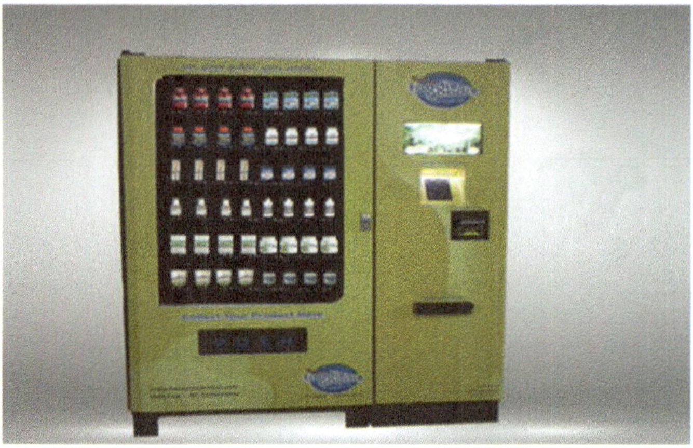

Fig. 15 The medicine vendor machine

required. It has a laserjet printer to print out the instructions and the descriptions of the pills. This bot has inbuilt tracker to track the expiration dates and will notify the authorities when any medicine will get expired or run out. It will have an input scanner to take the money from the user by whichever mode possible, be it using cards or cash.

This device will basically ease out the work pressure of the pharmacies and will help to deliver with much more accuracy and efficiency. Figure 15 shows a sample medicine vendor machine.

9.4 AI Diagnostics [15]

AI diagnosis may be the only task which will be the most useful when it comes to use machine learning in the medical department. Using machine learning scientists can now train a model by providing it with 1000 of examples and when the model is perfectly fitted then its diagnosis may also overcome the human diagnosis by eliminating the chance of error. Using computer vision technology doctors can now scan patients facial features to predict the diseases. It can successfully diagnose almost 8000 diseases and rare genetic disorders.

This technology has evolved to such extent that it can scan thousands of medical documents to separate out the patients who are more prone to diabetes, stroke, or heart problems. This technology will decrease the medical cost to great extent and it will only continue to get better with the experience because all the data is like a treasure for the software and will just keep training to get better at it. Soon chatbots will be available in place of real doctors meanwhile doctors will be attending the higher risk cases.

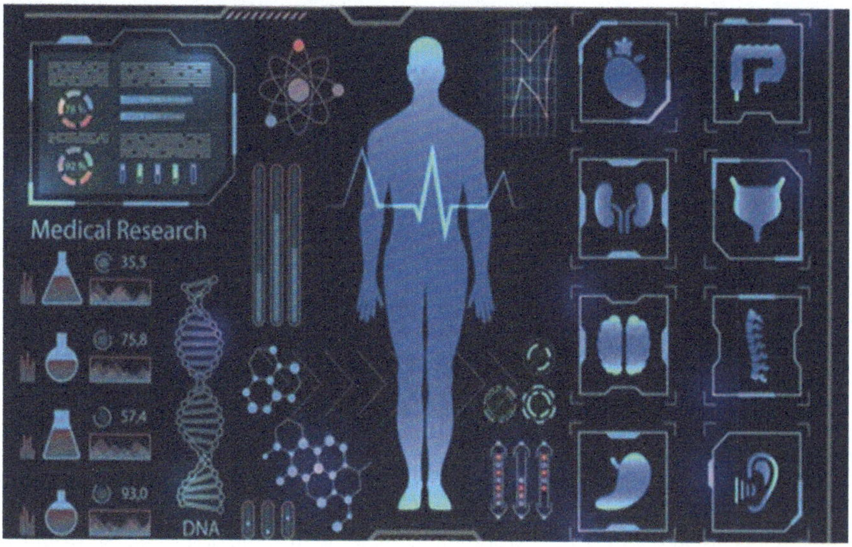

Fig. 16 Illustration of AI

Soon other features will include Brain–computer interface which will help people with speaking disorders, people with disabilities and spinal injuries by reading their neural signals. The most common thing we can predict in the near future is that virtual nursing assistants. They will be able to answer all the necessary but common questions of the patients to reduce the working load of the hospitals and also to reduce the unnecessary hospital visits. A sample illustration of AI is seen in Fig. 16.

9.5 Disinfectant Bots

No matter how good a hospital can be when it comes to treating patients but as long as it is not clean it will always remain a risk for all the personal as well as the patients being treated. The ground truth for the hospitals is that they need to be spotless. But that is not always the case when we look at the current scenario.

The solution to this was a bot that can move around freely and keep disinfecting all the surfaces without any human intervention. They keep on roaming around the corridor and whenever a patient checks out it moves into the room to disinfect it. They are equipped with very high powered UV beam emitters and they keep on beaming the rays for a few minutes until no microbe is left alive.

No matter how advanced a facility maty get but without proper sanitation it will only become the next breeding ground of the most deadly diseases of the world. Sanitation is the top priority and significant development has been made in this field and will keep developing. According to the studies by CDC one out of 25 patients in

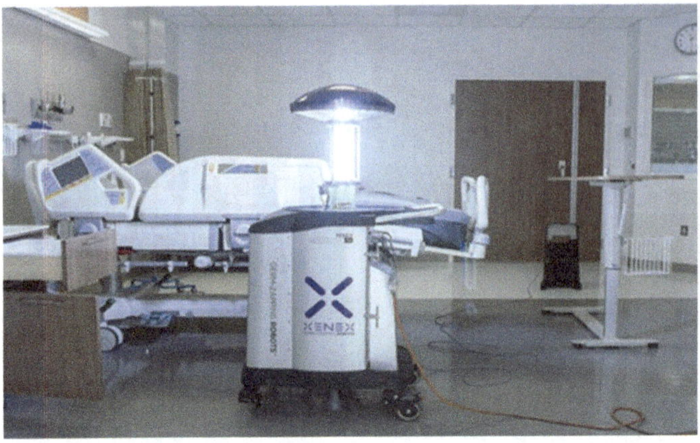

Fig. 17 Disinfect bot on duty

a hospital is always at high risk to come in contact with some other disease from the hospital due to improper sanitation. UV disinfectant bots will play an revolutionary role to bring a change and will make the hospitals a better place to get treated from. A disinfect bot is seen in Fig. 17.

9.6 *AI Epidemiology*

One thing which AI is best at is to recognize patterns and making predictions from the data which will be over complicated for humans to understand and decode and hence this led to a new AI system which can predict disease outbreaks. Figure 18 shows an illustration of virus.

The doctors supply the data to the system and then it cross-checks with all the available medical data and will predict when the outbreak will occur and help us to contain the spread.

There are many new products in the market doing the same but AIME system has proved to be one of the most successful so far. It had been deployed during the dengue outbreak in Malaysia and correctly predicted with an accuracy of 85% and had saved the life of millions of people as well as millions of dollars.

AIME stands for Artificial Intelligence and Medical Epidemiology and its goal is to aid in the prevention of diseases by utilizing the power of AI and machine learning to predict the outbreak before it becomes a pandemic. This is originally set up in Malaysia by Dr Dhesi Raja in collaboration with two computer scientists, Dr Peter Ho and Dr Choo-Yee Ting. It works by analyzing tons of data to predict the outbreak of the dengue fever. The system keeps on analyzing not only public health data, but also other data from outsources like the weather, wind speed, previous outbreaks.

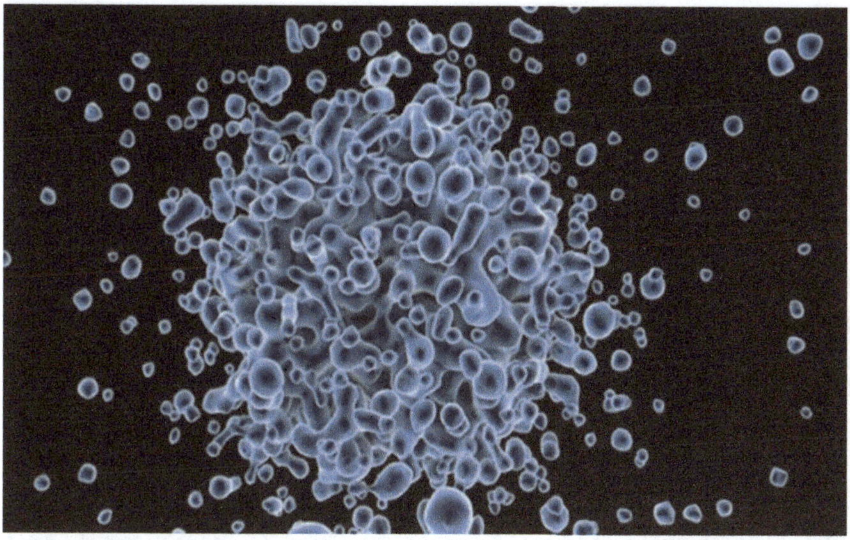

Fig. 18 Illustration of a virus

They claim to provide with the exact location and the date of the next dengue outbreak almost 3 months in advance.

9.7 Antibacterial Nanobot

This is perhaps the most advanced of all the bots out there. Antibacterial nanobots are extremely small machines made of gold nanowires which are then coated with platelets and RBC and are capable of clearing out the bacterial infection from the entire blood of the patient.

They actually perform this miracle using a very old concept of trojan horse. They mimic the bacteria and the toxins and when the bacteria approaches they trap them using the mesh. They can be used to clear out localized areas only by directing them using the ultrasound. The biggest advantage is that this method used no medicine to flush out the bacteria so there will not be any impact to the body's self immunity system and also prevents the development of antibiotic resistant diseases. A nanobot is seen in Fig. 19.

This army of bacteria trapping bots was developed at the University of California San Diego, the outer gold body reacts to the ultrasound and it helps them to swim around without the need of any extra fuel or power. This is the reason this bot can co easily entrap the bacteria and detoxify the blood without any side effects.

The bots are twenty-five times smaller than a human hair and can travel up to thirty-five micrometers per second in blood. This project is still in its early phase and major developments are yet to be done.

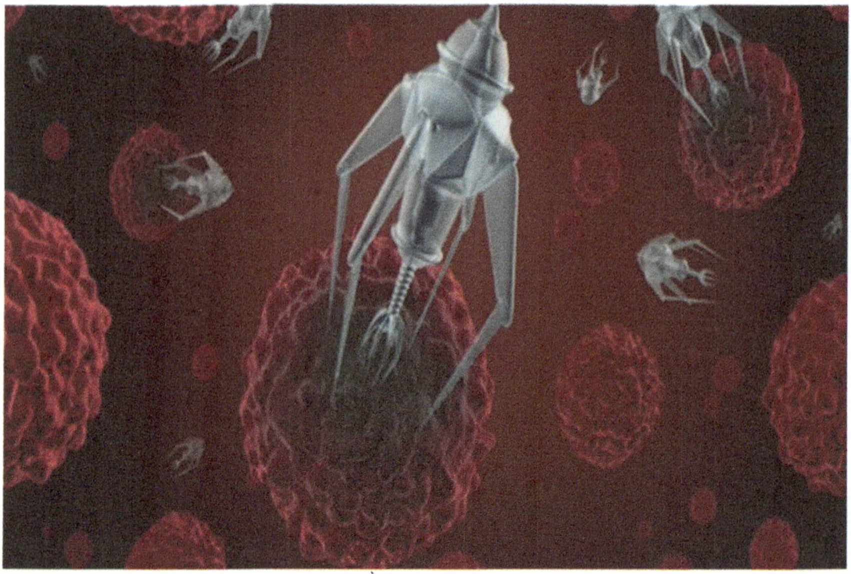

Fig. 19 Illustration of nanobots

10 Current Research and Development in Medical Robotics

Development of better and more effective methods to handle the operations of medical department is always going on. Many new promising researches have been going on to benefit both the patients and the industry.

10.1 RAVEN

These are the two most impressive robot-assisted systems which are currently being used for telesurgery. The RAVEN is a teleoperated laparoscopic system whose main goal is to maximize the surgical performance.

This bot has two arms with each seven degrees of freedom and is cable-driven. The kinematics of the arms are based on a spherical mechanism which enables the tools with zero inaccessible area to operate on. The mechanism is cheaper and more advanced than the DaVinci bot. They are equipped with haptic feedback which means that the operator can receive feedback on their hands. Figure 20 shows a Raven.

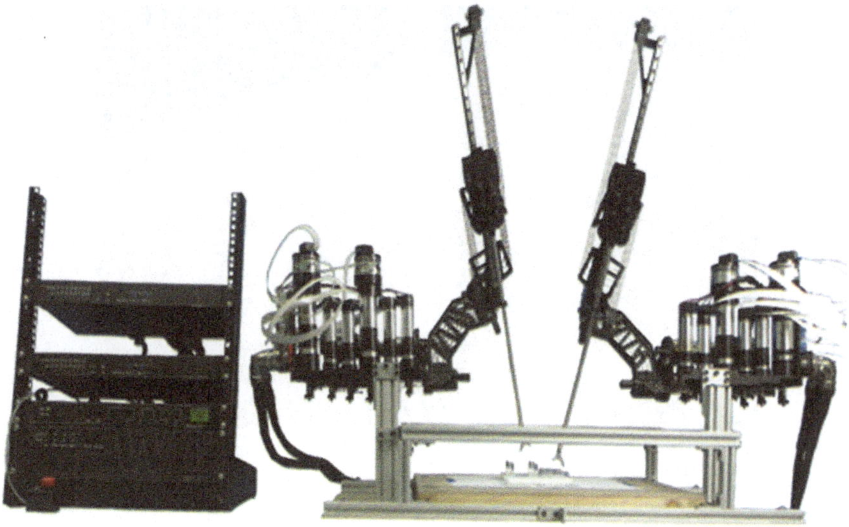

Fig. 20 Raven illustration

10.2 NeuroArm

The neuroArm is a two-armed neuro surgical device which uses MRI guidance. The neuroArm end effectors have three degrees of freedom and are precise up to tens of micrometers.

10.3 Trauma Pod

Trauma Pod is a semi-automatic remote-controlled system designed for surgeries. The surgical cell consists of a surgical robot, Scrub Nurse Subsystem, Tool Rack System, Supply Dispensing System, Patient Imaging System, predecessor of the aforementioned LS-1, and Supervisory Controller System.

10.4 Heart Lander

HeartLander is a worm type robot which uses suction to crawl around as seen in Fig. 21. The main purpose was to treat cardiac diseases when the heart keeps on beating His is a minimally invasive bot which keeps crawling on the surface of the heart.

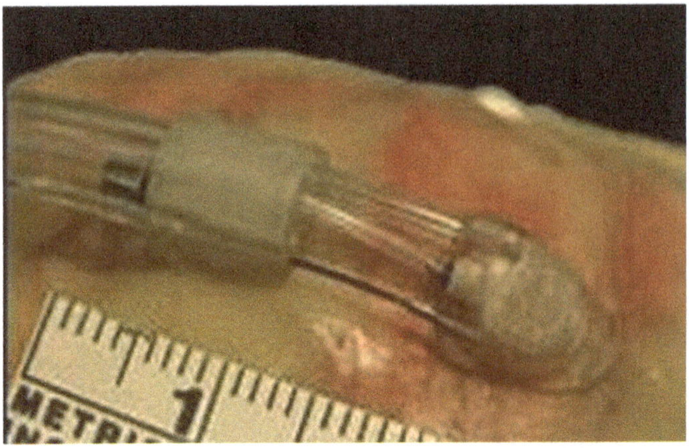

Fig. 21 Heartlander on duty

11 Key Technology

Major technologies used in medical bots include the following:-

- The technology used for the fabrication of medical bots and devices is MEMS. It can fabricate the tools which are suitable for micro-(sensing/actuation/manipulation) of samples. Until now they have either been using IC fabrication or micro-machining techniques.
- The software of programs which can efficiently map out a patient body before the bots performs surgeries is very crucial for the efficiency and safety.
- Reliable and efficient system integration of off-the-shelf components and devices for specific biological and medical operations.
- To develop the mathematical model to engineer the behavior and structure of the bot as a biological system. This is probably one of the most challenging portion of the industry because of the very complex nature of the biological systems.
- Engineers with solid concept of biology or the AI system for the medical application because making each motor and actuator work according to an algorithm which in turn will work according to the condition and feedback from the patients.

12 Biggest Challenges in Medical Robotics

There have always been challenges when something revolutionary has been invented. This is no exception. Robotics has a long list of never ending problems faced but let us pinpoint a few which has been one of the major drawbacks for the industry. Table 1 highlights the major issues in this domain.

Table 1 Major challenges faced in this domain

Serial number	Challenges faced	Description
1	**Developing new fabrication methods with new materials**	Developing new power efficient soft artificial muscles to replace the motors, servo, and actuators
2	**Creating bio-inspired robots**	The ultimate challenge faced is to create a device which will get inspiration from the nature but the drawbacks are still the same as they have been since the last 30 years:- 1. Better battery 2. Better actuators 3. Better memory 4. Better vision
3	**Better power sources**	Robots have always been a battery monster which has led to one of the biggest problem when it comes to make it a portable bot-POWER SOURCE Research is still being done to invent a battery which will not only support quick charging but also will be able to store large capacity with low discharging
4	**Better AI architecture**	Yes AI can outperform human in few domains but one thing AI is yet to develop is to develop understanding and reasoning when it comes to do heterogeneous tasks. They are yet to develop critical thinking capabilities
5	**Socially attractive idea of a Robot**	Robots are not socially friendly when it comes to interaction. Humans are great social beings but robots are not. Robots are good at short and to the point interaction but that is not what we humans do
6	**Ethics**	WE have all seen movies where it has been portrayed robots as a being ready to kill all humans to be the ONE Let us face the fact that day is centuries apart but the idea just can't be displaced so easily A robot without any ethics will be meaningless when it is being deployed in the medical industry

13 Conclusion

Medical robotics, and particularly autonomous surgical robotics, is still in an embryonic stage. To conclude, there are several steps that must be taken in order to further the use and development of robots in surgery (and in medicine in general). These are: The development, and international adoption, of safety standards the aim of task-specific, as opposed to general-purpose, robots the education of the medical community in the acceptance and integration of Robots. The economic and social advantages to be gained from the mass-use of robotics in medicine (and particularly surgery), as already expounded, are enormous. If all of the above steps are taken, then the full potential of robotics can be exploited in the medical sector, as it has been in industrial applications, for the improved welfare of society everywhere.

So now after we have discussed the basic of medical bots and the types of bots we can now conclude that medical bots will surely be a major help in the medical industry given the circumstances that major parts of the world are still lacking proper medical professionalism. Medical bots have yet to be upgraded more for a full autonomous experience but once implemented there will be no going back. Be it with or without AI but they have played an important part to revolutionized the medical industry in terms of safety, deliverance, efficiency, and trust. Doctors can now relax a bit but to win the battle of man VS machines we need to look from a new perception and turn it around as man with machines. Yes there are few setbacks but there is not a single great thing which has not seen failure. They have not only helped to prevent upcoming epidemics but also in other fields such as drug discovery and such.

One of the major advantages will be they will not only be able to save lives but also to save in a given constrained environment with constrained time and budget.

In time of emergencies they can outperform the humans when it comes to deal with stress and fatigue. They can perform surgeries in remote places in an ambulance which will not only help to save the critically injured but also reduce the number of deaths which happens on the way to hospitals.

Once the bots have been deployed in every corner of the world we can see a major upliftment in the economic and social aspects of society. We need to break the barrier between man and machine to envision a future with better health care marvels and standards.

References

1. Brighton, H., Selina, H.: Introducing artificial intelligence: a graphic guide, ser. Introducing... Icon Books Limited (2015). [Online]. [2] Available:https://books.google.com.pk/books?id=4GxGCgAAQBAJ
2. Bai, J., Wu, Y., Zhang, J., Chen, F.: Subset based deep learning for rgb-d object recognition. Neuro Comput. **165**, 280–292 (2015)
3. Xu, R., Xiong, C., Chen, W., Corso, J.J.: Jointly modeling deep video and compositional text to bridge vision and language in a unified framework (2015)

4. Narasimhan, K., Kulkarni, T., Barzilay, R.: Language understanding for text-based games using deep reinforcement learning (2015). arXiv preprint arXiv:1506.08941
5. Turan, M., Ornek, E.P., Ibrahimli, N., Giracoglu, C., Almalioglu, Y., Yanik, M.F., Sitti, M.: Unsupervised odometry and depth learning for endoscopic capsule robots (2018). arXiv preprint arXiv:1803.01047
6. Levine, S., Pastor, P., Krizhevsky, A., Quillen, D.: Learning hand-eye coordination for robotic grasping with large-scale data collection. In: International symposium on experimental robotics, pp. 173–184. Springer (2016)
7. Yang, Y., Fermuller, C., Li, Y., Aloimonos, Y.: Grasp type revisited: a modern perspective on a classical feature for vision. In: Proceedings of the IEEE conference on computer vision and pattern recognition, pp. 400–408 (2015)
8. Dong, C., Loy, C.C., He, K., Tang, X.: Image super resolution using deep convolutional networks. IEEE Trans. Patt. Anal. Mach. Intell. **38**(2), 295–307 (2016)
9. Cruz, F., Twiefel, J., Magg, S., Weber, C., Wermter, S.: Interactivereinforcement learning through speech guidance in a domesticscenario. In: Neural Networks (IJCNN), 2015 International JointConference on. IEEE, pp. 1–8 (2015)
10. Doshi, J., Kira, Z., Wagner, A.: From deep learning to episodicmemories: creating categories of visual experiences. In: Proceedings of the third annual conference on advances in cognitive systems ACS, p. 15 (2015)
11. Mishra, S., Tripathy, H.K., Mallick, P.K., Bhoi, A.K., Barsocchi, P.: EAGA-MLP—an enhanced and adaptive hybrid classification model for diabetes diagnosis. Sensors **20**, 4036 (2020)
12. Mishra, S., Mallick, P.K., Jena, L., Chae, G.S.: Optimization of skewed data using sampling-based preprocessing approach. Front Public Health **8**, 274 (2020). Published 2020 Jul 16. doi:https://doi.org/10.3389/fpubh.2020.00274
13. Mallick, P.K., Krishna, P., Nagargun, A.N.: An image classification framework exploring the capabilities of extreme learning machines and artificial bee colony. Neural Comput. Appl. https://doi.org/10.1007/s00521-019-04385-5. (SCI & SCOPUS Indexed) [Accepted]
14. Mallick, P.K., Mishra, D., Patnaik, S., Shaw, K.: A semi-supervised rough set and random forest approach for pattern classification of gene expression data. Int. J. Reas.-Based Intel. Syst. **8**(3–4), 155–167 (2016)
15. Mishra, Sushruta, Brojo Kishore Mishra, Hrudaya Kumar Tripathy.: Significance of biologically inspired optimization techniques in real-time applications.In: Robotic systems: concepts, methodologies, tools, and applications, pp. 224–248. IGI Global (2020)

A Study on the Crisis Recognition Model Using Machine Learning-Based Bio-Signals

Joon-Yong Kim

Abstract Background/Objectives: The purpose of this study is to contribute to the expansion of the social safety net by studying a machine-learning-based model that accurately distinguishes specific bio-signals occurring in crisis situations, which are roughly classified as disease situations. **Methods/Statistical analysis**: In this paper I verified the suitability of the model by modeling and learning bio-signal data of crisis and disease situations using a binary classification technique. CCE (Categorical Cross Entropy) was applied as an optimizer suitable for binary classification, and Adam was used as the loss function, and the most effective model was found using four functions mainly used for classification as the activation function. In addition, Keras' Sequential model was applied as a learning model, and TensorFlow 2.0 was used as the framework. **Findings**: The conclusions obtained through the research model showed that the data on the crisis and disease situations according to the bio-signals accurately distinguished the situation through learning, and the loss of the model also converged gradually, resulting in a successful result. Among the activation functions mainly used in the classification model, the loss and accuracy of each model trained using ReLU, Sigmoid, tanh, and Softmax were identified. As a result, it was found that the ReLU function has less loss by 0.0861 than other functions and its accuracy is high by 0.0167. Thus, it was concluded that the model to which the ReLU function was applied is the most suitable. **Improvements/Applications**: In order to use this model empirically in the future, it will be necessary to collaborate with the medical community to accumulate more empirical data, and then continue research on the implementation of a comprehensive social safety system applicable to the security field.

Keywords Binary classification · Bio-signals · Tensorflow · Categorical cross entropy · Adam · ReLU

J.-Y. Kim (✉)
Department of Liberal Arts (Computer Science), Seoul Theological University, 52 Hohyeon-ro 489beon-gil Gyeonggi-do, Bucheon-si 14754, South Korea
e-mail: musimk@stu.ac.kr

H. K. Tripathy et al. (eds.), *Technical Advancements of Machine Learning in Healthcare*, Studies in Computational Intelligence 936,
https://doi.org/10.1007/978-981-33-4698-7_18

1 Introduction

Based on the development of ICT technology through the Fourth Industrial Revolution, the modern society is developing the lives of modern people are developing more abundantly and safely by connecting the atom world and the bit world as one in various fields. In particular, ICT convergence technology using machine learning is expanding its domain to an infrastructure that solves the needs of each field of society. It provides information that can accurately determine social issues through social media and solve social problems in advance [1], and research on systems applied to various fields using bio-signals [2, 3], and teleconferences or education systems useful in non-face-to-face society such as the Corona era are good examples [4, 5]. As shown above, we can easily encounter the examples of systems that derive better effects by converging ICT technologies in each specialized field around us. In this paper, we studied a model that can integrate the preventive medicine field using bio-signals and the security field that can further solidify the social safety net by detecting crisis situations and recognizing dangerous situations in advance to lower the crime rate among various specialized fields. As a research model, we created a classification model by classifying signals that occur during crisis and disease situations based on blood pressure, body temperature, and heart rate that can be easily collected using a wearable device, and then measured the prediction accuracy of the model made through learning. In order to verify the accuracy of the model, various activation functions were used to verify the model. As a result, it was found that the use of the ReLU function showed the best effect. The research model in this paper is expected to contribute to the establishment of a system for preventing social crimes, which are getting serious.

2 Materials and Methods

In the crisis situation recognition model using bio-signals studied in this paper, the bio-signals that occur differently during disease and crisis situations were modeled using binary classification among various analysis techniques of machine learning. Binary classification is the most suitable technique for processing data in two forms, and is very advantageous in making a simple but very accurate and flexible model [6]. Tensorflow optimized for machine learning was used as a platform processing data, and CCE (Categorical Cross Entropy), which is mainly used for classification, was used as the loss function [7, 8]. Adam, which shows a lower loss rate than other functions, was applied as an optimizer, and Kerase's Sequential was used for model construction. Among the activation functions mainly used for classification model learning, ReLU, Sigmoid, tanh, and Softmax algorithms were used to compare the loss rate and accuracy of the model constructed in this way to select the most appropriate model for the research model.

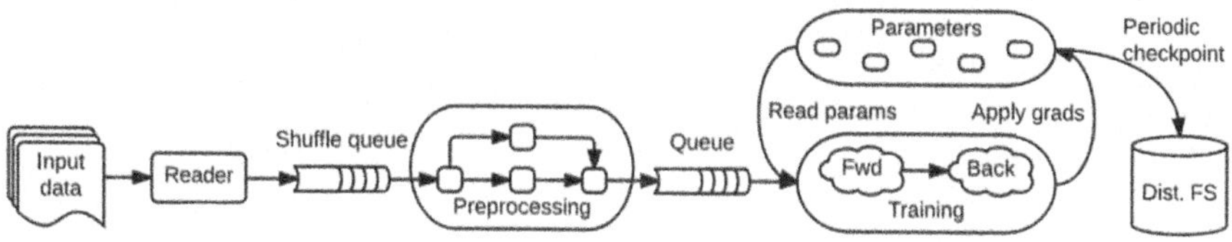

Fig. 1 Tensorflow dataflow graph

2.1 Tensorflow

TensorFlow is a learning algorithm optimized for machine learning and is an open source-based platform. It is a framework that solves problems such as Keras or PyTorch that was the mainstream in the early days of deep learning and is an algorithm that reads, separates, refines, analyzes input data, and learns it to derive a predicted value [9]. The following Fig. 1 is a TensorFlow dataflow graph for a training [10].

2.2 Optimizer Function

An optimizer function is an algorithm that iteratively differentiates the current value to obtain the optimal weight and bias, and various types of functions are used. Among them, Adam is optimized for a linear function, which is a form of binary classification. The following Fig. 2 shows the loss value of MNIST, a data set that collects handwriting, obtained by various optimizers, and Adam shows the smallest loss [11].

2.3 Activation Function

An activation function performs a task to obtain the organic learning effect of each density layer of the machine learning model. In addition, optimal results can be obtained only when the activation function of the last layer is applied according to the type of output data. In general, the best results can be obtained when using the Sigmoid function if the output is 1, while using the Softmax function if two results appear as in this study. In order to apply the optimal activation function to the learning model of this paper, four functions mainly used in artificial neural network analysis were selected [12–15]. The following Table 1 summarizes the formula of the activation function used to obtain model optimization.

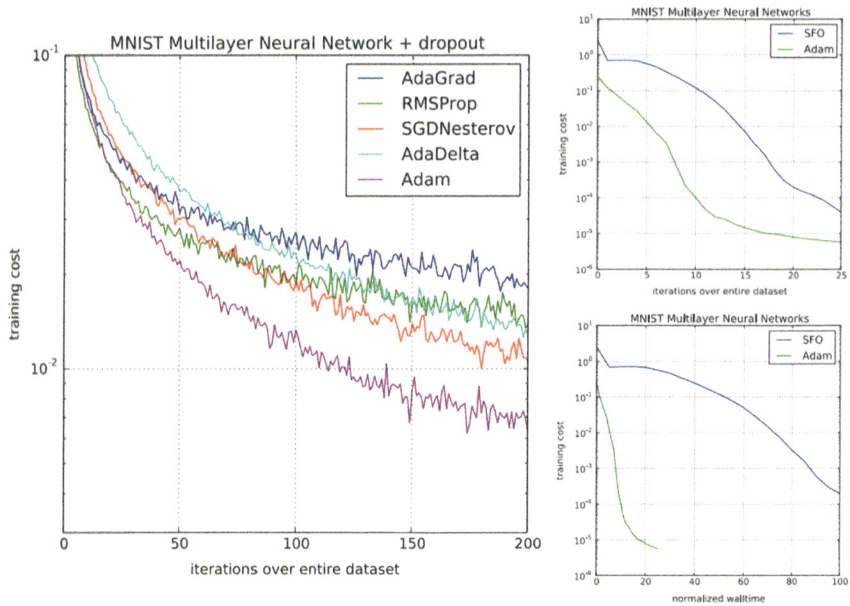

Fig. 2 Training of multilayer neural network on MNIST images

Table 1 Comparison table of activation functions

Activation function	Formula	Formula
ReLU	$R(z) = \max(0, z)$	• Output negative number as 0. Suitable for models with many hidden layers • Suitable for models with many hidden layers • Resolve the inefficiency of sigmoid with negative numbers
Sigmoid	$\sigma(z) = \frac{1}{1+e^{-z}}$	• A function with an S-shaped curve, which is mainly used in the early days of deep learning • Return output between 0 and 1 • When backpropagating an error, the value is getting smaller
tanth	$\tanh(x) = \frac{e^X - e^{-X}}{e^X + e^{-X}}$	• úúReturn output between -1 and 1 • A hyperbolic shape and used for learning RNN and LSTN
Softmax	$\sigma(z)_j = \frac{e^{zj}}{\sum_{k=1}^{k} e^{zk}}$	• A function that is used for multiple classification and makes the sum of the outputs 1

3 Results and Discussion

The model studied in this paper constituted a dataset by dividing data into data generated in a crisis situation and data generated in a disease situation based on blood pressure, body temperature, and heart rate among the bio- signals that can be easily obtained using a wearable device. After learning the configured data using machine learning, we verified the validity of the model by dividing whether the model is suitable into learning data and verification data, and checking the loss rate and accuracy.

The following Tables 2 and 3 shows bio-signal data of disease and crisis situations used in the research model.

As shown in Tables 2 and 3, a data set was constructed by collecting 150 bio-signals generated in each disease situation and crisis situation. The characteristics of the bio-signals for each situation are set that all three bio-signals deviate from the normal range in a disease situation, and that they rise together in a crisis situation

Table 2 Bio-signals in case of disease

	Blood pressure (mmHg)	Body temperature (°C)	Heart rate (bpm)
0	134	39.6	134
1	136	38.7	148
2	140	38.6	119
*	*	*	*
*	*	*	*
*	*	*	*
147	127	38.2	104
148	142	39.4	122
149	144	39.6	122

Table 3 Bio-signals in case of crisis

	Blood pressure (mmHg)	Body temperature (°C)	Heart rate (bpm)
0	129	36.0	119
1	146	36.3	141
2	128	36.6	149
*	*	*	*
*	*	*	*
*	*	*	*
147	142	36.1	117
148	132	36.9	135
149	134	37.0	142

because blood pressure and heart rate are correlated, and that body temperature does not deviate from the normal range.

The following Figs. 3 and 4 is a pre-processing step for learning each data. It is the result of randomly mixing the normalization process and the data to be learned and converting it to a numpy array.

Figure 3 above shows that all 300 data are normalized to values between min = 0 and max = 1.

As shown in Fig. 4, it can be seen that the normalized data is randomly mixed and reconstructed into an array.

```
<bound method NDFrame.head of      bood pressure  body temperature  heart rate  type
0          0.466667          0.904762    0.673469   0.0
1          0.533333          0.690476    0.959184   0.0
2          0.666667          0.666667    0.367347   0.0
3          0.300000          0.428571    0.204082   0.0
4          0.966667          0.904762    0.122449   0.0
..              ...               ...         ...   ...
145        0.300000          0.238095    0.653061   1.0
146        0.733333          0.285714    0.938776   1.0
147        0.166667          0.261905    0.795918   1.0
148        0.900000          0.166667    0.673469   1.0
149        0.366667          0.285714    0.183673   1.0

[300 rows x 4 columns]>
       bood pressure  body temperature  heart rate        type
count     300.000000        300.000000  300.000000  300.000000
mean        0.524000          0.424524    0.501020    0.500000
std         0.284065          0.284525    0.287620    0.500835
min         0.000000          0.000000    0.000000    0.000000
25%         0.291667          0.190476    0.244898    0.000000
50%         0.500000          0.345238    0.510204    0.500000
75%         0.766667          0.666667    0.755102    1.000000
max         1.000000          1.000000    1.000000    1.000000
```

Fig. 3 Data normalization

```
<bound method NDFrame.head of      bood pressure  body temperature  heart rate  type
48         0.366667          0.238095    0.551020   1.0
108        0.766667          0.571429    0.938776   0.0
42         0.300000          0.547619    0.571429   0.0
112        0.566667          0.047619    0.306122   1.0
26         0.766667          0.190476    0.551020   1.0
..              ...               ...         ...   ...
115        0.033333          0.309524    0.408163   1.0
39         0.333333          0.500000    0.204082   0.0
60         0.200000          0.047619    0.632653   1.0
116        0.766667          0.904762    0.387755   0.0
1          0.766667          0.095238    0.387755   1.0

[300 rows x 4 columns]>
[[0.36666667 0.23809524 0.55102041 1.        ]
 [0.76666667 0.57142857 0.93877551 0.        ]
 [0.3        0.54761905 0.57142857 0.        ]
 [0.56666667 0.04761905 0.30612245 1.        ]
 [0.76666667 0.19047619 0.55102041 1.        ]]
```

Fig. 4 Numpy array conversion

$$CCE = -\frac{1}{n}\sum_{i=1}^{n}(p(x)\log q(x))$$

n : Classification category

p(x) : Correct answer label

q(x) : Probability value of the label predicted by the classification network

Fig. 5 CCE formula

Since the research model can be divided into two cases, a crisis situation and a disease situation, the data was learned by applying a binary classification technique, and the learning model was divided into 4 layers using Keras' sequential model, and in-depth learning was conducted.

For the optimized learning effect, the optimizer used Adam. Training data and verification data were used by randomly mixing the two groups and dividing them in a ratio of 80:20.

As the activation functions, ReLU, Sigmoid, tanh, and Softmax were used to verify each efficiency. For the loss function of the last layer, Softmax was used because the learning model is a classification model.

For the loss function, Categorical Cross Entropy, which is effective in dividing the categories, was applied. The calculation formula of the loss function is as shown in Fig. 5, and is mainly used to distinguish two or more categories.

$$\text{CCE} = -\frac{1}{n}\sum_{i=1}^{n}(p(x)\log q(x))$$

n: Classification category.
$p(x)$: Correct answer label.
$q(x)$: Probability value of the label predicted by the classification network.

Using the above formula, we divided the crisis situation and the disease situation into 1.0 and 0.0, respectively, and obtained each predicted value through the process as shown in Fig. 6.

The following Fig. 7 is a Dense network graph of the learning model, showing that the MatMul and BiasAdd processes proceeded smoothly.

The following Figs. 8, 9, 10, 11 is a visualization of the result of verifying the model learned using the four activation functions and shows the loss and accuracy.

The following Table 4 is a table that summarizes the above results. The result of training the model using four activation functions mainly used in classification models showed that the ReLU function had a loss of 0.00861 less than other functions excluding the ReLU function and showed a high accuracy of 0.0167.

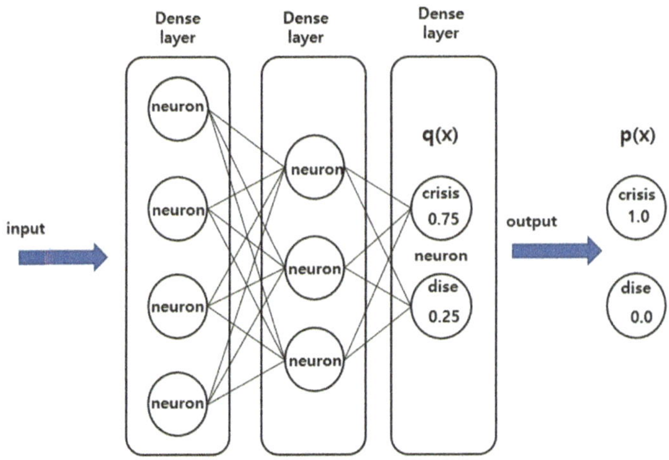

Fig. 6 Model network diagram

As shown in Fig. 8, the result of the above showed that the "Crisis Situation Recognition Model Using Machine Learning-Based Bio-Signals" studied in this paper shows a form that the loss value gradually decreases through learning and converges effectively, and that disease and crisis situations are classified without errors, with the accuracy of 1.0 (100%). Also, the result showed that it is best to complete the model by applying the ReLU function as shown in Table 4 as the loss function to be applied to the model.

4 Conclusion

The "crisis situation recognition model using bio-signals based on machine learning" modeled and verified in this paper expanded human services using bio-signals, which were mainly used in the existing medical and welfare fields, to the security field and verified whether it can contribute to making our society more secure. According to the verification result, the model of this paper, which is a classification model using machine learning, has excellent loss values and accuracy, and among various activation functions, the model using the ReLU function was found to be the optimal model by showing better results than other activation functions with a loss of 0.00695 and an accuracy of 1.0000. In order to use this model empirically in the future, it will be necessary to collaborate with the medical community to accumulate more empirical data, and then to continue research on the implementation of a comprehensive social safety system applicable to the security field.

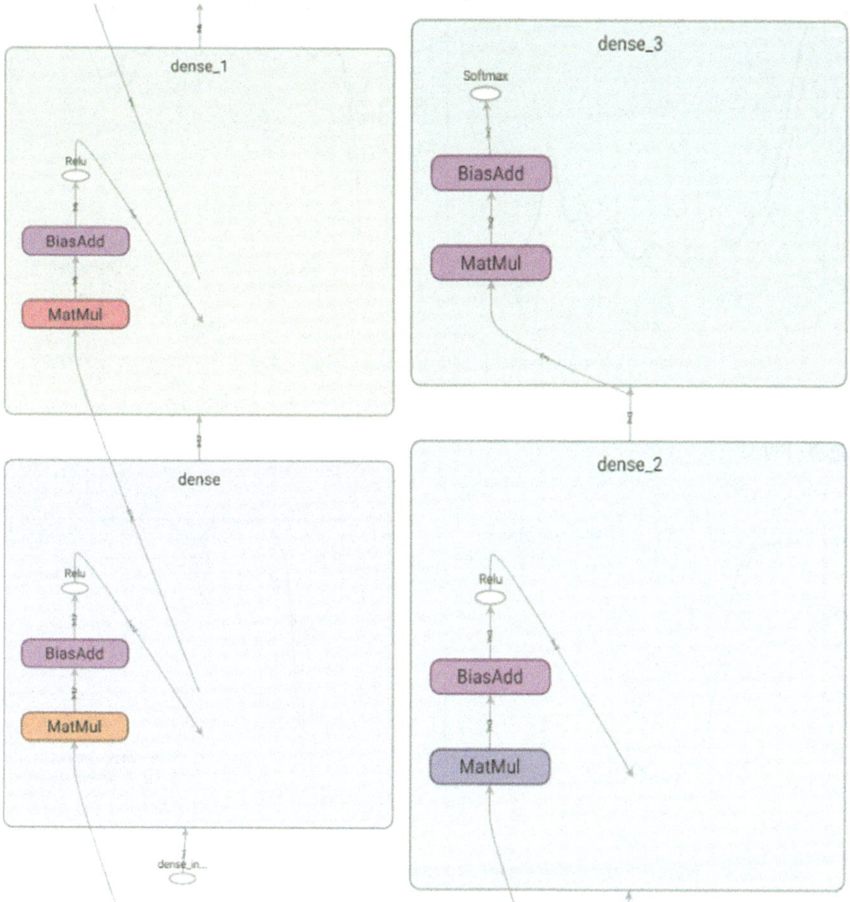

Fig. 7 Dense network

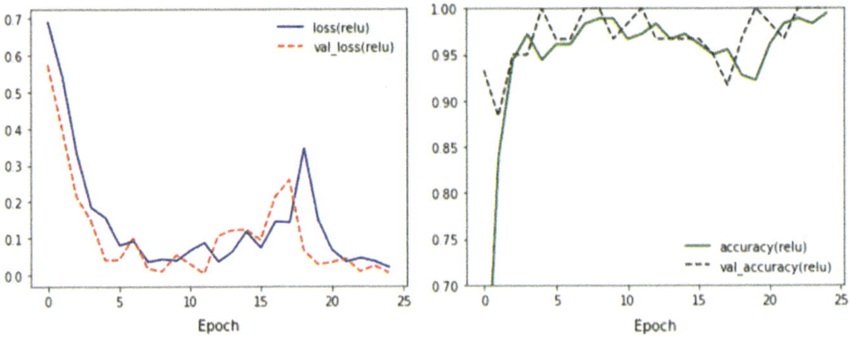


```
2/2 [==============================] - 0s 1ms/step - loss: 0.0070 - accuracy: 1.0000
[0.006950505543500185, 1.0]
```

Fig. 8 ReLU

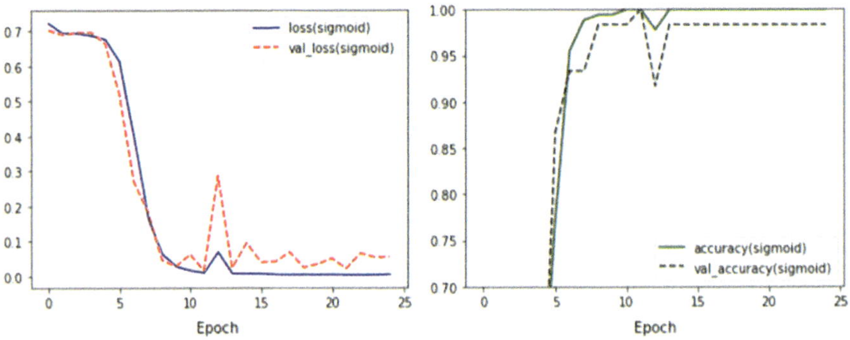


```
2/2 [==============================] - 0s 1ms/step - loss: 0.0393 - accuracy: 0.9833
[0.039339520037174225, 0.9833333492279053]
```

Fig. 9 Sigmoid

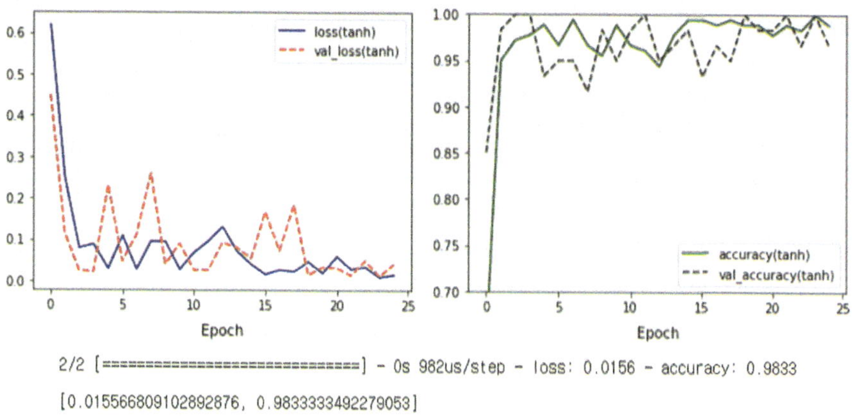

Fig. 10 tanh

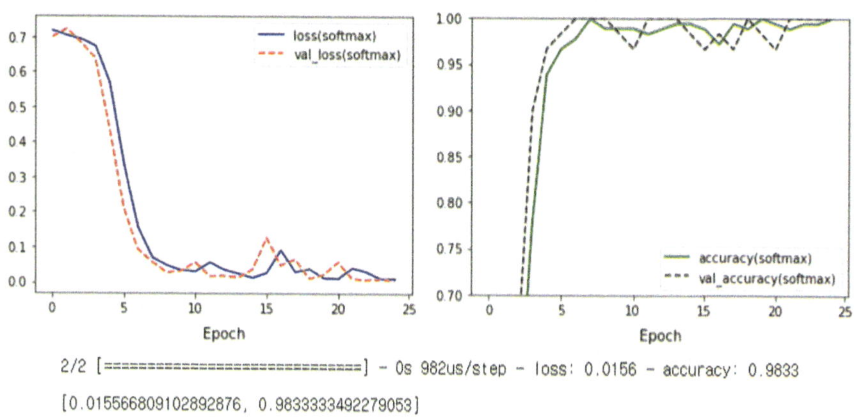

Fig. 11 Softmax

Table 4 Comparison table of loss and accuracy

	ReLU	Sigmoid	tanh	Softmax
Loss	**0.00695**	0.0393	0.1556	0.01556
Accuracy	**1.0000**	0.9833	0.9833	0.9833

Acknowledgements This study was supported by the Research Program funded by the Seoul Theological University.

References

1. Kim, T., Hong, J., Kang, P.: Box office forecasting using machine learning algorithms based on SNS data. Int. J. Forecast. **31**(2), 364–390 (2015)
2. Jung, D.K., Kim, K.N., Kim, G.R., Shim, D.H., Kim, M.H., Choi, B.C., Suh, D.J.: Biosignal monitoring system for mobile telemedicine. In: Proceedings of 7th International Workshop on Enterprise networking and Computing in Healthcare Industry, 2005. HEALTHCOM 2005, pp. 31–36. IEEE (2005)
3. Kelati, A., Dhaou, I.B., Tenhunen, H.: Biosignal monitoring platform using Wearable IoT. In: Proceedings of the 22st Conference of Open Innovations Association FRUCT, Petrozavodsk, Russia, pp. 9–13 (2018)
4. Halde, R.R.: Application of machine learning algorithms for betterment in education system. In: 2016 International Conference on Automatic Control and Dynamic Optimization Techniques (ICACDOT), pp. 1110–1114. IEEE (2016)
5. Bakare, J., Orji, C.T., Wogu, J.O., Ogbonna, C.A.: Effectiveness of teleconferencing in Nigerian universities: a descriptive approach. Int. J. u-and e-Service, Sci. Technol. **11**(3), 27–38 (2018)
6. Bellinger, C., Sharma, S., Japkowicz, N.: One-class versus binary classification: Which and when? In: 2012 11th International Conference on Machine Learning and Applications, vol. 2, pp. 102–106. IEEE (2012)
7. Lee, D.H., Fu, Y.: Cross-entropy optimization model for population synthesis in activity-based microsimulation models. Transp. Res. Rec. **2255**(1), 20–27 (2011)
8. Gómez, R.: Understanding categorical cross-entropy loss, binary cross-entropy loss, softmax loss, logistic loss, focal loss and all those confusing names. Retrieved 23 November, 2019 (2018)
9. Abadi, M., Agarwal, A., Barham, P., Brevdo, E., Chen, Z., Citro, C., Corrado, G.S., Davis, A., Dean, J., Devin, M.,Ghemawat, S.: Tensorflow: large-scale machine learning on heterogeneous distributed systems. arXiv preprint arXiv:1603.04467 (2016)
10. Abadi, M., Barham, P., Chen, J., Chen, Z., Davis, A., Dean, J., Devin, M., Ghemawat, S., Irving, G., Isard, M.,Kudlur, M.: Tensorflow: a system for large-scale machine learning. In: 12th {USENIX} Symposium on Operating Systems Design and Implementation ({OSDI} 16), pp. 265–283 (2016)
11. Kingma, D.P., Ba, J.: Adam: a method for stochastic optimization. arXiv preprint arXiv:1412.6980 (2014)
12. Karlik, B., Olgac, A.V.: Performance analysis of various activation functions in generalized MLP architectures of neural networks. Int. J. Artif. Intell. Expert Syst. **1**(4), 111–122 (2011)
13. Schmidt-Hieber, J.: Nonparametric regression using deep neural networks with ReLU activation function. Ann. Stat. **48**(4), 1875–1897 (2020)
14. Peng, H., Li, J., Song, Y., Liu, Y.: Incrementally learning the hierarchical softmax function for neural language models. In: AAAI, pp. 3267–3273 (2017)
15. He, Y.L., Zhang, X.L., Ao, W., Huang, J.Z.: Determining the optimal temperature parameter for Softmax function in reinforcement learning. Appl. Soft Comput. **70**, 80–85 (2018)

Exploration of Disease Occurrence Prediction Model Based on Clinical Pathology Results Using Machine Learning

Jai-Woo Oh and Jin-Kyu Kang

Abstract Background/Objectives: The purpose of this study is to perform predictive modeling for disease onset by automating the analysis of diagnostic test results using machine learning and big data analysis for small- and medium-sized hospitals. Methods/Statistical analysis: Methods/Statistical analysis: Excel and CatBoost algorithms were used for preprocessing and analysis of the collected data. 21,140 pieces of valid data consisting of 27 attributes were obtained, and they were classified into a training set and a test set necessary for the development and use of machine learning-based predictive models. The training set was used as input data to develop the predictive models, and the test set was used as input data to evaluate the performance of the developed models. A decision tree analysis algorithm was applied, and performance analysis was performed by using accuracy, precision, and the receiver operating characteristic (ROC) area as indicators. Findings: First, the predictive models developed for three diseases, i.e., diabetes, hypertension, and hyperlipidemia, were found to have a prediction accuracy exceeding 80 to 90% and a large AUC. Second, the collected data was useful in predictive modeling research, based on a cluster analysis of the data of patients who tested positive for metabolic syndromes (diabetes, hypertension, hyperlipidemia) and the data of patients who tested negative. Third, from the above study results, diabetes, hyperlipidemia, and hypertension were found to be adult diseases, with a high level of association with blood circulation, and it was determined that it would be possible to predict cases in which a single person had multiple diseases at the same time. Fourth, it was deemed that it would be possible to obtain useful results by changing the data structure into a form of test result data for time series analysis and data with a display of disease diagnosis time point. Improvements/Applications: Through the development of predictive models for diseases using machine learning technology, predictive modeling is expected to evolve to enable prediction of diverse diseases, thereby improving the

---

J.-W. Oh
Department of Health Management & Education, Kyungdong University, Wonju, Korea

J.-K. Kang (✉)
Department of Industrial and Management Engineering, Hanbat National University, Daejeon, Korea
e-mail: jkkang@hanbat.ac.kr; sbaby692001@naver.com

H. K. Tripathy et al. (eds.), *Technical Advancements of Machine Learning in Healthcare*, Studies in Computational Intelligence 936,
https://doi.org/10.1007/978-981-33-4698-7_19

clinical environment and enhancing the reliability and competitiveness of medical care by preventing potential diagnostic errors.

Keywords LIS (laboratory information system) · HIS (hospital information system) · Big data · Machine learning · AI (artificial intelligence)

1 Introduction

There has recently been a transition in medical advances and health concepts from being treatment-oriented to prevention-oriented, and there is growing interest in early detection and prevention of diseases to live healthier. This is reflected in the rising demand for health examinations, which help prevent diseases and early detection of diseases. To meet the demand, many medical institutions are offering a wide range of customized health examinations [1]. Due to industrialization, urbanization as well as improved nutrition, the average life expectancy has increased, which has made population aging more pronounced. In an aging society, some of the most prevalent diseases that threaten people's health are chronic, degenerative types. Chronic diseases arise from a combination of factors, require ongoing treatment and management, and lead to a financial burden due to the growing medical bill. Accordingly, a number of countries are interested in promoting mental, physical, and social health management as a way to help their citizens lead healthier lives, while people themselves are becoming more aware of the need to prevent diseases or at least detect them early in order to stay healthy as long as they can. As living standards improve, there is a stronger demand to be healthy, and to achieve this, various types of health promotion services are needed [2]. A health examination is a disease prevention strategy employed by medical institutions for early detection, treatment, and management of diseases as a way to prevent consequential disabilities, serious complications, and even death. The primary objective is early detection of cancer or chronic degenerative diseases [3]. As such, medical institutions are transforming into a medical environment tailored to user needs and characteristics, and this is key to qualitative improvement of medical services and enhanced competitiveness of the medical industry. Laboratory medicine, in particular, is playing an increasingly important role in diagnosis and treatment of diseases. The laboratory information system (LIS), intended to systematically manage and analyze massive amounts of data generated in laboratory medicine, must be considered a core component of the health information system (HIS) and be allocated equal resources as the HIS during establishment in order for it to be effective [4]. When it comes to apply new information and communications technology (ICT) such as big data analysis to diagnostic test results analysis and diagnosis, it is more effective to make decisions by analyzing clinical pathology results, and this is why it has become necessary to further advance the clinical pathology information system for clinical analysis [5]. According to previous research, a knowledge-based system using diagnostic test results or an expert system as a decision-making support system using the aforementioned system is useful for doctors [6]. While there is vigorous system development using big data analysis in the medical field, including clinical pathology, most of them are being developed in a fragmentary manner, and such systems remain as mere demonstration prototypes or research prototypes due to insufficient testing and modifications.

This study was carried out with the aim of creating a predictive model reflecting cause-and-effect relationships for an accurate judgment of diagnostic test results at small- and medium-sized hospitals that experience difficulty in employing medical specialists specializing in laboratory medicine and improving the reliability of the diagnostic test results through data analysis and machine learning.

2 Theoretical Consideration

2.1 Concept of Laboratory Information System

A laboratory information system (LIS) is an information system that serves to deliver and manage laboratory medicine information and diagnostic test information with excellent efficiency. It is capable of quickly and accurately performing all tasks associated with diagnostic tests from requesting tests to reporting results, and the information accumulated by the system can be used in medical care and research. The LIS is interconnected with the testing equipment so that the tests ordered for a patient, the results, and problem situations are inputted and notified. Although it cannot directly diagnose the patient's condition, it is a useful system for doctors providing treatment. The results from the lab are automatically entered into the patient registration system, and the patient's doctor can check them using the linked information system. The LIS has undergone considerable progress among all medical information systems, and it is expected to develop into a system that is integrated with an expert system with improved user convenience. There are three essential elements when it comes to the LIS: expertise in laboratory operations; software development tools and skills in order to develop a data management system; and knowledge of computer interfaces. The first two are already well-established, while medical equipment and computer interfaces are undergoing rapid advances as a result of the development of ICT advances and digital testing and examination equipment.

2.2 Concept of Big Data Analysis

A big data analysis system is arguably being most actively applied among various types of artificial intelligence (AI) technology. It involves representing the expertise or experiential knowledge of experts in a particular field in the computer so as to solve a problem without the help of an expert or to provide assistance when an expert attempts to solve a problem [7–10]. Big data began to garner attention at the turn of the twenty-first century. It emerged as vast amounts of data began to be accumulated and used as a result of a paradigm shift in technology caused by information revolution. By creating new value with the technology to process and analyze big data, it has become possible to gain more competitiveness for the future. Big data analysis methods include data mining, machine learning, natural language processing, and pattern recognition used in statistics. Meanwhile, text mining, opinion mining, social network analysis, and cluster analysis are on the rise due to an increase in unstructured data from social media and information accumulating as a result of smartphone use [11]. The big data analysis process is divided into data filtering, transformation, cleansing, conversion, integration, and reduction. Data filtering, transformation, and cleansing are preprocessing stages, and data conversion, integration, and reduction are post-processing stages. Data processing involves calculating certain data and showing the results to a human expert so that the human expert can make a decision, but big data processing takes a step further and presents a solution to a problem based on reasoning using knowledge from a knowledge base, and in the process may use the results of data processing. Cases where it is necessary to develop a big data analysis system to solve a problem in a certain field include when knowledge is becoming obsolete or information to be shared is scattered, when decision-making is complicated or there are a lot of data to be considered, when the demand for experts exceeds their supply, when the necessary education to be an expert in that field is costly and time-consuming, and when it is necessary to engage in knowledge-based reasoning rather than simply solving numerical calculation problems. Big data is expected to emerge as a source of new economic value, finding and making use of useful information amidst data will be the key, and companies that find this key will likely take leadership in the future.

2.3 Concept of Machine Learnings

Machine learning, a field of artificial intelligence, is a core technology applied for a computer to "learn" the accumulated data based on machine learning algorithms and predict what will happen in the future. This refers to a series of processing processes in which a computer that has not been preprogrammed learns patterns from data and then performs a task appropriately with respect to newly input data [12], as shown in (Table 1).

Table 1 Machine learning processing procedure

Step	Description
Representation	Determining how the computer will handle the input value
Evaluation	Judging whether the computer did its job accurately
Optimization	Finding the condition that best satisfies the evaluation criteria
Generalization	Predicting results by inputting new data into the completed predictive model

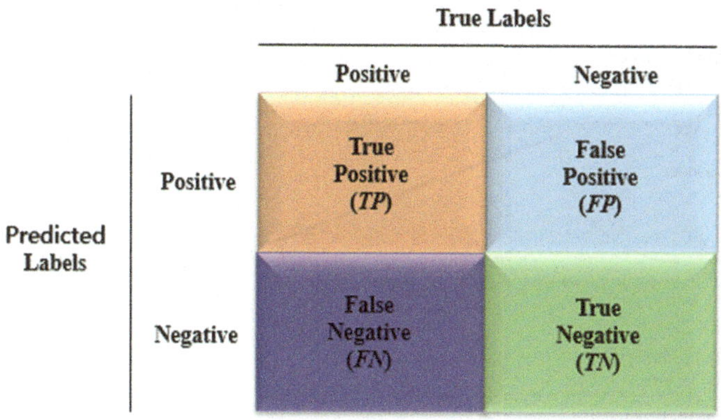

Fig. 1 Concepts of TP, FP, FN, and TN

The main objective of machine learning is to develop predictive models by inputting the data from the training set into classification, prediction, and clustering algorithms. It is thus useful for processing new data and predicting results, but it may be difficult to derive prediction results and determining the reason through analysis. In order to measure and analyze the performance of machine learning predictive models, it is necessary to understand the concepts of true positive (TP), false positive (FP), false negative (FN), and true negative (TN), which are shown in (Fig. 1) [13, 14]. Also, performance measurement can be performed by analyzing accuracy, recall, precision, F-measure [15], and receiver operating characteristic (ROC) area [13].

3 Research Method

3.1 Research Model

The purpose of this study is to develop a predictive model for metabolic syndromes (diabetes, hyperlipidemia, hypertension) using the results of diagnostic tests based on machine learning. To this end, a research model was developed using 23 basic test result factors such as hemoglobin, albumin, LDH, HDL, LDL, and HBA1C measured in a medical environment, and demographic characteristics of the examinees such as age and gender as shown in (Fig. 2).

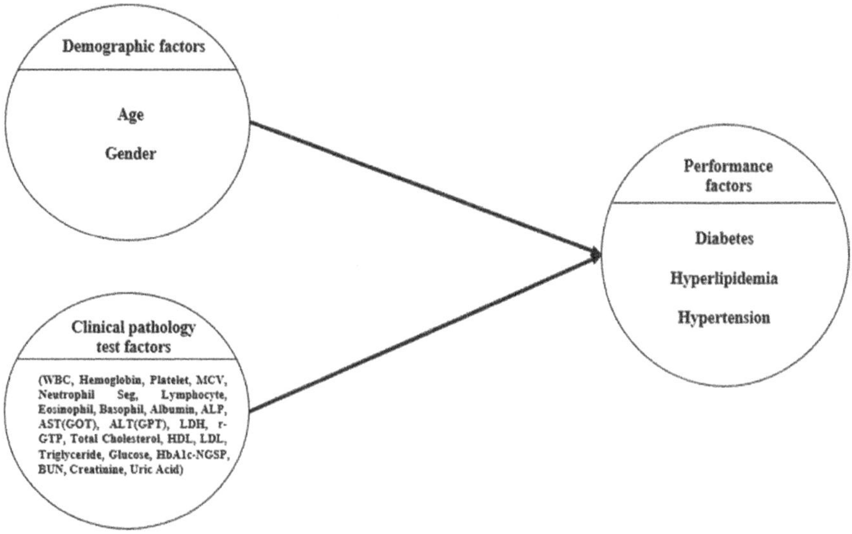

Fig. 2 Research model

3.2 Research Method

As for the method of designing the study for research model development and data collection, the following processes were carried out in said order: research model development, data collection and measurement, preprocessing of analytical data, analysis of descriptive statistics, predictive modeling, and validation of the predictive model. Also, in order to assess the performance of the predictive model, a detailed description of the data preprocessing method, the method of classifying the learning data and test data, and the method of predictive model performance evaluation were applied. In this study, Excel was used to perform preprocessing for data analysis, and the processed data was analyzed using CatBoost algorithm. For 27 attributes (2 demographic factors, 23 basic test factors, and 3 performance factors), 21,149 pieces of data were preprocessed. Missing data were excluded during preprocessing, and 21,100 pieces of data were secured as valid data after excluding missing values. Machine learning is very useful for processing new data or predicting results using a predictive model created based on data used in learning, and thus in this study, the previously collected data were converted into a training set and a test set necessary for predictive modeling and using the model developed. The training set was used as the input data to build predictive models, while the test set was used as the input data to evaluate the performance of the developed models. For predictive modeling, a decision tree analysis algorithm with 23 basic test factors and demographic factors was applied. For the predictive model performance analysis, the performance of each predictive model was measured and analyzed using the TP rate, FP rate, accuracy, precision, and receiver operating characteristic (ROC) area indicators. Among the indicators for performance evaluation of predictive models, accuracy was applied as the indicator for classification accuracy, while the ROC area was applied as the indicator for predictive validity.

3.3 *Predictive Model Analysis Results*

3.3.1 Analysis of the Predictive Model for Diabetes

In the dataset, positive cases of diabetes accounted for 18% of the total. It appears that the ratio of positive cases was intentionally increased for design purposes, and the data were deemed appropriate for use in predictive modeling. As a result of the preliminary decision tree analysis, the key predictors were clearly evident, and the model was created without major issues. See (Fig. 3) for information on the decision tree.

Among the various tests, HBA1C and LDH are two of the most important variables that distinguish the whole. It was found that if the HBA1C level is above a certain level, it is, in most cases, concluded that the person will have diabetes. This showed the need to develop a more sophisticated model (Refer to Fig. 4).

An evaluation was carried out by applying the CatBoost tree ensemble machine learning modeling method to use data for hold-out tests, and the results showed that the correct classification rate (accuracy) was 90.3% and the area under curve (AUC) of the ROC was 0.94, indicating a considerably high predictive power (see Fig. 5).

In the case of the predictive model for diabetes, the extent to which HBA1C contributed to the prediction was particularly high, but other variables also made significant contributions, indicating that the level of utility of the variables in this study was generally high from the aspect of data.

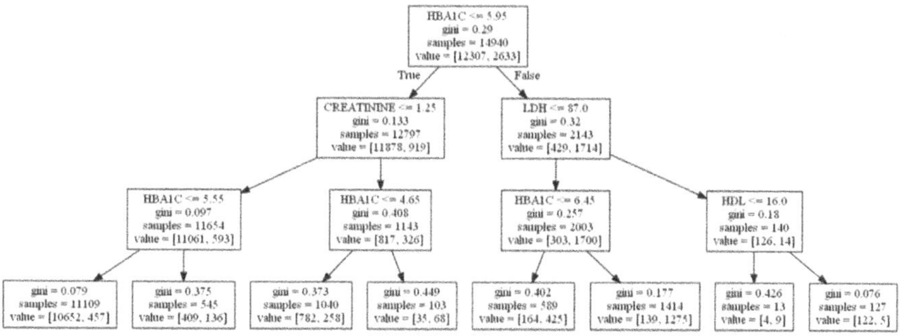

Fig. 3 Decision tree of the predictive model for diabetes

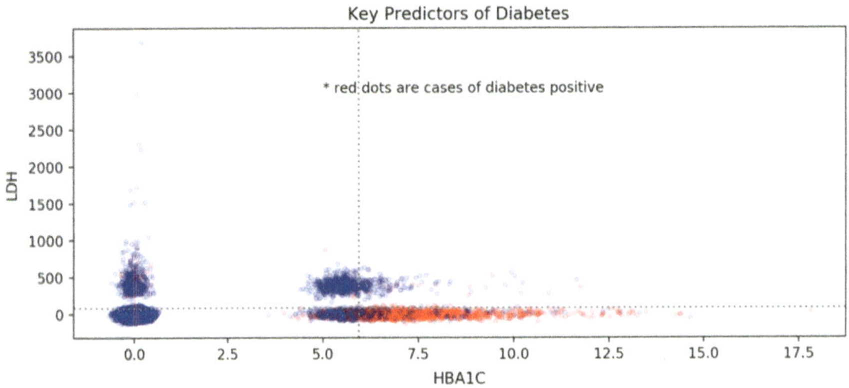

Fig. 4 Key predictors of diabetes

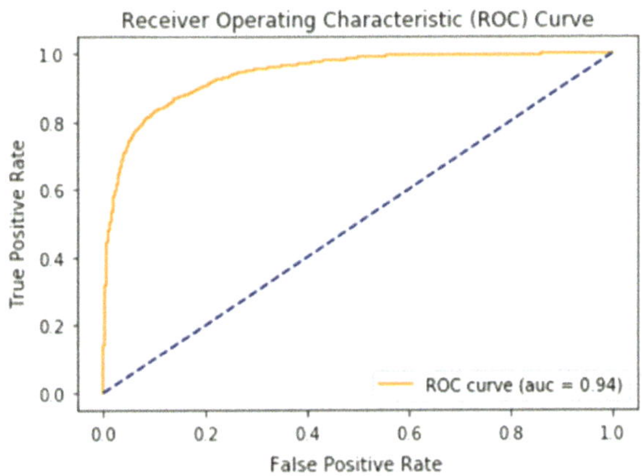

Fig. 5 Receiver Operation Characteristic (ROC) Curve (Diabetes)

3.3.2 Analysis of the Predictive Model for Hyperlipidemia

In the dataset, the percentage of positive cases of hyperlipidemia was 32%, and this ratio was found to be very advantageous in terms of design. It was deemed that the data were suitable for use in predictive modeling, and a decision tree analysis clearly identified key predictors, which made it possible to create a predictive model, as shown in (Fig. 6).

It was found that LDH and LDL were two variables with great importance in prediction, while age was the most important variable. That is, older people are exposed to a greater risk of hyperlipidemia. It also appears that diverse variables have similar levels of influence on predicting when the risk of hyperlipidemia (see Fig. 7).

CatBoost tree ensemble machine learning modeling method was applied and the data were used for hold-out tests. As a result, the correct classification rate (accuracy)

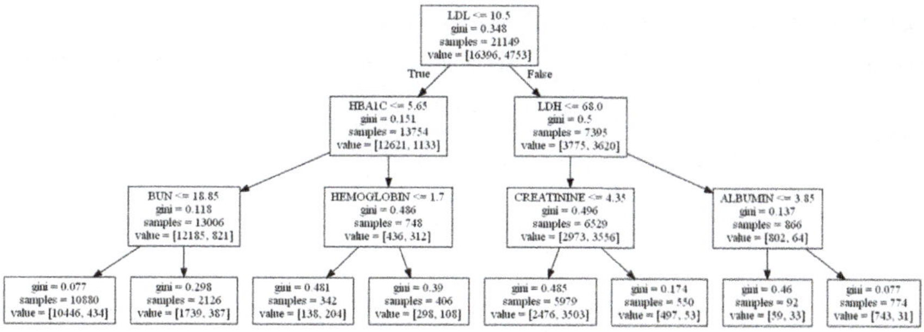

Fig. 6 Decision tree of the predictive model for hyperlipidemia

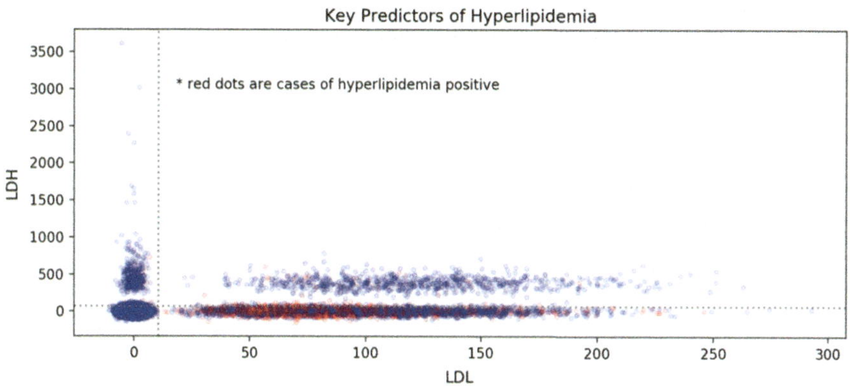

Fig. 7 Key predictors of hyperlipidemia

Fig. 8 Receiver operation characteristic (ROC) curve (Hyperlipidemia)

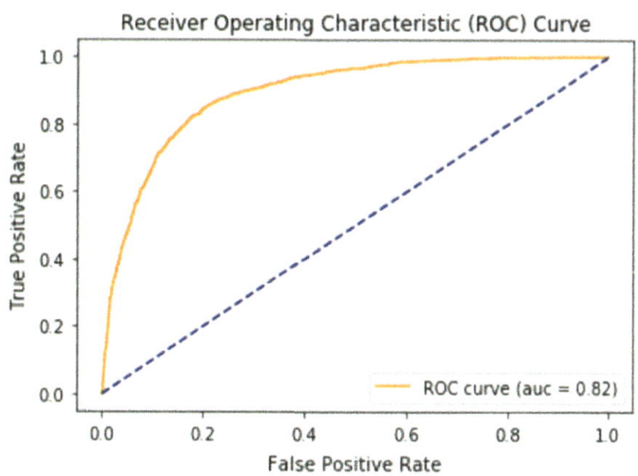

Table 2 Results of measuring the performance of the diagnostic models

Disease	Accuracy (%)	AUC (%)	Sensitivity (%)	Specificity (%)	Precision (%)	F1 score
Diabetes	90.3	95	82.7	92.0	70.5	76.1
Hyperlipidemia	84.9	90	69.5	89.0	66.3	67.9
Hypertension	83.1	83	57.7	85.2	27.9	37.6

was found to be 84% and AUC was determined to be 0.82, based on which it was determined that it was possible make relatively accurate predictions (see Fig. 8).

When it comes to the predictive model for hyperlipidemia, it appears that all variables have a fairly even level of utility, but age, a demographic factor, and LDH, a basic test factor, are particular more important.

3.4 Research Results

Accuracy, AUC of the ROC, sensitivity, specificity, and F1 score, which are commonly used to determine the accuracy of the classification model, were used as the indicators to determine the accuracy of the diagnostic test results. The results of evaluating the test set that was not used in the modeling set were applied to the evaluation of the performance of the model, and in order to determine the possibility of differences across samples, the standard deviation of the error was calculated by tenfold cross-validation, and it was used in a complementary manner. Table 2 shows the results of measuring the performance of the predictive models for diabetes, hyperlipidemia, and hypertension. The models were developed by applying the CatBoost boosting algorithms to input 23 test items, sex, and age in the raw form without generating additional derivative variables, and they can be used as baseline models for models to be developed in the future.

Even the results of similar academic studies have shown that a predictive model with ccuracy within the range of 85 to 95% has practicality for application on a commercial platform. As a result of developing a diagnostic model as a preliminary test for certain diseases using domestic data, the accuracy of the predictive models developed in this study was analyzed to within the range of 83 to 90%.

4 Conclusion

This study was carried out to help improve the reliability of small- and medium-sized hospitals facing difficulties in upgrading their clinical environment and to improve the accuracy of diagnostic tests. To this end, this study looked into predictive models for certain diseases using machine learning technology for the purpose of automatically determining the health condition of the patient or the diseases that he or she has, thereby preventing problems arising from erroneous test results, in addition to improving the clinical environment. Through this, implications for predicting diverse diseases were derived.

The conclusions based on the results and implications of this study are as follows:

First, the predictive models developed for three diseases, i.e. diabetes, hypertension, and hyperlipidemia, were found to have a prediction accuracy exceeding 80 to 90% and a large AUC. Second, the collected data was useful in predictive modeling research, based on a cluster analysis of the data of patients who tested positive for metabolic syndromes (diabetes, hypertension, hyperlipidemia) and the data of patients who tested negative. Third, from the above study results, diabetes, hyperlipidemia, and hypertension were found to be adult diseases, with a high level of association with blood circulation, and it was determined that it would be possible to predict cases in which a single person had multiple diseases at the same time. Fourth, it was deemed that it would be possible to obtain useful results by changing the data structure into a form of test result data for time series analysis and data with a display of disease diagnosis time point. Fifth, it was possible to enhance the utility by using visual information as a function of explaining the diagnostic results produced by the diagnostic models (that is, whether or not the patient had the disease) to the medical professionals and patients. Sixth, after calculating the degree to which each input factor contributed to making a correct diagnosis in the predictive model, the characteristics of few items with the greatest degree of contribution were summarized and visualized and the location of the patient to be diagnosed was provided.

A limitation of this study was that it was difficult to distinguish the time point at which the diagnostic test was run and the time point at which the disease (diabetes, hyperlipidemia, hypertension) was diagnosed using the collected data. It is hoped that a follow-up study will be conducted to analyze the effects of timeseries differences and seasonal errors by distinguishing the time points of collecting data for the model training set and the test set.

Acknowledgements This research was supported by the National Research Foundation of Korea (NRF) grant funded by the Korea government (MSIT) (NRF-2019R1G1A1099953)

References

1. Kim, H.S.: A Study on the Efficient Policy of Health Examination based on Comparing Private Health Sector with Public Health Sector. University of Kyunghee, Seoul (2010)
2. Kim, S., Lee, C.W.: Usage Intention of u-Healthcare Service Using Unified Theory of Technology Adoption and Usage. the Journal of the Korea Contents Association **13**(12), 379–388 (2013)
3. Cho, B.R., Ann, W.M.: Present Status and Problems of Health Screening Program in Korea. Health and Welfare Policy Forum **198**, 48–54 (2013)
4. Zheng, Z.: User Acceptance of Mobile Healthcare Applications: An Integrated Model of UTAUT and HBM Theory. Korean Policy Sciences Review **19**(3), 203–236 (2015)

5. Bartels, P.H., Thompson, D., Wedber, J.E.: Diagnostic and prognositc decision supportsystems. Pathologica **87**, 221–236 (1995)
6. Swets, J.A.: Measuring the accuracy of diagnostic systems. Science **240**, 1285–1293 (1998)
7. Waterman D. A.: A guide to expert systems. Addison-Wesley Publishing Company (1986)
8. James M., Steve O.: Building Experts Systems. Prentice Hall (1988)
9. Kamran P., Mark C.: Expert Systems for Experts. Wiley (1988)
10. John D.: Expert Systems : Design and Development. Macmillan (1994)
11. Choi H. R., Lee S. W., Kim Y. A., Lee J. H., K, H, Kim H. C.: The necessity and case analysis of bigdata quality control in medical institution. Korea J. BigData **2**(2) (2017)
12. Oh M. A., Choi H. S., Kim S. H., Jang J. H., Jin J. H., Chun M. K.: Study on social security big data analysis and prediction model based on machine learning. Korea Institute for Health and Social Affair (2017).
13. Davis, J., Goadrich, M.: The relationship between precision-recall and ROC curves. ICML '06: Proceedings of the 23rd international conference on Machine learning, vol.2006, pp. 233–240 (2006). https://doi.org/10.1145/1143844.1143874.
14. Lee, J.H.: Exploring the prediction model for middle school low-performing students ratio in mathematics using machine learning. University of Yeungnam, Daegu (2010)
15. Fritsch, J., Kühnl, T., Geiger, A.: A new performance measure and evaluation benchmark for road detection algorithms. 16th International IEEE Conference on Intelligent Transportation Systems (ITSC 2013) (2013). https://doi.org/10.1109/ITSC.2013.6728473

The manufacturer's authorised representative in the EU is Springer Nature Customer Service Centre GmbH, Europaplatz 3, 69115 Heidelberg, Germany. If you have any concerns regarding our products, please contact ProductSafety@springernature.com

Printed and bound by CPI Group (UK) Ltd, Croydon, CR0 4YY
30/09/2026
02225295-0010